Praise for *The Ketogenic Kitchen*

"The ketogenic diet can often be overwhelming. In *The Ketogenic Kitchen*, Kemp and Daly provide clear explanations and fantastic recipes delivered in a passionate and personal writing style. This book removes the difficulties and makes the integration of the ketogenic diet into one's life a rich and enjoyable process."

—**Travis Christofferson**, author of *Tripping Over the Truth*; founder and president, Single Cause Single Cure Foundation

"*The Ketogenic Kitchen* has quickly become my favorite resource for people with cancer who are transitioning to a ketogenic plan. This book is a neat package complete with meal plans, recipes, and nutrition info. The helpful advice and personal stories are a real bonus!"

—**Miriam Kalamian**, EdM, MS, CNS, www.dietarytherapies.com

"I awaited the release of *The Ketogenic Kitchen* with child-like anticipation, and it has not let me down. It is a toolbox 'must' for all my patients—to support and inspire them with the beautiful and delicious recipes that fill the pages. There are plenty of folks claiming to have written ketogenic cookbooks, many filled with underwhelming recipes and 'fake food' ingredients. *The Ketogenic Kitchen* focuses on real food, something harder to come by these days, as well as creative menu ideas. If you are looking to round out your cookbook collection, ketogenic or not, this book offers something for everyone."

—**Dr. Nasha Winters**, ND, LAc, FABNO

"There are many 'keto' cookbooks out there, but *The Ketogenic Kitchen* was specifically created for cancer patients by two people who have fought off cancer themselves. Many of the recipes were written to support the very low carbohydrate limits, which lower blood sugar and raise ketone levels quickly, an important goal for those diagnosed with cancer. This book will help so many patients and medical professionals learn how to implement the diet correctly, and it should be a standard in every oncology ward."

—**Ellen Davis**, MS, www.ketogenic-diet-resource.com

The
Ketogenic
Kitchen

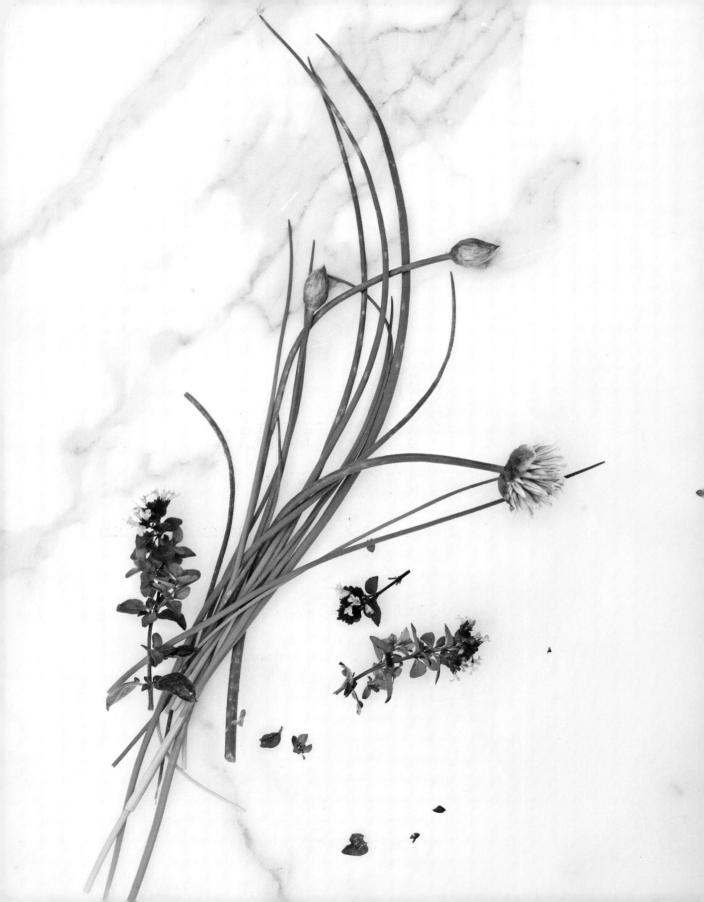

The Ketogenic Kitchen

Low carb. High fat. Extraordinary health.

Domini Kemp and Patricia Daly

Chelsea Green Publishing
White River Junction, Vermont

Originally published in Ireland by Gill Books in 2016.

Copyedited by Kristin Jensen
Structural editing by Gillian Fallon
Designed by www.grahamthew.com
Photographs styled by Orla Neligan of Cornershop Productions www.cornershopproductions.com
Assistant stylists: Susie Coakley and Lesielé Juliet
Nutritional information by Melissa Turner and Nutritics
All dishes cooked by Domini Kemp, Gillian Fallon and Patricia Daly
Indexed by Eileen O'Neill

This edition published by Chelsea Green Publishing, 2016.

Printed in the United States of America.
First printing August, 2016.
10 9 8 7 6 5 4 3 2   16 17 18 19 20

Our Commitment to Green Publishing
Chelsea Green sees publishing as a tool for cultural change and ecological stewardship. We strive to align our book manufacturing practices with our editorial mission and to reduce the impact of our business enterprise in the environment. We print our books and catalogs on chlorine-free recycled paper, using vegetable-based inks whenever possible. This book may cost slightly more because it was printed on paper that contains recycled fiber, and we hope you'll agree that it's worth it. Chelsea Green is a member of the Green Press Initiative (www.greenpressinitiative. org), a nonprofit coalition of publishers, manufacturers, and authors working to protect the world's endangered forests and conserve natural resources. *The Ketogenic Kitchen* was printed on paper supplied by LSC Communications that contains at least 10% postconsumer recycled fiber.

Library of Congress Cataloging-in-Publication Data is available upon request.

Chelsea Green Publishing
85 North Main Street, Suite 120
White River Junction, VT 05001
(802) 295-6300
www.chelseagreen.com

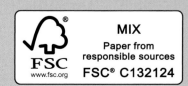

Information given in this book
is not intended to be taken as a
replacement for medical advice.
Any person with a condition
requiring medical attention
should consult a qualified medical
practitioner or therapist.

Acknowledgments

We would like to thank everyone in Gill Books who put so much hard work into making this book happen, especially Nicki Howard, Catherine Gough and Teresa Daly, and the inside-outsiders Graham Thew and Kristin Jensen.

We also owe a huge debt to photographer Joanne Murphy and stylist Orla Neligan, who did an amazing job. Thank you for making it all look so gorgeous.

Huge thanks to Gillian Fallon for her endless talents, from chopping and cooking to writing and editing. Gillian was the first person to really put some shape on all the writing, and we are extremely grateful for her brilliant editing skills. Thanks also to Melissa Turner for her nutritional analysis.

We also want to thank all the doctors, nurses and scientists that help people overcome this disease every day. We are both alive because of the excellent care that we received. Now it's our turn to try to give something back.

A huge amount of support and encouragement as well as excellent opinions in this book came from Professor Adrienne Scheck, Dr Colin Champ, Dr Mark Atkinson, Dr Georgia Ede and Susan Wood. We thank them sincerely for making the time to read the book, make suggestions and to contribute to the book. We cannot thank you enough.

Thanks also to many dear colleagues and friends, especially Alessandro Ferretti (www.chhp.com), Emily Maguire (www.lowcarbgenesis.com), Lily Nichols (www.realfoodforGD.com), Maev Creaven (www.nutritioncentre.ie) and Ivor Cummins (www.thefatemperor.com) for their continuous support, encouragement and sharing of knowledge.

And finally, special thanks to our families and friends. Throughout our treatment you were always there for us, and for that we are eternally grateful. Without you, there would have been no book. Thank you.

Domini Kemp and Patricia Daly, 2016
www.theketogenickitchen.com

Contents

Expert opinions

PUBLIC INTEREST IN ketogenic diets for the treatment of cancer and other challenging health conditions is growing rapidly – much faster, in fact, than the availability of high-quality resources people can use to apply these valuable dietary principles to their daily lives. That is precisely what makes *The Ketogenic Kitchen* such a timely treasure.

I follow a ketogenic diet myself, so I can tell you firsthand that it is safe, comfortable and effective. While it can be challenging to learn and adjust to at first, the benefits are well worth it. As a psychiatrist with a special interest in nutrition and metabolism who studies, writes about and prescribes ketogenic diets, I can tell you that they have uniquely powerful healing properties for the brain. Ketogenic diets have been used to treat a variety of complex neurological and psychiatric conditions, from epilepsy to Parkinson's disease to Alzheimer's dementia. There is even emerging evidence that people with bipolar disorder and other mood disorders may benefit from a ketogenic diet. These specially formulated low-carbohydrate, adequate-protein, high-fat diets rescue us from the invisible rollercoaster of blood sugar, insulin and stress hormones that most people ride all day long without even realising it. This dangerous pattern destabilises brain chemistry, causing spikes and crashes in energy, mood and concentration throughout the day. This is why I recommend low-carbohydrate/high-fat and ketogenic diets to my patients with mood and attention disorders.

Ketogenic diets are not just good for the brain, they are good for the whole body. Conventional carbohydrate-based diets flood our bodies with sugar and wreak havoc with our metabolism, which can lead to type 2 diabetes, obesity and other serious health problems, including cancer. It is firmly established that cancer cells thrive on glucose (sugar) and have a very difficult time burning fat, whereas most normal cells can easily burn fat for energy. Furthermore, excess glucose in the blood triggers insulin surges, which promote the growth and multiplication of all cells, including cancer cells. Ketogenic diets nourish normal cells with healthy fats and proteins and shield them from the damaging effects of excess sugar, starch and protein (all of which can turn into glucose) while simultaneously depriving cancer cells of the fuel they need to grow and spread. There is no other nutritional approach that can do all of these wonderful things.

Patricia Daly and Domini Kemp have written an authoritative guide that will help you put the powerful science of ketogenic principles to work in your daily life. Their hard-earned wisdom coupled with their culinary expertise set this book apart from other health-oriented cookbooks. For issues ranging from mental health disorders to diabetes to cancer, *The Ketogenic Kitchen* will be indispensable to those seeking to incorporate a powerful, science-based nutritional approach into their comprehensive treatment plan.

Georgia Ede, MD
Psychiatrist and Nutrition Consultant
www.diagnosisdiet.com

THERE IS A growing awareness among oncologists that cancer is primarily a mitochondrial metabolic disease according to the original theory of Otto Warburg. A gradual damage or protracted insufficiency of cellular respiration eventually causes cells to adapt a fermentation metabolism in order to survive. Fermentation is a primitive form of energy metabolism that predominated in most organisms before oxygen appeared in the atmosphere some 2.7 billion years ago. Like many cancer cells, unbridled proliferation was a key feature of organisms that fermented. Only those cells that can transition from respiration to fermentation have the potential to become cancer cells. Cells that cannot make this energy transition will die and can never become cancer. Glucose and glutamine are prime fermentable fuels for cancer cells. The regulation of these metabolites can be effective in cancer management.

The large numbers of gene mutations discovered in the various cancers arise as secondary effects of insufficient respiration with compensatory fermentation. Insufficient respiration produces reactive oxygen species that cause mutations in the nuclear genome. The oncogene and tumor suppressor gene mutations are not the cause of cancer but arise as effects of destabilized energy metabolism. This fact cannot be overemphasized, as the cancer industry believes that cancer arises from genetic mutations that must be targeted to obtain resolution. The misunderstanding that cancer is a genetic disease rather than a mitochondrial metabolic disease has significantly delayed progress towards development of effective therapies.

As damage to mitochondrial respiration with compensatory fermentation is the origin of cancer, protection of mitochondrial energy metabolism can prevent cancer. Patricia Daly has done an excellent job debunking myths about fats, proteins, and carbohydrates. Healthy diets can protect cellular mitochondria from damage and thus reduce risk of cancer. We also showed that the ratio of blood glucose to blood ketone bodies—i.e. the Glucose Ketone Index (GKI)—could predict survival in preclinical mouse models of invasive brain cancer and in advanced systemic metastatic cancer (Meidenbauer et al. *Nutrition & Metabolism* (2015) 12:12). Patricia Daly also discusses the utility of the GKI in cancer management.

We consider GKI index values of 1.0 or below as effective for either the management or prevention of cancer. Cancer patients can therefore measure their GKI to determine whether the specific diet they are consuming might be able to help manage their particular cancer. Some degree of dietary energy reduction is often required to help cancer patients enter the GKI therapeutic zone, as an unrestricted consumption of even fat-enriched diets are not likely to produce GKI values of 1.0 or below. It will therefore be necessary for cancer patients to carefully monitor their GKI values if diet therapy is considered for cancer management.

Thomas N. Seyfried, Ph.D.
Professor
Boston College
Chestnut Hill, MA
USA

BASED ON A plethora of preclinical data, trials are underway from the US to Germany. The benefits of a ketogenic diet have already been shown for weight loss and metabolic improvement, and we are hopeful that similar benefits will be seen in the cancer world. Perhaps most intriguing is that some of the data albeit based on preclinical animal studies, may suggest a preventative role of a ketogenic diet. While the diet has been shown to synergise with standard therapies like radiation therapy in preclinical studies, recent studies are underway to test this in humans.

Unable to wait for these results, many have chosen to engage in a ketogenic diet during their cancer treatment. It is our job to make sure this is done safely and effectively, and *The Ketogenic Kitchen* is a vital resource that we have been lacking in the clinic. This is a great source of information for both patient and physician, helping to ensure that the diet is done safely with a variety of healthy, delicious and nutrient-dense foods.

Dr Colin E. Champ
Assistant Professor, Pittsburgh Cancer Institute
Radiation Oncologist
University of Pittsburgh Medical Center
Author of Misguided Medicine
www.cavemandoctor.com

WHAT YOU EAT (and *don't* eat), how you eat, the amount you eat, the nutritional supplements you take, the way you manage your stress and emotions, the support you receive, the amount of rest, physical activity and sleep you get and the level of happiness, awareness and meaning you have in your life all play a vital role in the cancer recovery process.

Let's take the first one – what you eat (and don't eat). When I provide advice to clients with cancer, I talk about two very different diets: the pesco-vegetarian, Mediterranean-style diet and the ketogenic diet. Of course there are many other options, but these are the two I focus on. They both have pros and cons. If someone is highly motivated, willing to learn about the ketogenic diet and committed to being on the ketogenic diet (and has the support of those within their household), then this is often the best option – especially if that client has high fasting insulin/glucose levels and/or is overweight. If someone lacks motivation and doesn't really care about food, then we focus on cutting out sugar and processed foods, avoiding foods to which they are sensitive/intolerant and maximising nutrient intake.

Some clients start with a ketogenic diet and then transition to a Mediterranean diet after six months or so. Others will remain on the ketogenic diet. Why? Because they feel great! Until now, the challenge was a lack of access to ketogenic recipes that taste great. That has all changed with the arrival of *The Ketogenic Kitchen*. *The Ketogenic Kitchen* is a wonderful, practical resource for the person who wants to improve their health by shifting to ketone-based metabolism. This is the cookbook that my clients and I have been waiting for!

Dr Mark Atkinson, MBBS
Mind–Body Medicine Physician,
Cancer Recovery Advisor and Developer of the
Cancer Recovery by Design Programme
www.drmarkatkinson.com

CHOOSING TO ADAPT your diet to a lower-carbohydrate, higher-fat version involves an understanding of food composition and a creative flair for turning this into tasty, nutritious meals that suit YOU. One size certainly does not fit all, so it is refreshing to see a range of recipe ideas for the moderate carbohydrate eater through to options for the very low-carbohydrate ketogenic approach, all in one book.

Lower-carbohydrate, higher-fat diets are most widely used by comparatively well adults looking to improve weight control, moderate blood glucose levels or perhaps alter body composition and improve sports performance. Medical use in disease management is mainly confined to drug-resistant epilepsy where there are treatment protocols, experienced clinical teams and a wealth of published evidence endorsing the effectiveness. Medical use as a component of tumour management is very much an outsider, only just being considered with a small number of human trials (mainly in relation to brain tumours) just getting started. It's an exciting time, but also a frustrating time for those of us supporting this clinical sector. Public interest is increasing but clinical trials exploring the effect of lower-carbohydrate or ketogenic diets are slow to get off the ground, and clinical support, experience and understanding can be frustratingly hard to come by. Patricia and Domini's book explains the precautions, the practicalities, the theories and the uncertainties and will be of value to individuals, their families and the clinicians supporting their treatment pathway. Thank you, Patricia and Domini, for your considerable endeavours in creating such an informative and deliciously practical book.

Sue Wood
Specialist Ketogenic Dietician,
Matthew's Friends Clinics, UK

WORK IN OUR laboratory and others has demonstrated that a ketogenic diet can slow the growth of brain and other tumours in preclinical models. In addition, it has been shown that a ketogenic diet can enhance the effectiveness of radiation and chemotherapy in these same models. We now have scientific evidence demonstrating that it is not just the reduction in glucose that has a beneficial effect; it is also the increase in ketones. For this reason, the proper use of a ketogenic diet is likely to have a multitude of beneficial effects in the fight against cancer. This is now being recognised by patients and clinicians alike.

Published case reports and a large body of as yet unpublished information from reputable sources are demonstrating the utility of a ketogenic diet in people with brain tumours and other cancers. This has led to the opening of clinical trials designed to demonstrate efficacy; however, the available data combined with the demonstrated safety of a properly managed ketogenic diet from the epilepsy community has made this approach desirable even before the clinical trial data is available.

The proper design of a ketogenic diet that is both palatable and safe is not common knowledge, even among registered dieticians. *The Ketogenic Kitchen* will be an invaluable resource for those wanting to follow a ketogenic diet under the direction of their medical professionals, and it will be an equally useful resource for medical professionals who want to add this to their patients' therapeutic regime.

Adrienne C. Scheck, PhD
Associate Professor
Neuro-Oncology Research
Barrow Brain Tumor Research Center
Barrow Neurological Institute
Phoenix, AZ

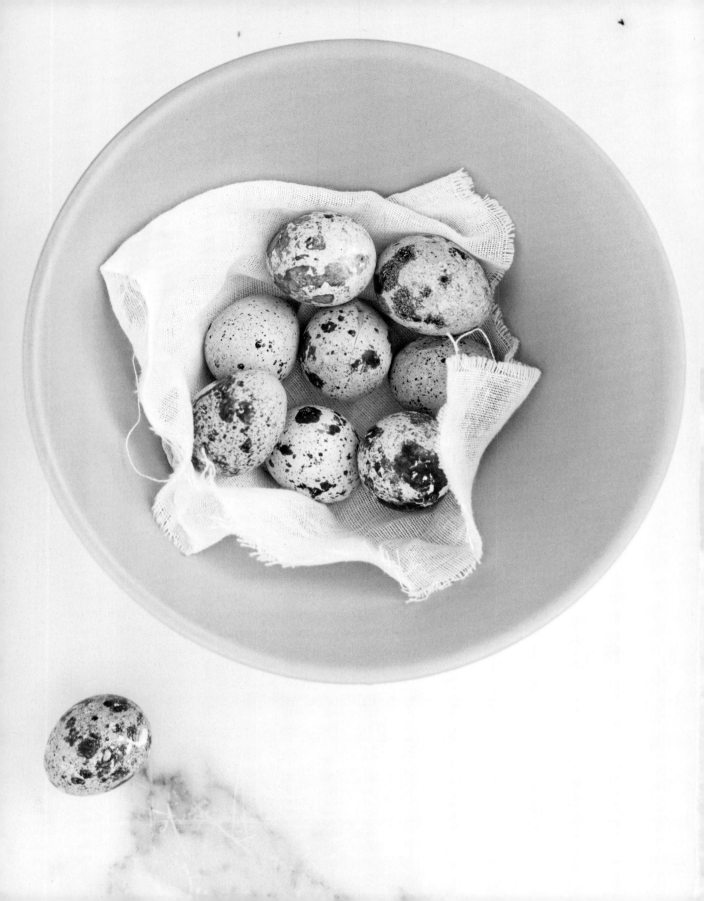

Part 1: Introduction to the Ketogenic Kitchen

Introduction from Domini and Patricia

Welcome to our ketogenic kitchen!

We have written this book because we've both experienced the very real health benefits of a new way of eating – in our cases, to support our treatment for cancer when we had it and to support our (and our families') health more generally now that treatment is over. The results have been so astonishing that we feel we simply have to share it with more people.

The clue, really, is in the title. But what is a ketogenic diet? And what benefits does it offer that would make you want to try it? Essentially, it is a way of eating that is low in carbs and high in fat – an idea that sort of flips the food pyramid on its head. It's a way of eating that people have been talking a lot about lately, but in fact keto has been around for millennia.

In simple terms, a ketogenic diet is one that, over time, switches the body from burning sugar (glucose/carbs) for energy to burning fat (ketones). After you've consumed them, all carbohydrates – whether it's a spud or a slice of bread – turn to glucose, or sugars, in the blood. But if you eat a very low amount of carbohydrates and instead replace them with lots of fats and a moderate amount of protein, the cells in your body will switch from burning glucose to burning fat for their energy. The diet that causes this switch to be made is called *ketogenic*, and when it happens, the body enters a state called *ketosis*.

The ketogenic diet has been around as long as humans have been roving the planet, simply because when certain foods (carbs) weren't available – due to seasonal shortages or crop failure, for example – our bodies had to adapt and switch to burning fat for energy instead.

There are many people who credit a ketogenic way of eating for successful weight loss and management, but what is really exciting for us is the emerging evidence of the benefits of this way of eating for our health. For example, for decades the diet has been used very successfully to treat epilepsy, especially in children (Groesbeck, Bluml and Kossoff, 2006). But the most exciting developments have been seen in the last decade or so, when this way of eating – the keto lifestyle – has been shown to be beneficial in the management and treatment of illness, particularly cancer (which we've both had, twice) and many chronic illnesses (Paoli et al, 2013).

Patricia has followed the ketogenic diet for over four years, while Domini takes a more 80:20 approach. Thankfully (and currently) we are both well. **We attribute our health not only to the conventional cancer treatments and excellent care we received, but also to the support that our diets and lifestyle gave our systems both during and after treatment. It was a good combination.**

And while we're on the subject of cancer, a word about conventional treatments. First and foremost, the benefits of the ketogenic diet have been shown when it is used *alongside conventional treatments*. There is currently no data to support the idea that the diet by itself can treat, cure, maintain or manage cancer. We're both huge lovers of food and firmly believe in its potential to improve (or indeed damage) health.

The recipes have their roots in our very different professional backgrounds. Domini is a chef, food writer and businesswoman. Patricia is a nutritional therapist helping people around the world manage and overcome illness, and support their treatment, through the life-giving qualities of honest, good food and the nutrients it contains. Both of us are busy women (mothers, wives, friends, colleagues) with heavy work schedules. And yes, both of us have had cancer. So between us we believe we've found a balance that works: food that tastes good, gets you cooking, supports your health (especially when sick) and makes you feel great not just in the moment – at the dinner table – but in the long term. In Domini's case that means low-carb meals, and in Patricia's, fully ketogenic meals.

The food in this book is not faddy or flashy. This is food that functions – it energises, nourishes and supports you – without being merely (or boringly!) functional. And while we give a lot of attention to flavour, the emphasis is very firmly on the nutritional side of things and on the magic that nutrients work in the body.

But this book is not just for people with cancer. The recipes in it celebrate food's ability to make us feel good *in* rather than *about* our bodies. It's about simple, truly nutritious food that makes you feel great. And once you feel great, there's no going back.

How to navigate the confusing world of nutrition

Where have we gone wrong?

Have you been told to do or follow at least one of the following?

- Have at least 1 litre of fresh juice a day, but not too much fruit.
- Stop eating dairy, but make sure you have enough calcium in your diet.
- Have some red meat, but not too much.
- Eat a healthy, balanced diet. Follow the food pyramid.
- Avoid foods you might be intolerant to, but have lots of variety in your diet.
- Make sure you don't have too much mercury from fish, but get enough omega-3s.
- Don't drink coffee.
- You must drink coffee, but only decaf coffee.
- You don't need supplements if you have a balanced diet.
- Take supplements.
- Stick to low-fat options.
- Raw diets are the best for health.
- Eggs cause high cholesterol.

Inevitably you will have followed the advice of at least one of the above and then seen the arguments for and against eventually unravel.

Let's face it: nutrition is a controversial, confusing and at times frustrating topic. Eating food affects each and every one of us, whether we like it or not, and more and more people are taking an active interest in what, how and why they eat. Yet many of us can easily get overwhelmed by all the information out there.

You may have noticed that the outcomes of nutrition studies tend to attract more media attention than most other areas of science. Hardly a day goes by that you don't read about a specific food or diet claiming to cause or prevent certain diseases. For the general public, it's hard to see the big picture amidst all those messages making different, often competing claims.

One thing has become clear: whatever guidelines we as a population have followed since the mid-1970s, it's not working. Whether in the developed world or in low- and middle-income countries, today we are sicker and heavier than ever before. While improvements in sanitation, medical services and access to food have led to a sharp decline in deaths from malnutrition and infectious disease over the past decades, chronic disease is on the rise. The World Health Organization (WHO) presents some insightful statistics:

- Chronic (also called 'non-communicable') diseases like cardiovascular disease, cancer, respiratory diseases and diabetes were the leading cause of death globally in 2012.
- Chronic disease now accounts for more than two out of every three deaths worldwide, up from just over half in 1990.
- Worldwide obesity rates have more than doubled since 1980, and the scary thing is that they have increased particularly fast in children.
- The number of new cancer cases is expected to rise by about 70% over the next two decades.

In the UK, one in two people will develop cancer at some point in their lives, according to Cancer Research UK. According to the National Cancer Registry of Ireland (NCRI), one in three people in Ireland will develop cancer during their lifetime. In Ireland, an average of 30,000 new cases of cancer are diagnosed each year. The number is expected to rise to over 40,000 per year by 2020.

Of course, we could attribute these developments to the fact that life expectancy has improved nicely and that we simply become more susceptible to developing a chronic disease the older we get. But we can't deny that cancer rates are also on a steady rise in children and young adults (see www.cancerresearchuk. org/cancer-info/cancerstats/teenage-and-young-adult-cancer/incidence/#Trends).

Research shows that cancer and other chronic diseases could be preventable by making major lifestyle choices. Poor dietary choices, for instance, can increase the risk of developing cancer by 30–35% (Anand et al, 2008).

But the big question remains: which dietary choices are poor? In recent times, many well-established and accepted nutrition 'facts' have been turned upside down and revised. Foods that we have avoided for decades make a comeback overnight and we're told that they've been wrongly accused of being troublemakers. Here are a few highlights from the Academy of Nutrition and Dietetics, the world's largest organisation of food and nutrition professionals:

- Eggs are good and are not to be blamed for causing high blood cholesterol levels.
- Cholesterol has been dropped from the 'nutrients of concern' list.
- Saturated fats are 'de-emphasized from nutrients of concern, given the lack of evidence connecting it with cardiovascular disease'.
- There are also concerns over sodium restrictions because there is 'a growing body of research suggesting that the low sodium intake levels recommended by the DGAC (Dietary Guidelines Advisory Committee) are actually associated with increased mortality for healthy individuals'.
- 'The identification and recognition of the specific health risks posed by added sugars represents an important step forward for public health.'

In short, many of the guidelines we've been following for decades, like limiting cholesterol and saturated fat intake, not adding salt to food and loading our plates with carbohydrates and sugars, are now being revisited. This is incredibly confusing for the general public, but in actual fact the data has been here for a good while.

Let's take an example. Most mainstream health organisations recommend that we restrict dietary fat to less than 30% of our total calorie intake, but a large number of randomised controlled trials (the gold standard in science) confirm that a high-fat diet is more effective for weight loss than low-fat (for example, see Tobias et al, 2015). In addition, high-fat diets also significantly improved important biomarkers like insulin, triglycerides or fasting blood glucose. Many of these studies were done in 2003 and 2004, more than 10 years ago, and yet the guidelines the general public are given remain the same.

The same applies to the saturated fat debate. For more than five decades we've been told that saturated fat causes heart disease. Many people think they have a healthy diet because they eat margarine instead of butter, replace their beloved full-fat Greek yoghurt with low-fat versions or cook their spuds in vegetable oil instead of duck fat.

A review of large, well-designed studies published in 2010 (Siri-Tarino et al, 2010) questions the relationship between saturated fat intake and the incidence of heart disease or stroke. Similarly, a Japanese study showed that saturated fat intake can actually lower your risk of stroke (Yamagishi et al, 2010). This relatively new information is now starting to make its way into mainstream dietary recommendations, which is good to see.

Navigating your way through the nutrition jungle

But why is it so difficult to find reliable information on nutrition? What's the reason for so many disagreements even among the most prominent experts and researchers? Why do they seem to change their minds so quickly? Let's shed some light on the challenges of nutrition and research.

- First and foremost, there's the so-called 'biochemical individuality'. It's something every nutrition student learns in one of their first lessons: we are all different! There is no one food, supplement or diet that suits everybody because we all have different genetic predispositions, we grew up in different climates, under more or less stress and are influenced heavily by our environment. This obviously doesn't only apply to nutrition science. Just because a study shows positive outcomes for a drug, for instance, doesn't mean it will work for everybody.
- Many nutrition studies rely on past self-recalled nutrition data to draw conclusions on medical outcomes and health conditions. In other words, these studies rely on what people can remember about what they've eaten. To be honest, this approach can't possibly be evidence based. Do you remember what you ate three days ago, a month ago or even a year ago? We certainly don't, and food plays a vital role in our lives.
- Confounding factors (exercise, smoking, sun exposure, alcohol, psychological aspects) can have an impact on nutrition

Epigenetics

The emerging concept of epigenetics will also shed more light on why and how we react differently to diet and lifestyle changes. As we all know, DNA contains the instructions for building all the parts of the body. All cells in the human body contain an identical copy of DNA, with the potential for producing more than 20,000 proteins.

We don't have any influence on our genome, the genetic instructions that we inherited from our parents. And up until recently, scientists were convinced that a person's genetic characteristics were set in stone at the moment of conception. But we now know that this isn't entirely true and that the chemical environment in the womb can determine which genes are expressed and which ones are silenced in various parts of the body. And most importantly, gene expression is regulated by environmental factors like stress, diet, behaviour and toxins. In short, it matters what we eat (and drink and do!).

Epigenetics therefore refers to changes in gene expression through our environment. Research into this discipline is still in its infancy, but it shows promise when it comes to preventing and managing chronic degenerative disease.

study outcomes. If one study participant makes other lifestyle changes on top of the dietary change that he is supposed to do, it can obviously have either positive or negative effects on health markers.

- The first thing we check when studying a research paper is who funded the study and what possible conflicts of interest the authors might have. There can be political and economic interests involved in some of those studies, so we're extra cautious when taking on board the results of a possibly biased study.
- Nutrition is a very young and multifaceted field of science that is constantly changing and advancing rapidly. Not all studies are rigorous randomised controlled trials (RCTs), but rather are correlational studies that show preliminary results and give guidance on starting points for further studies.

So what can you do to navigate this nutrition jungle? At the risk of repeating ourselves, you know yourself better than any doctor or nutritionist does. If you eat a food – even if it's super nutritious – or follow a certain regime but don't feel well on it, chances are it's not for you. Also, try to follow practitioners, scientists and reputable sources of information that you know and trust. Believe us, it's a full-time job learning about research, combing through the most recent studies and drawing the correct conclusions from them. If you can lean on somebody who can give you guidance and support and then combine this with the knowledge of your own body, you're on the right track.

How to use this book

This is really two books in one, and there's a serious reason we decided to do it together: because we've both had amazing results with this way of eating.

Both our sections are about low-carb eating and its potential to offer significant health benefits. Even a moderate carb restriction has proven to be beneficial for many individuals (Ebbeling et al, 2012) and **Domini's recipes** are all about moderate carb restriction. So if you've never heard of the ketogenic diet and haven't a clue where to start, these recipes will be just the gentle learning curve you need: low-carb most of the time and low-ish some of the time. And if you find it's a lifestyle that suits you, you can stick to it rather than go the whole way to being fully ketogenic.

Patricia's recipes, on the other hand, are carefully put together to meet the precise requirements of the ketogenic diet, which should consist of no more than 4% carbs at any time and, often, over 70% fat(s). For most people this represents a dramatic reduction in carb intake, but the book is full of advice on how to successfully make that transition in your own time and at your own pace, without being overwhelmed (see the Before You Start and Clean Up Your Diet sections on pages 238 and 241 respectively). And that's important if you are already dealing with the very real change (and challenges) that serious illness can bring. In essence, then, keto is metabolic therapy – it fundamentally changes the way our cells generate energy. And that includes cancer cells.

Of course, it has to suit you, which is why the book includes details of contraindications (see pages 239–240) as well as information on what to expect when you start the diet. There are also important notes in the appendix on pantry essentials and kitchen equipment to make life easier; on the particular blood tests you need to do before embarking on the keto diet; and on monitoring yourself to ensure optimal health while you follow the diet, particularly if you are receiving treatment for cancer.

Our approaches are slightly different. Patricia's recipes and meal plans are designed for periods during and post-cancer treatment or when you're feeling poorly and are fully ketogenic. They are carefully designed to maximise the effectiveness of treatment and to support your system to recover quickly and be more resilient in the longer term.

Domini takes a looser approach: her recipes are low-carb but allow for times when you need to let your hair down – and the carbs in. This is food for people looking to eat more wholesome, healthy grub that packs in a greater amount of plants and good fats and lower amounts of carbohydrates than we are used to. Designed as a way to eat every day, it's for people who want to keep their weight under control by following a low-carb diet; for cancer patients in long-term management; for people who want to get to know low-carb recipes; or for people who can't/don't want to go the whole hog with keto. While some people, for instance, thrive on being in ketosis during cancer treatment and indeed find that it helps keep side effects at bay, others find it so challenging and restrictive that they prefer the more moderate approach of a low-carb diet. This book offers you choice and information.

References

Anand, P. et al (2008) 'Cancer is a preventable disease that requires major lifestyle changes', *Pharmaceutical Research*, 25(9), pp. 2,097–2,116.

Ebbeling, C.B. et al (2012) 'Effects of dietary composition during weight loss maintenance: A controlled feeding study', *Journal of the American Medical Association*, 307(24), pp. 2,627–2,634.

Paoli, A. et al (2013) 'Beyond weight loss: A review of the therapeutic uses of very-low-carbohydrate (ketogenic) diets', *European Journal of Clinical Nutrition*, 67(8), pp. 789–796.

Siri-Tarino, P.W. et al (2010) 'Meta-analysis of prospective cohort studies evaluating the association of saturated fat with cardiovascular disease', *American Journal of Clinical Nutrition*, 91(3), pp. 535–546.

Tobias, D.K. et al (2015) 'Effect of low-fat diet interventions versus other diet interventions on long-term weight change in adults: A systematic review and meta-analysis', *The Lancet Diabetes & Endocrinology*.

Yamagishi, K. et al (2010) 'Dietary intake of saturated fatty acids and mortality from cardiovascular disease in Japanese: The Japan Collaborative Cohort Study for Evaluation of Cancer Risk (JACC) Study', *American Journal of Clinical Nutrition*, 92(4), pp. 759–765.

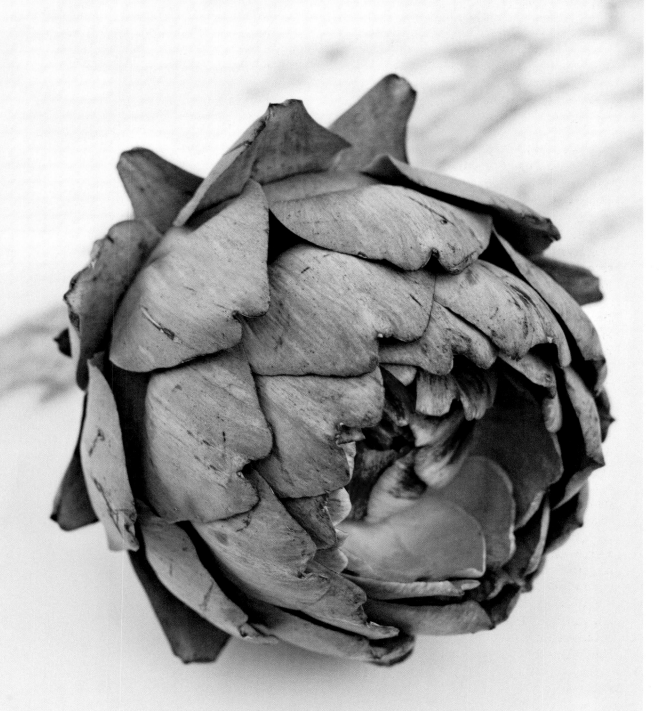

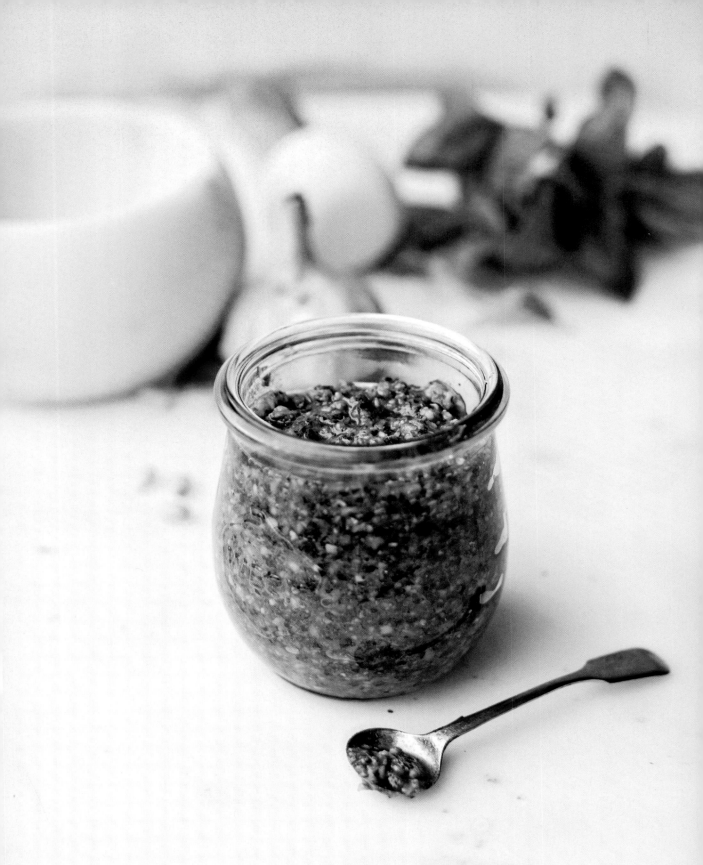

Part 2: The Low-Carb Way

Introduction to the low-carb way

Let's make one thing clear: there is no one perfect diet for everyone. Although low-carb diets can be incredibly beneficial for many – especially chronically ill – people, this doesn't imply that all high-carb foods are 'bad'. There is no doubt that some foods high in carbohydrates have amazing health benefits and provide lots of essential nutrients, like buckwheat, quinoa, oats, bananas, beetroot, oranges, sweet potatoes, kidney beans or chickpeas. **We encourage you to reduce the high-carb foods that are refined and processed, like white breads and pastas**. But your body needs to know what to do with carbohydrates and how to use them efficiently to reap any benefits, otherwise carbohydrate-rich foods can wreak more havoc with your body despite all the nutrients. In order to understand how this happens, let's look at the role of insulin in the body.

The role of insulin

Insulin is a crucial hormone with many functions. Without it, we simply wouldn't survive. Insulin tells our cells to pick up glucose from the bloodstream if levels become too high. It's also the 'fat-storing hormone' that triggers our cells to store energy, either as glycogen (the stored form of glucose) or fat. Dr Robert Lustig, an American paediatric endocrinologist, sums it up nicely in 'The Cause of Obesity' video on YouTube: 'Insulin shunts sugar to fat. Insulin makes fat. More insulin, more fat. Period.' And by this, he means chronically elevated insulin levels.

Across the span of human evolution, insulin production became the mechanism by which the body could choose which form of energy to burn, fat or glucose, depending on what foods were available. When we have a healthy metabolism, the body produces sufficient amounts of insulin to remove any excess glucose from the bloodstream so that it can't harm us. In times of starvation (winter, in ancient times), this enables us to switch into a fat-burning mode to provide more energy. But when there's lots of food available, we become insulin resistant in order to store extra food as fat.

The problem is that in modern society we have access to, and consume, far more carbs than our ancestors – even our parents! And in combination with a high carbohydrate intake, insulin resistance can lead to major issues. Glucose isn't getting into the cells, so it builds up in the bloodstream. The pancreas is getting signals that there's still too much glucose and therefore keeps producing insulin. Eventually, this can cause type 2 diabetes and other metabolic disorders.

Elevated insulin and disease

The evidence is mounting that chronically elevated insulin levels are implicated in causal pathways in many modern diseases such as diabetes, cancer, cardiovascular disease and neurological issues. In his book *What the Fat?*, Professor Grant Schofield emphasises that it's not only dietary factors that affects our level of insulin resistance, but many other lifestyle aspects like stress, poor sleep, smoking, sun exposure, pollutants, toxins, our activity levels or genes. But reducing insulinogenic foods (i.e. foods that raise insulin, like sugar, carbohydrates and certain proteins) from our diet, keeping an eye on our ratio of omega-6 to omega-3 and correcting micronutrient deficiencies is the first step to managing – or indeed, hopefully preventing – some of the most prevalent chronic conditions.

Are you sensitive to carbohydrates? How can you find out whether you could benefit from a low-carb approach if you haven't been diagnosed with a chronic illness? On her website www.diagnosisdiet.com, Dr Georgia Ede has a good tool called the 'Carbohydrate Sensitivity Quiz' that might give you a good insight. She asks the following questions:

1. Do you feel sleepy or foggy two hours or less after eating a meal or snack that contains sugars or starches?
2. Do you tend to gain weight around your middle instead of in your hips and thighs?
3. Does your weight fluctuate a lot?
4. Do you feel hungry when you shouldn't need any more food?
5. Do you frequently crave sweets, starches or dairy products?
6. Do you wake up in the middle of the night and have a hard time getting back to sleep unless you eat something sweet or starchy?
7. Do you get irritable, restless, tense or anxious in the early evening before dinner?
8. Do you have a hard time controlling how much sugar or starch you eat?
9. Do you have symptoms of hypoglycaemia if you don't eat every two or three hours? (Typical hypoglycaemic symptoms include feeling shaky, panicky, irritable, anxious or lightheaded when you're hungry.)
10. Are you an 'emotional eater'?
11. Do you gain weight easily?
12. Do any of the following diseases run in your immediate family?
    • Obesity
    • High cholesterol
    • Type 2 diabetes
13. Do you often binge on sweets, starches or dairy products?
14. Are you obsessed with food?
15. Do you prefer sweets and starches over all other types of food?
16. Do sweets and starches make you feel temporarily less depressed or less anxious?
17. Do you feel you need to carry food with you wherever you go?
18. Are you very hungry first thing in the morning?
19. Do you tend to get panicky or hungry while exercising?
20. Women only: Do you feel much more emotional in the days prior to your period?

The more questions you can answer 'yes' to, the more it indicates that you may be sensitive to carbohydrates and would perhaps benefit from lowering your intake. If you're concerned that you may be on the way to developing some health problems, you can ask your doctor to do a glucose tolerance test, a fasting insulin level or a haemoglobin A1C test.

If you're like us and you suffer from a so-called 'chronic degenerative disease' (sounds lovely, doesn't it?) and you'd like to take a proactive role in the management of your condition, we strongly suggest you consider a low-carb/ketogenic diet. Below is an overview of the current evidence for various diseases. As you can see, some of the evidence is only emerging but research papers are published on a regular basis that confirm the benefits.

The benefits of fat: The evidence is mounting

After reading all this, you might ask why more people aren't adopting this dietary approach and, more importantly, why more doctors aren't recommending it. We believe that it will take time to shift the current mindset of 'fat is bad and carbs are good' and to move away from the food pyramid/healthy eating plate that is at the core of most government policies across the globe. Most mainstream health organisations recommend restricting dietary fat to less than 30% of total calorie intake, but in the past 12 years, an increasing number of randomised controlled trials (the gold standard of science) have successfully challenged the low-fat dietary approach (Yancy et al, 2004).

Well-designed longitudinal studies are expensive and complex but are necessary to cause a paradigm shift in the medical establishment. Most current studies on the benefits of low-carb diets are short term, although we know that it is safe to be in ketosis for long periods of time (Dashti et al, 2014).

But things are starting to change, albeit slowly. In June 2014, *Time Magazine* published an article called 'Ending the war on fat' and the Academy of Nutrition and Dietetics, the world's largest organisation of food and nutrition professionals, has decided to remove cholesterol from the 'nutrients of concern' list and saturated fat will be ' "de-emphasised" from nutrients of concern, given the lack of evidence connecting it with cardiovascular disease' (Siri-Tarino et al, 2010). That there is increased interest in the topic is demonstrated by research papers like 'Dietary carbohydrate restriction as the first approach in diabetes management: Critical review and evidence base' (Feinman et al, 2015), which has been the most downloaded nutrition article from Science Direct for some time now.

There is also a steadily growing number of motivated and talented doctors and researchers on the case who are keen to make a difference in people's lives. This will help provide the research and expertise we need to make the low-carb/ketogenic lifestyle a recognised approach in the treatment of many chronic illnesses alongside conventional therapies.

We used Nutritics software and the help of a nutritional therapist, Melissa Turner, to do Domini's recipes. Patricia used Nutritics (www.nutritics.com) to do her own analysis. Sometimes the portion or serving amount looks odd. That's because for dishes like the tapenades or dressings, it's hard to say how much someone will use. Therefore, we have

STRONG EVIDENCE

HEART HEALTH:
- IMPROVED BLOOD LIPIDS
- LOWER HMG-COA ACTIVITY (THE TARGET OF STATINS)

WEIGHT LOSS:
- REDUCTION IN CRAVINGS
- INCREASED FAT BURNING

DIABETES:
- REDUCED BLOOD GLUCOSE LEVELS
- SYMPTOMS OF INSULIN RESISTANCE IMPROVE

EPILEPSY:
- INFLUENCE ON NEUROTRANSMITTER ACTIVITY
- ANTICONVULSANT EFFECT OF KETONE BODIES

KETOGENIC DIETS

EMERGING EVIDENCE

CANCER:
- REDUCED BLOOD GLUCOSE AND INSULIN LEVELS
- LOWER IGF-1 LEVELS
- LOWER SYSTEMIC INFLAMMATION

NEUROLOGICAL DISEASE:
- IMPROVED MITOCHONDRIAL FUNCTION
- NEUROPROTECTIVE EFFECTS OF KETONE BODIES

ACNE:
- LOWER IGF-1 LEVELS
- LOWER GLYCAEMIC LOAD

PCOS (POLYCYSTIC OVARY SYNDROME):
- SYMPTOMS OF INSULIN RESISTANCE
- IMPROVED REDUCTION OF BODY WEIGHT

reduced the serving size to something resembling a tablespoon or two, with the idea that you will pay attention to the portion amounts if that's what you are interested in. For the ketogenic section of the book, quantities and serving sizes obviously become a lot more important. A tablespoon of olive oil doesn't weigh the same as a tablespoon of mustard, for example, and coconut oil can be hard to measure in anything other than grams. These varying quantities will inevitably cause confusion. In the low-carb section, you will see the number of grams in brackets afterwards. This is what the nutritional information is based on, because half an avocado is not exact enough. You might also notice that sometimes the percentages in the pie charts do not exactly add up to 100% – this is due to rounding.

References

Dashti, H.M. et al (2014) 'Long-term effects of a ketogenic diet in obese patients', *Experimental and Clinical Cardiology*, 9(3), pp. 200–205.

Feinman, R. et al (2015) 'Dietary carbohydrate restriction as the first approach in diabetes management: Critical review and evidence base', *Nutrition*, 31(1), pp. 1–13.

Siri-Tarino, P.W. et al (2010) 'Meta-analysis of prospective cohort studies evaluating the association of saturated fat with cardiovascular disease', *American Journal of Clinical Nutrition*, 91(3), pp. 535–546.

Yancy, W.S. Jr et al (2004) 'A low-carbohydrate, ketogenic diet versus a low-fat diet to treat obesity and hyperlipidemia: A randomized, controlled trial', *Annals of Internal Medicine*, 140(10), pp. 769–777.

Domini Kemp
My story

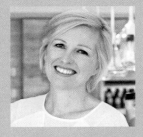

The following recipes represent the way I eat now. For me, it's about living simply, making some changes that will help you feel better about what you're cooking at home and giving you plenty of ideas for foods that will really benefit you when you are feeling poorly. It's about lowering your carbohydrate intake, making sure you get plenty of vegetables and that your diet remains predominantly plant based with moderate amounts of protein thrown in. It's moderate but at the same time plainer, with an emphasis on the nutritional side of things and how we can pack more nutrients into us without feeling cheated when it comes to flavour and tastiness.

The tricks and hints I used to indulge in, like adding a pinch of sugar to combat acidity and blandness or to help with caramelisation, or not being concerned by a squirt of ketchup to enhance marinades that needed a kick, are no longer part of my advice when cooking for everyday eating. None of these cheeky tricks are encouraged in this book. You see, I have mended some of my old carb ways. Having trained as a chef and developed food businesses with

my sister, I thought I knew a lot about food. And to an extent, I did. I just didn't know how much I didn't know, if you see what I mean. Until I got cancer, that is, and had to do some serious research into the effects of food on my body.

The fat battle
Like many in my generation as well as my parents', I grew up regarding fat as an enemy. As long as every dinner was home cooked and contained very little fat, then I was sure I was on the right track. I used to happily eat toast for breakfast – with no butter, of course, but lashings of honey or jam. Then I'd eat more carbs at lunch and a bowl of pasta for dinner with a tomato sauce or sautéed vegetables, again with no fat, which therefore implied it was healthy, right? Wrong!

Following the standard advice at the time – which was to embrace a low-fat diet without really mentioning all those processed carbs – I thought I was doing great. But it's clear looking back on it that it was skewed towards one main food group. I have always been against heavily processed foods, so although you could say the diet was weighted towards one food group, on the plus side at least I was cooking. But I thought nothing of sugar and how it cropped up in practically everything we eat.

But as I have learned more over the years, I realise this information is being turned on its head.

For example, our understanding of the role of fat is definitely changing. For years we were told fat was bad, or at best to be eaten only in moderation. But 'good' fats (no icky trans fats or hydrogenated fats, thank you) play a crucial role in keeping our bodies, digestion and brains supple and responsive. Some nutrients, including vitamins A, D, E and K, are fat soluble and therefore can be absorbed only if eaten with fat. Fats also do some seriously heavy lifting – in energy production, cell building, oxygen transport and blood clotting, for starters. No mean feat, I reckon. But it wasn't always this way with fat. It used to be Public Enemy No. 1.

So although I was restrictive when it came to eating fat, I have always detested the processed spreads and low-fat convenience foods that are often touted as 'healthy'. What nonsense some of those food companies peddle. To try to figure out what we should be doing, I listened to folks like Michael Pollan, whose sage advice includes snippets like 'don't eat anything your grandmother wouldn't recognise as real food', then branched out into nutritional experts who have overturned the status quo, like Sally Fallon, who embraces fats with a vengeance and is vociferous about our use of seeded oils and our underuse of organ meats and fresh food.

My sister-in-law Doris Choi, a best-selling author and raw food chef from New York whom I met in 2008, really started to open my eyes about raw food, juicing and general well-being. Every summer we get to spend two weeks in the kitchen cooking for our husbands' families (handy, huh? two of the brothers married chefs) and swapping tips and ideas.

Another important person also came into my life around this time: Susan Jane White, whose best-selling book, *The Extra Virgin Kitchen*, is all about wheat-free, dairy-free and sugar-free cooking. Over many dinners with Doris and Susan Jane, I began to learn about nutrients – which abound in natural foods – and also about the use of home remedies.

More and more, I started to see that diet was becoming increasingly confusing for those of us who are not in the business of full-time nutrition as more and more information became available. I liked parts of what everyone said, but found they couldn't all agree on everything. But they did agree on lots of things, so it was really a question of trying to figure out what and how I could convert that into what I wanted to cook at home for my family for everyday nutrition and well-being.

Cancer

Then suddenly my world was turned upside down. The year 2013 began badly for me. I had been sick with adult whooping cough at the start of the year and then found a small lump in my left breast, which I got checked out by my GP. I was then referred to go to the breast check clinic for triple assessment.

I went to get the results and unfortunately (but actually, fortunately!) they found two more tumours in the same breast as the small lump I had found. I was given chemo first – six sessions in total, or one every three weeks. But I made it my mission that instead of getting 'match fit', I was going to get 'chemo fit'. This meant keeping up with work, exercise and going on a healthy eating binge like no other.

Changes to our lives

Back in 1998, I'd had a malignant melanoma, had surgery and was treated with a drug called Interferon. It was chalked up to the fact that I was born in the Bahamas with Celtic skin in an era when no one wore sun block; I'd had numerous sunburns as a child. Pregnancy kick-started the growth of the melanoma. Skin cancer is extremely dangerous, as it can spread so quickly and people can be slow to notice they have a mole or growth that needs attention. I was lucky, but the fright made me look into the idea of staying healthier in life and looking at things that were 'anti-cancer'. I read books by Dr Andrew Weil and Dr Servan-Schreiber and followed advice where and when I could. I was no angel, but I was certainly aware, so when my breast cancer diagnosis came, I knew what I wanted to do.

For the most part, that meant lots of green juicing, reducing carbohydrates, avoiding sugar or anything processed plus drinking wheatgrass shots every morning and using turmeric, garlic and ginger as much as possible. Bone broths and miso soup became staples. Fermented foods were introduced and I inadvertently ended up fasting a bit during chemo. It was around this time that I not only really started to rely on my foodie friends Doris and Susan Jane for advice, but it was also when I met Patricia. I entered a new phase of eating and was keen to see how it worked.

Don't get me wrong: I do not eat a perfect diet and on occasion I take a more relaxed approach. Naturally, I would break out and celebrate if out with friends, but I tried to eat better 80–90% of the time. I know this wouldn't appeal to many people, but I certainly was able to keep exercising, working and living life as normally as possible. I would be wiped out for a few days post-chemo and then would slowly bring myself back up. I do believe my diet and exercise were major contributors to my well-being and that this helped my treatment. I wanted to support my immune system and not do anything to jeopardise treatment. I was keen to see if what I did was going to make everything more effective. I believe it did.

I don't like jogging or running, but I tried to get out every day for 30 minutes at some stage for a shuffling run. It wasn't to get tight buns, but rather to 'kill cancer'. I just wanted to fight rather than wail 'why me'. This was my way and I would do it again if I had to.

I had the mastectomy after chemo; the thought of it is so much worse than the reality. I also had an immediate reconstruction. I then went through six weeks of radiation and one final operation. All in all, it took close to a year before I was well and truly done.

When you look at websites, you see words like 'long-term survival rates' and 'outcomes'. These are very hard words to read and even harder for your loved ones to hear. But I guess the magic number is to try to get to five years without the disease coming back. You have to take it one step at a time, but the statistics are there: one woman in 10 will develop breast cancer in Ireland, according to www.cancer.ie.

I would have been aware of what to avoid in life and what to do to 'prevent' cancer in very general terms – don't smoke, avoid getting sunburn, eat healthily, exercise, eat a balanced diet – but it does feel like a really crap lottery.

The more I am learning, the more it seems so clear and obvious that although there are a few common mistakes with the dietary advice patients are being given, I think patients want to do more to help themselves and healthy people want to do as much as possible to prevent disease. Trying to stay fit and lean helps. Exercise is vital. And stress levels need to be kept in control – one of the trickiest things, I find.

It's also about making some small changes, seeing how you get on and then if it feels good, following that path further. My recipes are about getting started on that path. If you're keen to pursue it further, just keep turning the pages to get to Patricia's section.

Today's advice

Now, I do not claim to be a nutritionist, but I am a chef with a keen interest in nutrition. I do know a reasonably small amount, but in the last few years I have made it my business to learn more, not just about how to cook, but about how to cook in ways that maximise nutritional uptake so our bodies make the most of what we put into them – all those vitamins, minerals and suchlike.

It can take time to introduce new flavours and textures to your weekly menu, however. Training your palate is a process, especially if your diet has been high in processed foods full of sugar, unhealthy fats and salt for a long time, as few foods can match the brain's appetite for these substances; they send our pleasure receptors haywire. Really, then, you're retraining your brain as much as your taste buds.

Or at least that's the gist of it. Many of my recipes are more like guides, really. This is because many ingredients, such as herbs and spices, can be successfully swapped for something else if that's what you like and it works for you. Don't like kale? Use spinach instead. Don't like goat's cheese? Sure, feta will do, and if you want to ease up on cheese, mash an avocado and season it up and you'll get the required creaminess we often crave. It's all about figuring it out as you go along.

Gaining the confidence to cook in this way takes a bit of time, and if you're a novice cook it can feel important to stick to recipes as it builds your confidence. But as your skills and confidence grow, well, in theory the world is your culinary oyster.

Hopefully these small steps will help you and your loved ones to feel brighter, healthier and stronger.

– Domini Kemp, 2016

Breakfast

It's no secret that I buy a lot of cookbooks, and I do mean a lot. The recent shift towards healthier books with lots of things reduced – namely, sugar and processed carbohydrates – means that authors have to get mighty creative with their breakfast offerings. While I love looking at these dishes, there is no way in hell that I am going to make buckwheat, apricot and banana pancakes with a vegan cream. I just don't have the time or energy.

My breakfast is usually full-fat live yoghurt (or vegan coconut yoghurt) with some berries, maybe a spoonful of applesauce, some bee pollen plus my 'sprinkles', which are usually chia seeds, hemp seeds and goji berries. Before this, I knock back a shot of wheatgrass and lemon juice (yuck!). I advise anyone embarking on this ritual to hold their nose and think of all the good it's doing you rather than focus on the taste of silage infiltrating your taste buds.

I also have a cup of tea with some almond milk. Yes, regular old Barry's tea. I'm not a huge coffee drinker, but when I do have it, I like a flat white from a coffee shop. I would never bother making it at home. You see, I can't do everything, so I have to pick and choose what stuff I *can* do.

I don't allow my kids to have any processed carbs in the morning, as they both eat bread or some form of carbs for lunch. But I can control what they eat in the morning and for dinner. Battling with them about what they eat during the day is tough, but encouraging better choices for lunchtime and during the day – eating brown bread instead of white sliced pan, choosing breads like pitta, which are less carby, and avoiding processed meats as fillings – are things I can get them to follow through with. Staying away from fizzy drinks or straight fruit juices are also things they can do.

This all becomes trickier when they get older and have some buying power. I have seen kids whose parents are too strict about their food (in the best way) totally rebel and go crazy when presented with a smorgasbord of sweets and treats at a kids' birthday party. I have friends whose parents used to make them go to parties with their own packed lunch and strict instructions to the mum in charge forbidding their child to eat any cake. As my pal recalls, this led to an unhealthy gorging on junk as soon as their parents' backs were turned; such is the desire to fit in and taste the forbidden. I have another friend whose mum used to feed her to the brim before she went to parties so that she would be too stuffed to indulge, but she said she turned to terrible eating habits as a teenager instead. What to do?

Kids, like adults, *love* junk food. We try not to buy rubbish at home, and when there is a party, well, I think you have to turn a bit of a blind eye. Prohibition failed miserably back in the 1920s. In my opinion, taking the same approach to all occasions can backfire, but I do appreciate that not everyone will agree. At most parties these days, you see parents making an effort to at least have a few bits of fruit available. The fruit skewers may not get touched, but at least it's there. Rarely do you see kids getting colas or other fizzy drinks; everyone accepts this is a no-no, especially from a sanity point of view.

Once they get older, the list of banned foods gets shorter as they reach that phase of inevitable teenage rebellion. My only real dietary request for my teenager is that she stays away from sodas and endless amounts of choc-bars or crisps, but especially the fizzy drinks. I hint that some fruit during the day is a good thing, but so is a small handful of nuts or the odd bit of dried fruit.

Again, I believe that if you strangle their choices too much, they secretly rebel and make poor choices just to give you the two fingers. You've got to achieve the right balance and educate them so that they can make smart choices when they have purchasing power. Until then, you have more say in what they eat than they do. But don't be a complete pain.

Like most parents I know, we water down fruit juice heavily and try to encourage drinking water when thirsty as opposed to quenching thirst with juice, which is loaded with sugar. Dinner is always about getting as much veg into them as I can, plus some good fats and a little protein too. I don't buy biscuits or crisps, because if they were in the house, we (and probably mainly me!) would eat them. We don't have ready meals but do allow the odd take-away pizza or sushi. The thing is that when you wean yourself off processed food and eat better more often, the lure of salty, greasy, industrialised food wanes. You start craving the good stuff. And surely that has to be a good thing, right?

So, back to breakfast. You'll find that this section is simple and no-nonsense. I make an effort with dinner; not so much with brekkie. Some days I like to fast during the day, drinking plenty of filtered water with raw cider vinegar, or maybe a light soup or a green juice. Then there are some days when I could eat the entire fridge. Fasting is easier when you are truly on the run all day. I find it impossible to do when on my computer, especially when writing about food. I find myself making endless trips down to the fridge trying to satisfy my insatiable hunger that comes from dreaming up new recipes.

Beetroot smoothie

Beetroot is amazing in juices and smoothies. In smoothies, you get the benefit of all that fibre. I had to tweak it a bit, but this smoothie is delicious. You'll need a powerful blender, but the results are worth it – a week's worth of virtue in one glass.

1 medium fresh beetroot, trimmed and peeled (80g)
1 avocado (180g)
1 apple (100g)
½ cucumber (300g)
Flesh of 1 whole lemon (130g whole)
Flesh of 1 whole lime (72g whole)
Good knob of ginger, peeled (10g)
200ml (⅞c) water (200g)

Makes 2 generous portions

Put all the ingredients into a powerful blender and blitz until it's as smooth as you can get it. Serve in the firm knowledge you are doing yourself proud on the nutrition front.

PER PORTION

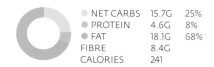

NET CARBS	15.7G	25%
PROTEIN	4.6G	8%
FAT	18.1G	68%
FIBRE	8.4G	
CALORIES	241	

Stewed apples

Now this is something I do all the time, and it couldn't be easier. Allow two apples per person so you have a few days' worth. This is great for your gut and makes boring old yoghurt taste a little bit more exotic. I would happily pour a jar of honey onto Greek yoghurt every day, but I'm not allowed. This is the poor relation, but I have to save my brownie points for something else!

2 apples (200g)
100ml (⅜c) water (100g)
½ tsp ground cinnamon (1g)

Serves 1

Peel and chop the apples and stick them in a small saucepan with a little water (about 2cm [¾in] worth) and the cinnamon, and even some vanilla if you fancy. Cook very slowly for about 20 minutes with a lid on, until mushy.

PER PORTION

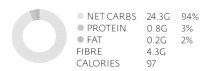

NET CARBS	24.3G	94%
PROTEIN	0.8G	3%
FAT	0.2G	2%
FIBRE	4.3G	
CALORIES	97	

If I had to name my favourite ingredient in the world, it would quite possibly be eggs. I adore them, especially soft-boiled with a knob of butter, flaky sea salt (preferably Maldon) and a drizzle of olive oil. Divine. I love this delicious egg-style salad made with soft-boiled eggs and plenty of tasty additions, which is lovely served on some Biona rye bread. Naturally you could serve it on your favourite brown bread, but there is something nice and Scandinavian about these flavours.

Put the eggs in a large saucepan and cover them with cold water. Put the pan on the heat and bring up to a simmer for 6 minutes, then turn them off and plunge into cold water. When cold, peel the eggs and grate them into a bowl, adding the celery, red onion, chilli and seasoning. Mix together the mayonnaise and curry paste and add it to the eggs. Add the dill, check the seasoning and set aside. It'll be fine in the fridge for an hour.

Spread some egg onto each piece of bread and top with sliced tomatoes. Serve with lots of black pepper.

Curried egg salad on rye

8 eggs (456g)
2 sticks of celery, very finely diced (120g)
1 small red onion, very finely diced (60g)
1 red chilli, seeded and very finely diced (20g)
Salt and pepper (3g)
Approx. 3 tbsp mayonnaise (66g)
2 tsp Indian curry paste (24g)
Small bunch of fresh dill, finely chopped (8g)
4 slices rye or brown bread (288g)
2 ripe tomatoes, sliced (260g)

Serves 4

PER PORTION

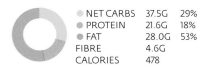

NET CARBS	37.5G	29%
PROTEIN	21.6G	18%
FAT	28.0G	53%
FIBRE	4.6G	
CALORIES	478	

Baked beans with chorizo, egg and feta

1 chorizo sausage, diced (200g)

2 large onions, finely chopped (300g)

4 garlic cloves, finely chopped (12g)

Few sprigs of thyme or rosemary, chopped (4g)

80ml (⅓c) red wine vinegar (80g)

4 tbsp tomato purée (204g)

2 × 400g cans (28.2 oz) of chopped tomatoes (800g)

Salt and pepper (3g)

1 × 400g can (14.1 oz) of cannellini beans, drained and rinsed (drained weight 246g)

8 large eggs (544g)

Splash of olive oil (4.2g)

200g pack (7 oz) of feta (approx.) (200g)

Serves 4

This is also excellent for dinner and is usually my 'OMG, there's no food in the house' kind of supper.

Preheat the oven to 180°C (350°F).

Sauté the chorizo in a large frying pan that can go into the oven until the chorizo is starting to caramelise. It does release lots of fat, which you can leave in there for extra unctuousness. Add the onions and continue to sauté until they too are just starting to colour. Add the garlic, herbs, red wine vinegar, tomato purée and tomatoes. Mix well, season and cook for another few minutes.

When everything feels well blended, take it off the heat and mix in the cannellini beans. Make eight wells or holes in the beans and crack an egg into each well. Drizzle with a little olive oil, crumble the feta on top, season with lots of black pepper and bake for 15 minutes or so, until the eggs are just cooked.

PER PORTION

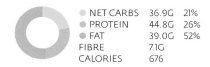

NET CARBS	36.9G	21%
PROTEIN	44.8G	26%
FAT	39.0G	52%
FIBRE	7.1G	
CALORIES	676	

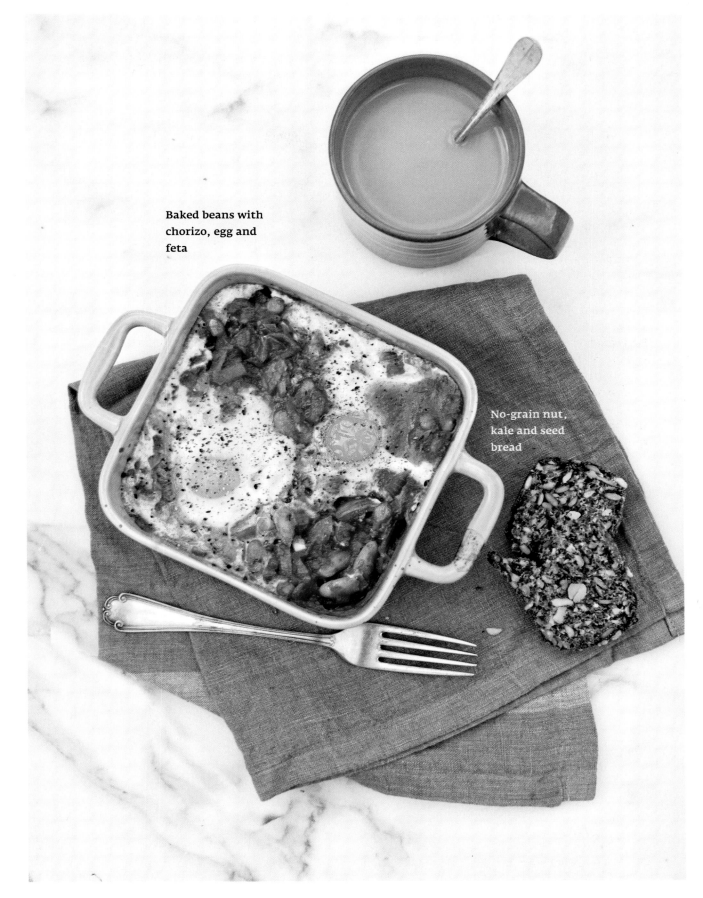

Baked beans with chorizo, egg and feta

No-grain nut, kale and seed bread

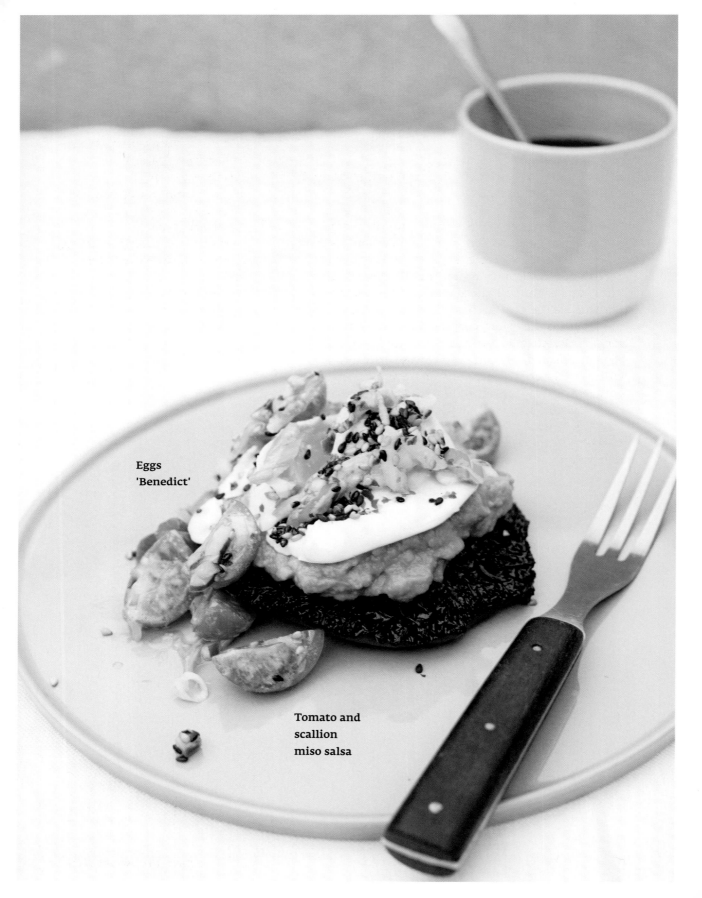

Eggs
'Benedict'

Tomato and
scallion
miso salsa

Preheat the oven to 180°C (365°F).

Peel the mushrooms but leave them whole. Put them in a roasting tray, sprinkle with the sherry vinegar and season. Roast for 15–20 minutes, until they are soft and juicy.

Mix the mashed avocados with the tamari, sesame oil and hot sauce and set aside.

Now poach your eggs. If I was doing this in a large batch, then I would just plop them in without worrying too much about swirling the water and so on, so just get on with it. Get a frying pan and fill it with water. Bring it up to the boil and add the white wine vinegar, then reduce the heat so that it's barely bubbling. Crack the eggs into the water, keeping the water simmering very gently. After 1½–2 minutes, lift the eggs out of the saucepan with a slotted spoon and pat them dry with some kitchen paper. Top the warm mushrooms with the avocado cream, then the poached eggs and some furikake seasoning, which is available in health food stores, good delis and Asian markets. It's a mix of toasted sesame seeds and seaweed and is quite delicious, especially sprinkled on avocados.

Eggs 'Benedict'

4 Portobello mushrooms (336g)
2 tbsp sherry vinegar (23g)
Salt and pepper (3g)
2 ripe avocados, mashed (360g)
1 tbsp tamari (18g)
1 tsp sesame oil (4g)
Few shakes of hot sauce (no sugar) (5g)
Splash of white wine vinegar (2g)
4 eggs (228g)
Furikake seasoning

Serves 4

PER PORTION

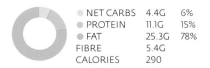

NET CARBS	4.4G	6%
PROTEIN	11.1G	15%
FAT	25.3G	78%
FIBRE	5.4G	
CALORIES	290	

Spring scrambled eggs

2 ripe avocados (360g)
1 garlic clove, crushed (3g)
Juice of 1 lime (20g)
Good splash of hot sauce (no sugar) (10g)
40g (3tbsp) butter (40g)
Small bunch of scallions, finely chopped (50g)
8 eggs, beaten (456g)
About 10 cherry tomatoes, quartered (120g)

Serves 4

First mash the avocados in a bowl. Add the garlic, lime juice and hot sauce and set aside.

Next, melt the butter in a large frying pan over a medium heat. Add the scallions and soften for a minute or two before adding the eggs and tomatoes. Cook until soft, remembering that the eggs will continue to cook once they're off the heat, so don't overdo it. Serve with a good blob of the mashed avocado on top.

PER PORTION

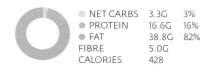

NET CARBS	3.3G	3%
PROTEIN	16.6G	16%
FAT	38.8G	82%
FIBRE	5.0G	
CALORIES	428	

Spinach scrambled eggs

40g (3tbsp) butter (40g)
1 red onion, very finely diced (150g)
Salt and pepper (3g)
10 cherry tomatoes, chopped into quarters (120g)
8 eggs, beaten (456g)
100g (3.5 oz) baby spinach (100g)

Serves 4

This is a variation of the above, but it's another favourite and the type of dish I could have any evening.

Sweat the butter and onion together until very soft. Season well, then add the tomatoes, then the beaten eggs. When the eggs are starting to solidify, fold in the spinach. Take the pan off the heat and let the residual heat cook the spinach and finish off the eggs. Season again and serve.

PER PORTION

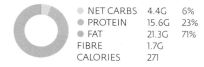

NET CARBS	4.4G	6%
PROTEIN	15.6G	23%
FAT	21.3G	71%
FIBRE	1.7G	
CALORIES	271	

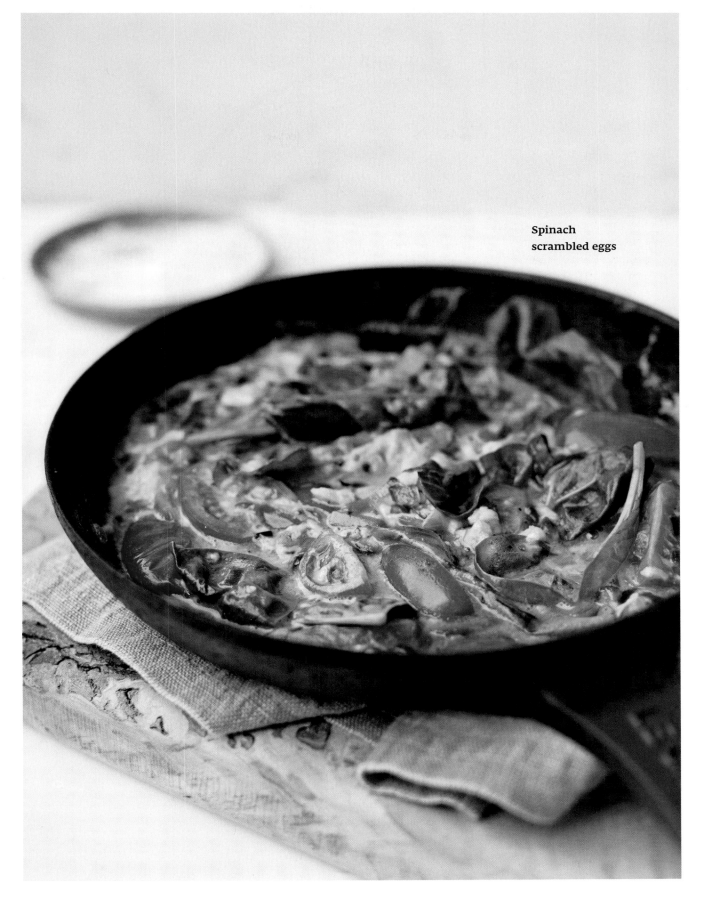

Spinach
scrambled eggs

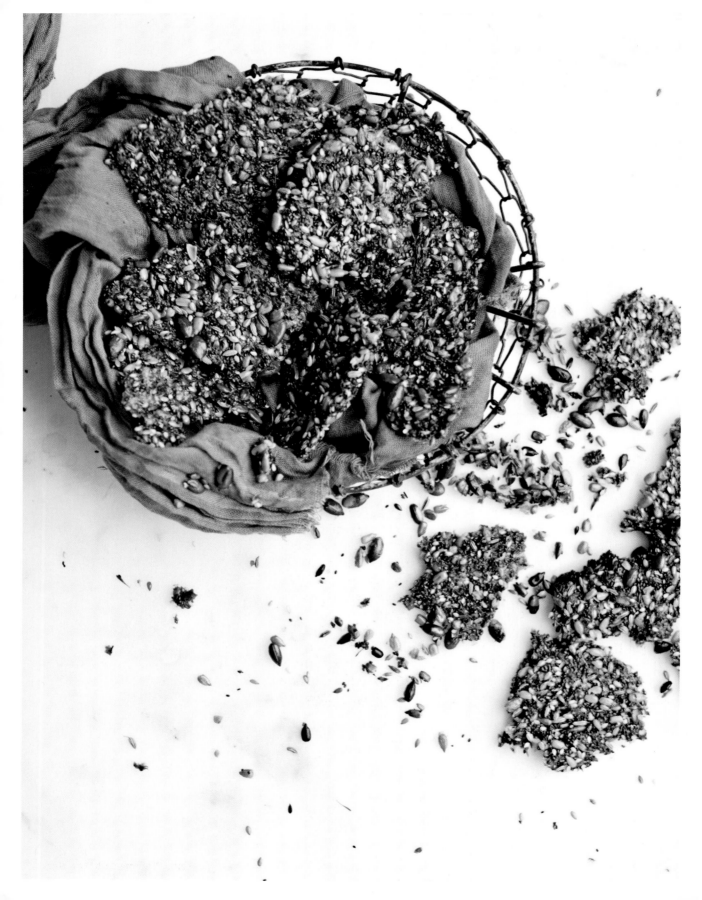

These crackers were adapted ever so slightly from the original recipe from Sarah Britton's book, *My New Roots*. The trick was to remove the oats. Oats in general are a great food, but they are mega high in carbohydrates. After many attempts, here they are: low-carb, grain-free and absolutely delicious.

Preheat the oven to 170°C (340°F). Line a baking tray with non-stick baking paper.

Put all the dry ingredients in a large bowl and mix well. Next, add the coconut oil to the boiling water so it melts. Once this has melted, add this to the dry ingredients and mix well to form a wet dough that's kind of cement-like.

Pour the sludge into the lined baking tray and smooth it out with a spatula. If the mix is being really uncooperative, sprinkle it with water so it gets a bit wetter and therefore spreads easier. It just means you'll have to cook them longer. Press down the mix roughly so it spreads out, then place a second sheet of non-stick baking paper on top of the cracker blanket and carefully apply pressure to make the mixture thinner and so that it covers the whole tray. It's easier doing it this way than with a rolling pin.

When that's done, remove the top piece of baking paper and bake the crackers for 30 minutes. If you can, use a flat surface to flip them over (like you would one half of a cake) and bake for another 20 minutes. If you find the outside bits are going nice and brown but the inside is still a bit raw, break off the cooked bits and keep cooking the middle. They need to be really crisp and golden brown, not raw and wet or soft. Turn off the oven and leave them to cool fully and dry out before breaking up into rough squares or rectangles for serving.

If after a day or so you find they need to be crunchier, stick them back in the oven for a blast. The main thing is to let them truly cool down before you store them, or any residual heat will make them sweaty and soggy. Ewww.

Cracking crackers

75g (2.6 oz) sunflower seeds (75g)
60g (2.1 oz)chia seeds (60g)
45g (1.6 oz) psyllium seed husks (most health stores have these) (45g)
45g (1.6 oz) flaxseeds (45g)
30g (1.1 oz) pumpkin seeds (30g)
20g (0.7 oz) sesame seeds (20g)
2 tsp fennel seeds (10g)
1½ tsp sea salt or Himalayan pink salt (8g)
1 tsp dried thyme (1g)
3 good tbsp coconut oil (81g)
200ml (⅞c) boiling water (200g)

Makes about 12 crackers

PER CRACKER

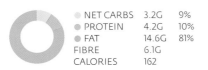

NET CARBS	3.2G	9%
PROTEIN	4.2G	10%
FAT	14.6G	81%
FIBRE	6.1G	
CALORIES	162	

Banana and coconut pancakes

2 ripe bananas (320g with skins)

3 eggs (171g)

40g (1.4 oz) rice flour (40g)

25g (0.9 oz) desiccated coconut (25g)

½ tsp ground cinnamon (1g)

1 punnet (5.3 oz) blueberries (150g)

1–2 tbsp olive oil or butter, to fry
  (19g)

**Makes 8 small but thick pancakes,
which would serve 4–6**

These pancakes were too eggy initially, but the rice flour helps to keep them real.

Mix the bananas and eggs in a blender until smooth. Whisk in the rice flour, coconut and cinnamon, then fold in about half of the blueberries. Let it sit for about 10 minutes and get a frying pan ready. Heat up some olive oil or butter and ladle or pour in blobs of batter from a jug. Let them set on one side, then turn them over. Cook on both sides and then pile up all of the cooked pancakes on a platter. Scatter with the remaining blueberries and serve.

PER PANCAKE

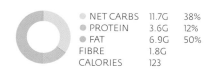

NET CARBS	11.7G	38%
PROTEIN	3.6G	12%
FAT	6.9G	50%
FIBRE	1.8G	
CALORIES	123	

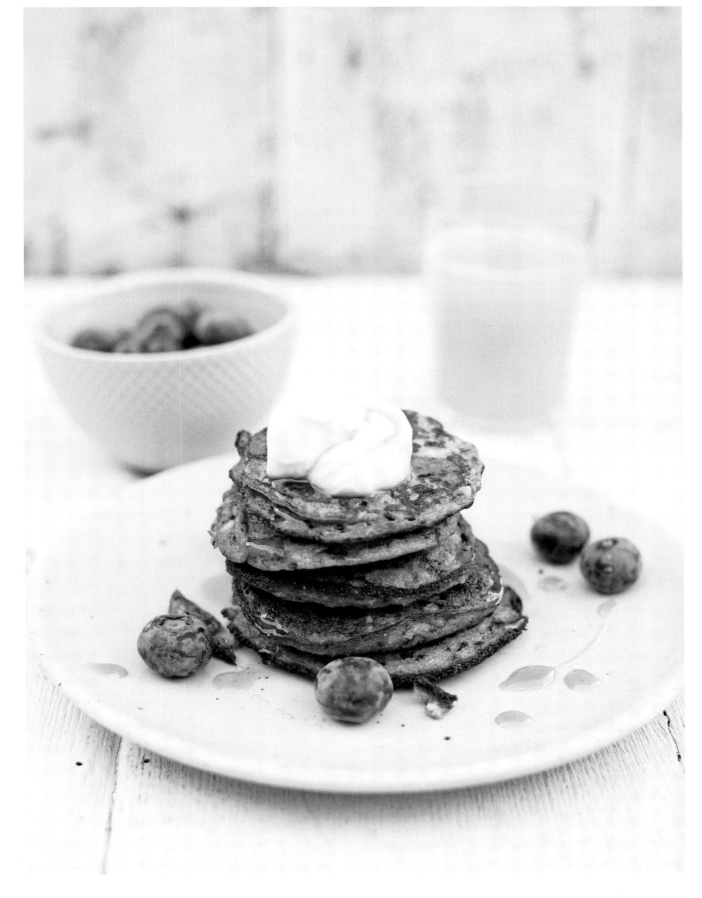

Soup and good things to go with it

Soup: it's a bit of a letdown as far as words go, but truly, a bowl of soup when you're feeling a bit under the weather or in need of a food-hug cannot be overstated. I'm often ashamed of how reluctant I am to make a batch of soup, as the rewards are so great – it's nutritious, and truly delicious, and sometimes it can keep you going for days. Go on, make some. You can thank me later.

Chicken and cilantro soup

2 leeks, washed and chopped (340g)

2 onions, chopped (300g)

4 garlic cloves, crushed (12g)

Big knob of butter (25g)

1½ litres (6⅓c) chicken or vegetable stock (1.5kg)

2 big bunches of fresh cilantro (50g)

4 skinless chicken breasts, diced (520g)

Serves 4–6

In a large saucepan on a medium heat, sweat the leeks, onions and garlic in the butter for about 10 minutes, until they're soft. Add the stock and cilantro and blitz with a blender until smooth. Add the raw (or cooked) diced chicken and poach gently for 10 minutes, until cooked (or if it's already cooked, just until it's warmed through).

PER PORTION (¹⁄₆ OF THE RECIPE)

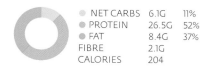

NET CARBS	6.1G	11%
PROTEIN	26.5G	52%
FAT	8.4G	37%
FIBRE	2.1G	
CALORIES	204	

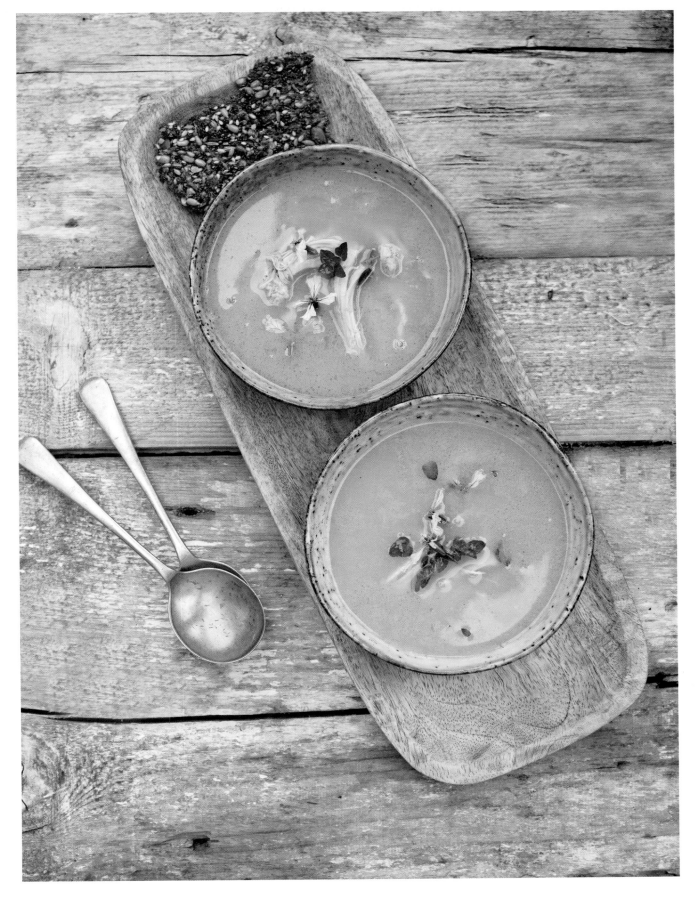

Beetroot soup with avocado aioli

1 tbsp olive oil (13g)
1 onion, diced (150g)
1–2 carrots, peeled and diced (150g)
2 celery sticks, diced (120g)
4 garlic cloves, chopped (12g)
600g (1.3lbs) beetroot, peeled and
   diced (600g)
750ml (3⅛c) vegetable stock (750g)
Fresh horseradish to grate into it
   (optional)

Avocado aioli:
1 avocado (180g)
Juice of 2 lemons (80g)
2 garlic cloves, crushed (6g)
2 good tbsp olive oil (26g)
1 good tbsp Dijon mustard (28g)
Salt and pepper (3g)
Splash of water if necessary

Serves 4

Luscious and rich, the avocado aioli gives a smooth richness to take away from the earthy beetroot. It's delicious with everything, to be honest.

To make the avocado aioli, whizz everything in a blender until light and creamy.

Heat the oil in a good-sized saucepan that has a lid and sweat all the vegetables in it for about 10 minutes, until softened. Add the stock, put the lid on and let it cook gently for about 25 minutes, until the vegetables are tender. If you don't have a lid the water will evaporate, so when you blend the soup you'll just need to add more water. Do make sure the vegetables are tender before blitzing in a blender or food processor, and if you need to add more liquid to get it moving in the machine, that won't be a problem.

If it tastes a little earthy or bland, remember that the aioli will give it a good punch. A little grated fresh horseradish is always nice, or else just serve a sliver of the cured salmon from page 128 on the side, which also goes superbly with the aioli.

PER PORTION (SOUP ONLY)

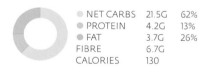

NET CARBS	21.5G	62%
PROTEIN	4.2G	13%
FAT	3.7G	26%
FIBRE	6.7G	
CALORIES	130	

PER 30G PORTION OF AIOLI (APPROX. 1 TBSP)

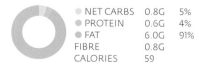

NET CARBS	0.8G	5%
PROTEIN	0.6G	4%
FAT	6.0G	91%
FIBRE	0.8G	
CALORIES	59	

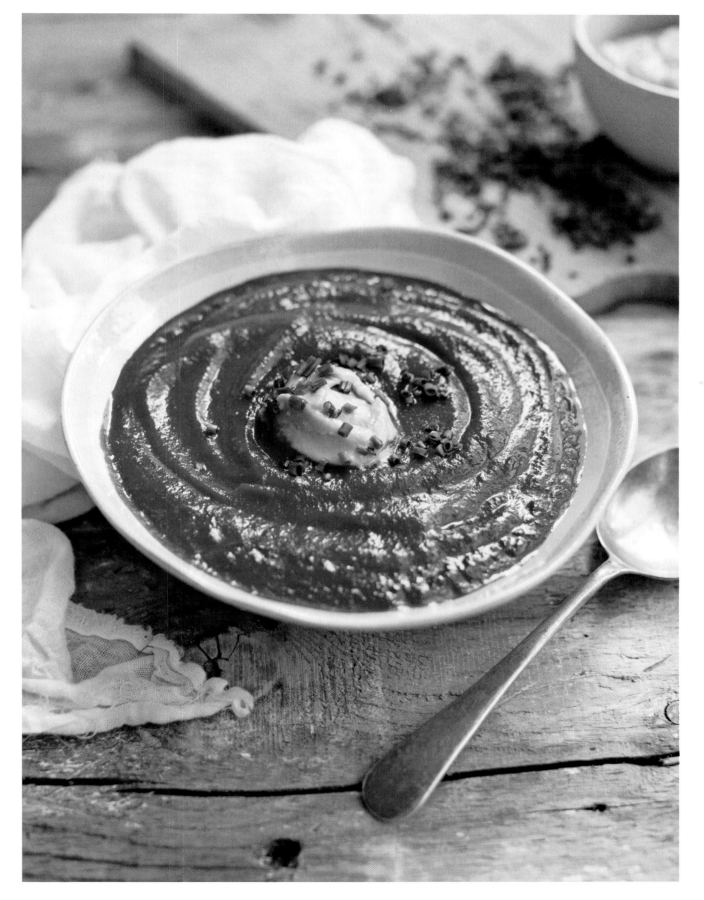

Harira chicken soup

8 chicken pieces (thighs, legs and
   breast, skin on) (1kg)
1 tbsp allspice (6g)
1 tsp ground turmeric (2.2g)
1 tsp saffron (1g)
½ tsp cardamom (1g)
Few gratings of nutmeg (1g)
Salt and pepper (3g)
Big knob of butter (25g)
2 onions, chopped (300g)
2 carrots, peeled and chopped
   (200g)
2 celery sticks, chopped (120g)
6 garlic cloves, chopped (18g)
1 × 400g can (14.1 oz) of chopped
   tomatoes (400g)
1 × 400g can (14.1 oz) of chickpeas,
   drained and rinsed (230g drained)
250g (8.8 oz) brown or red lentils
   (250g red)
½ 200g tube (⅜c) of tomato purée
   (100g)
3 bay leaves
3 cloves (1g)
2 cinnamon sticks
Big bunch of cilantro or parsley,
   chopped (20g)

Serves 6–8

This soup is North African in inspiration but 100% universally appealing. And don't be put off by the long list of ingredients – all those spices just get chucked in together with the chicken before the joints are stewed along with the rest of the ingredients, mainly vegetables and pulses. And truly, chuck in what's available spice wise. No allspice? Then ground cinnamon (but maybe just 1 teaspoon) and more of everything else will do. Please don't fret; this, along with most of my recipes, is very forgiving. And don't forget: this is a stew masquerading as a soup, and all the better for it.

Toss the chicken pieces with all the spices in a large bowl and mix well.

Next, heat the butter in a large saucepan and brown the chicken pieces. When done, remove the whole lot from the pan. Turn down the heat and sweat the onions, carrots, celery and garlic in the remaining fat until soft. Add the chicken back in and all of the remaining ingredients except for the fresh herbs. Add 2–3 (8½–12½c) litres of water, organise everything with a wooden spoon so it's well mixed, put the lid on and simmer for 1 hour over a low to medium heat. Remove the lid for the last 15 minutes and raise the heat to reduce the soup if it's too liquid.

To serve, remove the bay leaves, cloves and cinnamon sticks, spoon the soup into large bowls and sprinkle with the fresh herbs.

PER PORTION (⅛ OF THE RECIPE)

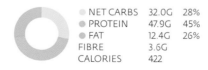

●	NET CARBS	32.0G	28%
●	PROTEIN	47.9G	45%
●	FAT	12.4G	26%
	FIBRE	3.6G	
	CALORIES	422	

This is quite rich but is perfect as a shot of something delicious. It's also ideal if you don't want to have a starter, but still want something to take the edge off everyone's hunger.

To make the garnish, just mix everything together and chill until ready to serve.

To make the soup, cut the avocados in half, remove the stones and scoop out the flesh. Blend everything in a blender or food processor until silky smooth. Season and chill until ready to serve in glasses or bowls with some of the garnish sprinkled on top.

PER PORTION

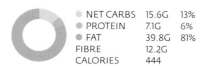

● NET CARBS	15.6G	13%
● PROTEIN	7.1G	6%
● FAT	39.8G	81%
FIBRE	12.2G	
CALORIES	444	

Chilled avocado soup

Soup:

4 very ripe avocadoes (720g)

4 garlic cloves, crushed (12g)

Juice of 4 limes (80g)

400ml (1⅝c) cold vegetable stock (400g)

Few tablespoons yoghurt or cream (100g yoghurt)

1 tsp hot sauce (no sugar) (10g)

Garnish:

4 ripe tomatoes, finely chopped (520g)

3 celery sticks, very finely sliced (180g)

1 red onion, very finely diced (150g)

1 tbsp olive oil (13g)

2 tsp lime juice (10g)

Salt and pepper (3g)

Feeds 4

Lazy fish soup

3 tbsp olive oil (39g)

2 onions, chopped (300g)

4 garlic cloves, chopped (12g)

2 leeks, chopped (340g)

½ head of celery, thickly sliced (220g)

1 fennel bulb, diced (87g)

1 bay leaf (1g)

½ tbsp hot sauce (no sugar) (15g)

½ tbsp Worcestershire sauce (9g)

½ tsp cayenne pepper (1g)

Pinch of dried chilli flakes (2g)

2 × 400g cans (28.2 oz) of chopped
   tomatoes (800g)

Zest and juice of 1 orange (1g + 55g)

1 litre (4¼c) vegetable stock (1kg)

Salt and pepper (3g)

500g (1.1lb) monkfish or cod, cut into
   chunks (500g)

200g (7 oz) frozen prawns (optional)
   (200g)

200g (7 oz) mussels (200g)

Chopped parsley (4g)

Rouille:

4 egg yolks, at room temperature
   (72g)

Approx. 200ml (⅞c) olive oil (200g)

3 garlic cloves, crushed (9g)

Thyme leaves, finely chopped (4g)

½ tsp tomato purée (9g)

Good pinch of cayenne pepper (1g)

Salt (2g)

Serves 4 generously, plus leftovers

I love bouillabaisse and classic fish soups, but bouillabaisse takes a lot of loving. This recipe is a kind of soupy stew and does not involve bones, stock and hours of your time. It's lazy, but tasty and satisfying and very much a meal in itself. Feel free to play around with whatever fish you want to add.

Heat the olive oil in a big, heavy-based saucepan and sweat the onions and garlic till soft. Add the leeks, celery, fennel, bay leaf, hot sauce, Worcestershire sauce, cayenne pepper and chilli flakes. Mix well and sweat for a few minutes, until well coated. Add the tomatoes, orange zest and juice and stock. Cook on a gentle heat for about 45 minutes to let the flavours develop. Taste and season with salt and pepper. You can cool it down and refrigerate it at this stage or else chuck in the fish and cook for another 10 minutes on a gentle heat. Make sure the mussels are well rinsed and scrubbed before you put them in and that they are fully closed. After cooking for 10 minutes, discard any mussels that haven't opened up.

Make the rouille while the soup is cooking. Whisk together the egg yolks with a few drops of olive oil. Gradually and very slowly add the oil – when it has started to thicken, you can add it a bit more quickly. After adding about 150ml (⅝c) oil, add the rest of the ingredients and taste. You may want to add the rest of the olive oil or you may prefer to keep the rouille thicker and stronger. This will make a lot more than you need, but it's always handy to have with grilled chicken or fish.

Scatter some chopped parsley on top of the soup and serve with a blob of rouille.

PER PORTION (¹/₆ OF THE SOUP RECIPE WITHOUT ROUILLE)

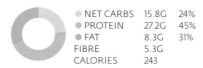

NET CARBS	15.8G	24%
PROTEIN	27.2G	45%
FAT	8.3G	31%
FIBRE	5.3G	
CALORIES	243	

PER 20G PORTION OF ROUILLE

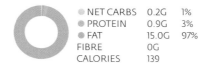

NET CARBS	0.2G	1%
PROTEIN	0.9G	3%
FAT	15.0G	97%
FIBRE	0G	
CALORIES	139	

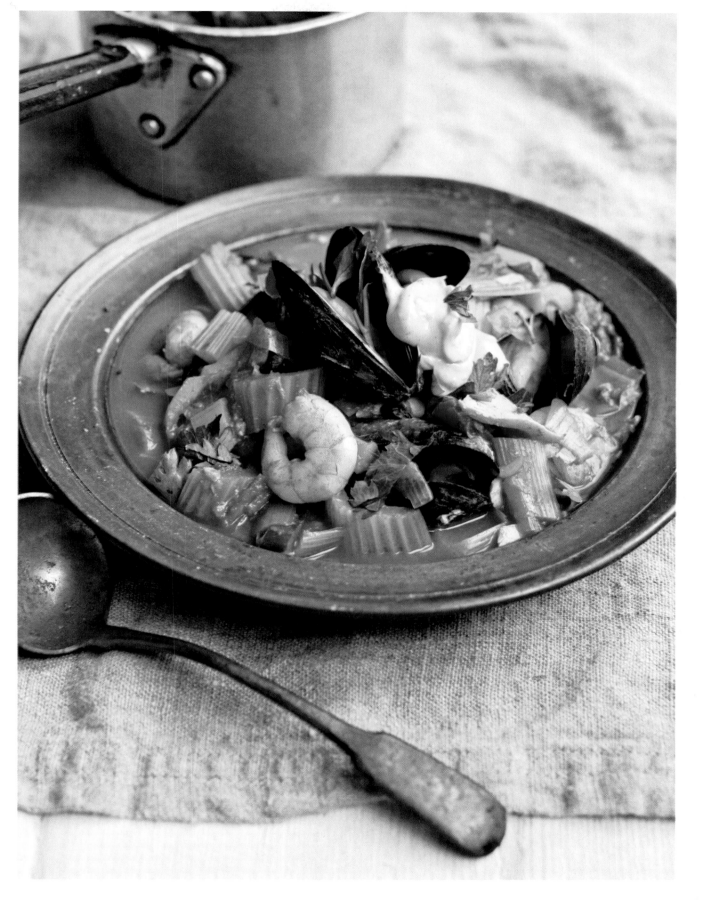

Cauliflower, leek and garlic soup

2 leeks, cut into chunks (340g)
½ head of cauliflower, broken into
    florets (500g)
4 garlic cloves, crushed (12g)
2 tbsp olive oil (26g)
Salt and pepper (3g)
Freshly grated nutmeg (1g)
600ml (2½c) vegetable or chicken
    stock or water (600g)
1 bay leaf
200ml (⅞c) cream (200g)

Serves 4

This is a straightforward, no-nonsense, rib-sticking soup.

Preheat the oven to 200°C (400°F).

Toss the leeks, cauliflower and garlic in the olive oil. Season well and grate some nutmeg on top. Roast in the oven for 25 minutes, until starting to go golden brown.

Chuck into a saucepan and add the stock and bay leaf. Bring up to the boil, then reduce the heat and simmer for 10–15 minutes. Remove the bay leaf, purée with a hand-held blender or in a regular blender, then pour it back into the saucepan and add the cream. Check the seasoning and adjust if necessary. This can be served straight away or made a few days in advance and reheated.

PER PORTION (¼ OF THE RECIPE)

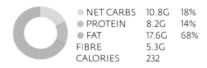

NET CARBS	10.8G	18%
PROTEIN	8.2G	14%
FAT	17.6G	68%
FIBRE	5.3G	
CALORIES	232	

'Therapies that reduce glucose and elevate ketones can starve glucose-dependent cancer cells while protecting and fueling healthy cells. There is no other cancer therapy that can do this.'
Dr Thomas Seyfried

A creamy, filling soup of cauliflower and leek with a warm hint of fennel seed. The original version used coconut oil but it was more pronounced than I expected, so we decided to ditch it for butter or olive oil instead. Supper in a bowl.

Melt the butter or heat the olive oil in a large saucepan and gently sauté the onion, garlic and fennel seeds until they've softened a bit. Next, add the leeks and leave to soften for 5 minutes before adding the cauliflower and water. Season very well, put the lid on and simmer until everything is just done – about 15 minutes. Check the seasoning again and adjust to your taste before whizzing the whole lot with a blender or using a soup gun to make it smooth. If you want to jazz it up further, you can top it with some grated cheese (Parmesan or Cheddar is great), crisp bacon or even a handful of chopped parsley.

PER PORTION (¹/₆ OF THE RECIPE WITHOUT TOPPINGS)

NET CARBS	9.2G	35%
PROTEIN	7.4G	29%
FAT	4.0G	36%
FIBRE	4.9G	
CALORIES	101	

Cauliflower, leek and fennel soup

1 tbsp butter or splash of olive oil (15g)
1 onion, roughly chopped (150g)
2 garlic cloves, roughly chopped (6g)
2 tsp fennel seeds (4g)
2 leeks, washed well and roughly chopped (340g)
1 cauliflower, roughly chopped (1kg)
1 litre (4¼c) water (1kg)
Salt and pepper (3g)

Serves 4–6

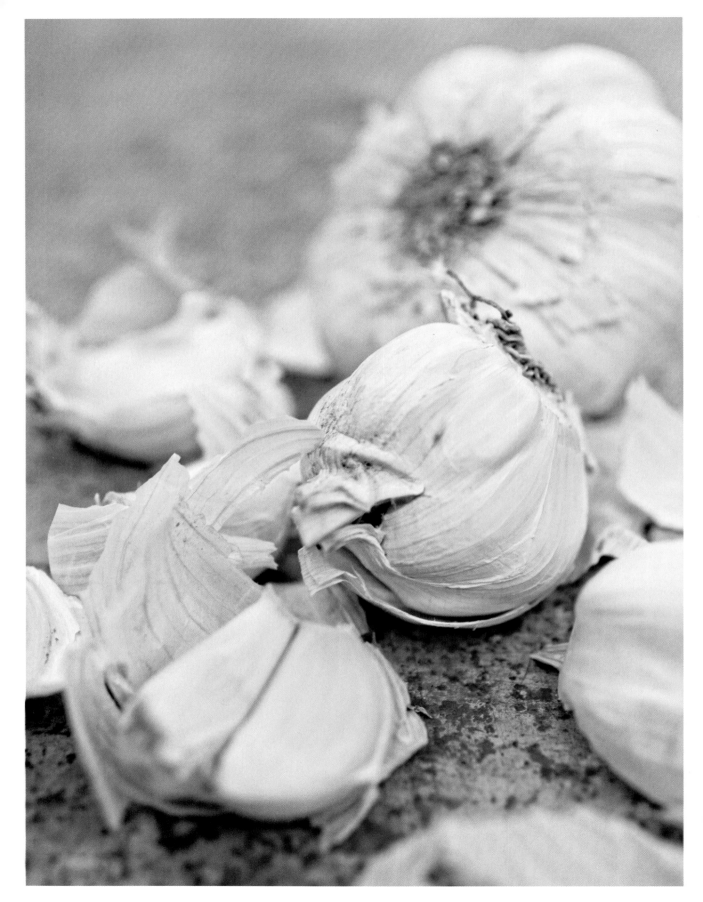

Quick tomato soup

This 'quick' tomato soup is the perfect larder lunch: there's nothing in it that you won't find in your store cupboard. And don't skip the anchovies. You won't taste them but they add some umami oomph to this 15-minute wonder.

Sweat the onion, anchovies, garlic and fresh herbs in the butter over a medium heat for about 5 minutes, until soft, then add the tomatoes and vinegar. Simmer for about 10 minutes before blitzing until smooth in a blender. Season well and serve with a drizzle of olive oil, some fresh parsley and the flaxseed bread on page 47.

PER PORTION

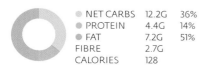

● NET CARBS	12.2G	36%
● PROTEIN	4.4G	14%
● FAT	7.2G	51%
FIBRE	2.7G	
CALORIES	128	

1 large white onion, chopped (240g)
6 anchovies, drained and chopped (18g)
6 garlic cloves, chopped (18g)
Few sprigs of fresh rosemary or thyme (or both), chopped (12g)
1 good knob of butter (20g)
2 × 400g cans (28.2 oz) of chopped tomatoes (800g)
2 tsp sherry vinegar (8g)
Salt and pepper (3g)
Olive oil, to garnish (8g/½ tsp per portion)
Parsley, chopped, to garnish (4g)

Serves 4

Butternut squash soup with coconut, lime and miso

1 large or 2 small butternut squash
   (1.3kg)
2 tbsp olive oil (26g)
1 onion, diced (150g)
2 garlic cloves, crushed (6g)
1 good knob of ginger, peeled and
   diced (10g)
1 small tsp chilli flakes (2g)
1 tsp ground turmeric (2g)
1 good tbsp miso paste (35g)
1 × 400ml can (14.1 oz) of coconut
   milk (400g)
Juice and zest of 2 limes (40g + 2g)
Approx. 500ml (2⅛c) water (500g)
Salt and pepper (3g)
Big bunch of cilantro, roughly
   chopped (20g)

Serves 4–6

A good soup is always delicious and desirable. Miso and lime work fantastically well with sweet butternut squash.

Peel the butternut squash, then cut the top cylindrical shape off and chop it. Cut the bottom wider bit in half lengthways, scoop out and discard the seeds and hairy bits, and roughly chop the flesh.

Heat the olive oil in a large saucepan and sweat the squash along with the onion, garlic, ginger, chilli and turmeric for at least 10 minutes. You can keep a lid on, give it regular stirs and just let everything soften and meld together, flavour wise. Add the miso and mix it around, then add the coconut milk, lime zest and juice. Simmer gently until the butternut squash is tender and add enough water to make sure you can blend it with one of those soupy gadget things, or else put it in a food processor in batches and blend. Add enough water until you are happy with the consistency. Stir and taste. Adjust the seasoning and add some cilantro. Serve hot or cool down and reheat as necessary, adding some extra water to loosen if it goes too thick.

PER PORTION (¹⁄₆ OF THE RECIPE)

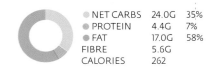

NET CARBS	24.0G	35%
PROTEIN	4.4G	7%
FAT	17.0G	58%
FIBRE	5.6G	
CALORIES	262	

You will need a 20cm (8in) square pan for this, lined with non-stick baking paper and buttered or oiled. This is based on the original Hemsley and Hemsley recipe, but I upped the acidity and added more seasoning. A lovely recipe.

Preheat the oven to 170°C (340°F).

You'll need a food processor for this. Place all the ingredients in the processor bowl and blitz to mix together. The result resembles brown porridge, but don't despair. Pour it into the lined pan and bake for 45 minutes. Leave to cool before slicing and serving with the quick tomato soup on page 45.

PER PORTION (¹/₁₀ OF THE LOAF)

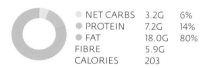

● NET CARBS	3.2G	6%
● PROTEIN	7.2G	14%
● FAT	18.0G	80%
FIBRE	5.9G	
CALORIES	203	

Flaxseed bread

250g (8.8 oz) flaxseeds – use a
   mixture of ground and whole
   (150g ground, 100g whole)
80g (2.8 oz) ground almonds (80g)
50g (3½tbsp) butter or coconut oil
   (50g butter)
100ml (⅜c) water (100g)
2 tbsp cider vinegar (23g)
2 tsp fennel seeds (4g)
1½ tsp baking soda (6g)
1 tsp chopped fresh rosemary (2g)
Few scrapes of lemon zest (1g)
1 pinch of flaky sea salt (preferably
   Maldon) (3g)

Makes 10 slices

No-grain nut, kale and seed bread

100g (3.5 oz) quinoa (100g)
60g (2.1 oz) coconut oil (60g)
350ml (1½c) water (350g)
1 tbsp maple syrup (20g)
100g (3.5 oz) kale (100g)
125g (4.5 oz) whole blanched
   almonds, toasted and chopped
   (125g)
85g (3 oz) linseeds (85g)
70g (2.5 oz) pumpkin seeds (70g)
45g (1.5 oz) sunflower seeds (45g)
25g (0.8 oz) chia seeds (25g)
3 tbsp psyllium husks (54g)
1 tbsp coconut flour (9g)
Good pinch or so of sea salt (3g)

Makes 1 loaf

The flaxseed bread recipe on page 47 is one option that I now make regularly, but I can't stop experimenting, so here's a recipe I've adapted from Natasha Corrett's book, *Honestly, Healthy, Cleanse*. I fiddled about to make it simpler, swapping oats for quinoa to avoid the gluten and reduce the carbs (a little) and wilting the kale in the oven (since it has already been preheated for baking the loaf) rather than faffing about with a steamer. The list of ingredients looks a bit long, but this is more assembly than baking – no kneading or proving required – which in my book is reason enough to cook it.

First soak the quinoa for an hour in water, then drain.

Preheat the oven to 170°C (340°F). Line a 22cm × 11cm (9in × 4in) loaf pan and butter or oil it.

Melt the coconut oil, then add the water and maple syrup and mix well. Wash and chop the kale but don't dry it. Just spread it on a tray and leave it in the oven until it's wilted – about 5 minutes.

Next, drain the quinoa and put it into a large bowl along with all the other dry ingredients and mix well before adding the chopped, wilted kale and then the liquid ingredients. The chia seeds will swell quickly, helping the ingredients to come together into a stiff, dough-like consistency.

Transfer the dough to the lined loaf pan. Press it well into the corners and flatten the top. Cook for 45 minutes before removing from the pan and cooking it on a wire rack for another 15 minutes to dry it out.

PER PORTION (¹⁄₁₀ OF THE LOAF)

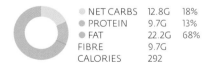

● NET CARBS	12.8G	18%
● PROTEIN	9.7G	13%
● FAT	22.2G	68%
FIBRE	9.7G	
CALORIES	292	

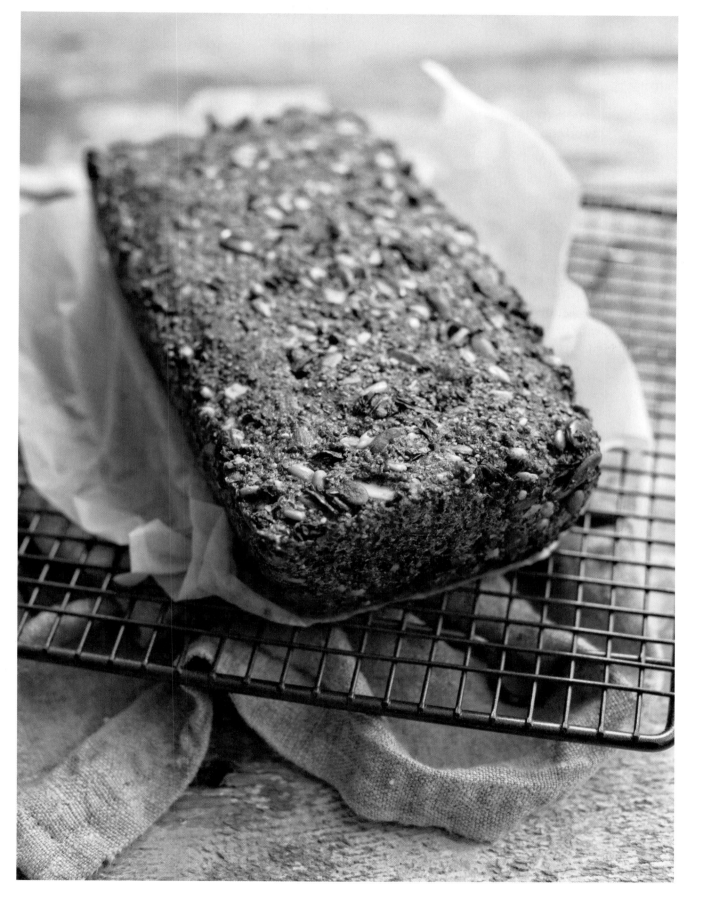

Mains

How do you redefine dinner when it's so often thought of as a plate with meat and two veg, with our quintessential 'two veg' always including potatoes? Nowadays, my plate looks different. I sometimes roast sweet potatoes for dinner, mainly to bulk out the kids' meals, but more often the 'two veg' means just that: two portions of non-starchy, low-carb vegetables.

There are fancier things to do with vegetables later on in the book, but keep it simple if you're making a nice main dish. If you're making a stew, say, then some gently steamed or boiled broccoli with a knob of butter is perfect. We don't need spuds and stew and a snazzy veg dish for an easy supper. Cut down on what you cook and eat and everyone will be happy.

Having some starch for kids is the easiest way to bulk out dinner because no one wants to be cooking two or three different meals for one evening, so some rice, wild rice, baked sweet potatoes or even regular boiled potatoes are all perfect for them. I've included recipes for some lentil and quinoa dishes because I love them and eat them in moderation, and I do try to prepare them in the traditional way (more of that later). I'm also a fan of black rice, but again, I have changed my portion sizes. I think of eating carb side dishes in terms of ice cream scoops. If I limit it to that, I find it easier to

manage my weight and health, but it does take a while to readjust.

So how many carbs should you eat to officially be 'low-carb'? There seem to be plenty of caveats to recommending an official amount of grams per day to achieve 'low-carb' status. Age, gender and the amount of exercise you do all seem to be factors, especially the degree of carbohydrate intolerance you have (you can take the test on page 13). For example, a type 2 diabetic who, on a 'balanced' diet of 300g of carbs a day, requires several shots of insulin a day to keep glucose values under control might have to lower carbohydrates a lot more to reduce medication than someone who wants to lose some extra pounds but has no health issues otherwise. Generally, however, most experts seem to agree that staying around 50–100g per day is good. This would allow for sensible meals, some fruit per day and a small amount of starchy carbohydrates. Most of the meals in my section fall into this range, taking into consideration other things you will be eating throughout the day. For example, if you eat the spring scrambled eggs on page 28 you'll have more room to play with later in the day, but eating the moong dal on page 80 will mean you have to be conscious of your other meals and keep them more fat and protein based.

Get your blender or food processor out for this one. If you forget to buy lemongrass, for example, don't worry. Just add in more of the other stuff, like garlic and ginger. Double the recipe and freeze half of it. Serve with any kind of rice you fancy. I like the cauliflower rice on page 297.

Whizz all the curry paste ingredients together until it resembles green sludge. If your food processor jams, add a little water to help it along.

Chop the chicken into bite-sized pieces and chuck into a large bowl. Wash your hands, chopping board and knife carefully! Pour the green gloop on top. Mix so the chicken is well coated and leave for anywhere between 10 minutes and overnight, whatever you can manage.

Chop the onions and eggplants into bite-sized pieces. Heat a large saucepan and cook the onions over a high heat in the coconut oil until they are starting to colour. Add the eggplants and watch them suck up all the juice. Season with a little salt. Don't worry if they start to burn in patches. Add the marinated chicken, mix well and add the coconut milk. Bring up to a gentle boil, then leave to simmer gently for 30–40 minutes. Taste and serve with the cauliflower rice on page 180.

PER PORTION

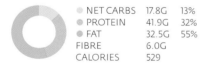

NET CARBS	17.8G	13%
PROTEIN	41.9G	32%
FAT	32.5G	55%
FIBRE	6.0G	
CALORIES	529	

Green and light Thai-ish, very lazy chicken curry

4 skinless chicken breasts (520g)
2 onions, peeled (300g)
2 eggplants (600g)
1 good tbsp coconut oil (27g)
Salt (2g)
1 × 400ml can (14.1 oz) of coconut milk (400g)

Green gloop:

1 onion, roughly chopped (150g)
4 garlic cloves, peeled (12g)
Big bunch of cilantro, rinsed lightly and stalks left on (20g)
1 green chilli, deseeded (20g)
1 giant thumb's worth of ginger, peeled (add more if you like it) (40g)
2 stalks of lemongrass, roughly chopped (9.6g)
Juice and zest of 2 limes (30g + 4g)
2 tbsp fish sauce (36g)
1 heaped tbsp dried curry leaves (6g)

Serves 4

Roast chicken

2 carrots, peeled and roughly
  chopped (200g)

2 onions, roughly chopped (don't
  peel them) (300g)

1 head of garlic, unpeeled (30g)

1 medium chicken, approx 1.5kg
  (3.3lb) (1.5kg)

1 lemon, cut in half (130g)

Few sprigs of thyme (4g)

Salt and pepper (3g)

1 tbsp Worcestershire sauce (18g)

Approx. 200ml (⅞c) chicken stock,
  water or a glass of white wine
  (200g wine)

Serves 4 plus leftovers

One of my all-time favourite dinners, and the best part is the bone broth, which is ready by day two or three. It's WD-40 for the soul and any aching joints.

You will see that the nutritional info below is dependent on the assumption that one average roast chicken will feed eight people. This seems way out of whack for many of us. I usually assume one roast chicken will feed four adults as well as leave a few bits for leftovers. While this might be fine if you are following a low-carb diet, it's important to note that if you are on a ketogenic diet, eating a quarter of a roast chicken (say, a full leg or breast) would be way too much protein. So if you are interested in how many grams of protein you are eating, bear in mind that you get quite a lot of protein from chicken.

Preheat the oven to 190°C (375°F).

Put the carrots, onions and garlic in the middle of a roasting tray, then place the chicken, breast side down, on top of the veg. Squeeze the lemon over the chicken, then stuff the lemon halves into the chicken. Season generously with thyme, salt and pepper.

Cover with tin foil and roast for about 35 minutes, then remove the foil and turn down the oven to 180°C (350°F). Flip the bird over and douse with the Worcestershire sauce on top and the glass of wine in the bottom. Season again and cook for another 40 minutes.

At this stage, take it out and leave for a few minutes. Give the legs a wiggle: they should move about freely. If you aren't sure, slice between the leg and the breast and check what colour it is. It shouldn't be too pink and the juices should definitely be clear.

PER PORTION (⅛ OF THE RECIPE)

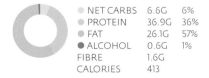

NET CARBS	6.6G	6%
PROTEIN	36.9G	36%
FAT	26.1G	57%
ALCOHOL	0.6G	1%
FIBRE	1.6G	
CALORIES	413	

In this recipe, kale turns up in an unusual place – a dip. Not just any dip, perfect for carrot or celery sticks or even used as a spread on brown bread for school lunch boxes, but one that doubles as a stuffing for chicken joints. The kale is cooked briefly and then blitzed with cheese, capers and garlic to create a moreish stuffing that, when baked, becomes a golden, bubbling pool of flavour. I've tried this with a bit of chorizo too and it works brilliantly. Maybe it's easy to be green after all.

Preheat the oven to 180°C (350°F).

To make the dip, blanch the kale for 20 seconds in a saucepan of boiling water before draining and refreshing under cold running water until it's cool. Drain it well – you may need to squeeze it – then put the kale and all the other ingredients in a food processor and blitz till smooth-ish. You can now use it either as a dip or as a stuffing for the chicken.

Use your fingers to lift the skin away from the flesh of the chicken, but without removing it entirely. You want to create a pocket for the stuffing. Use your hands to smear generous quantities of the stuffing under the skin – it doesn't matter if it drips down the side a little.

When all the thighs are stuffed, place them in a large roasting pan, season well and get the crisping started by drizzling with a little olive oil. Roast for 45 minutes in the hot oven, until golden and bubbling. Serve with a green salad.

Roast chicken with green feta stuffing

8 chicken thighs, skin on (800g including bone)
Salt and pepper (3g)
2 tsp olive oil (8g)

Green feta dip:
50g (1.8 oz) kale, destalked and washed (50g)
100g (3.5 oz) feta (100g)
1 small garlic clove, crushed (2g)
Small bunch of dill (8g)
3 tbsp Greek yoghurt (135g)
1 tbsp olive oil (13g)
1 tsp capers (3g)

Serves 4

PER PORTION (¼ OF THE CHICKEN RECIPE)

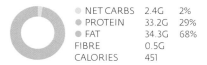

	NET CARBS	2.4G	2%
	PROTEIN	33.2G	29%
	FAT	34.3G	68%
	FIBRE	0.5G	
	CALORIES	451	

PER PORTION (¹⁄₆ OF THE FETA DIP OR 52G)

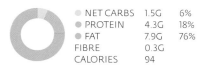

	NET CARBS	1.5G	6%
	PROTEIN	4.3G	18%
	FAT	7.9G	76%
	FIBRE	0.3G	
	CALORIES	94	

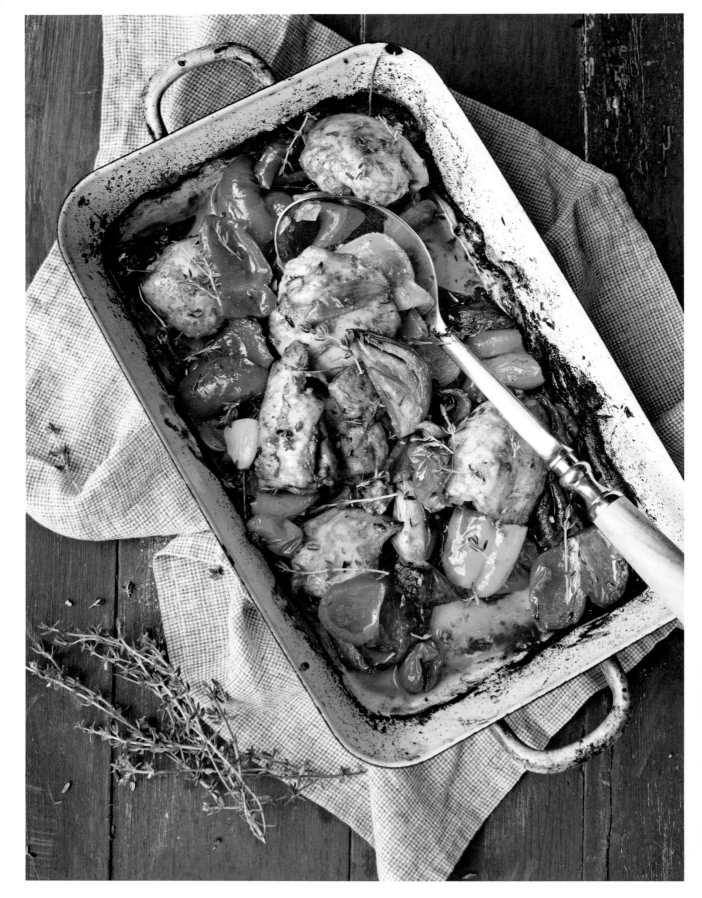

This roast chicken bake is a bit more Mediterranean in feel – a reminder of summer when you most need it. And if you get your butcher to debone the thighs as part of your order, this dish takes less than 10 minutes to prepare. It's almost ludicrously easy. You simply mix all the ingredients together in a bowl, transfer onto a tray, bung it in the oven and *voilà*! It really is the ultimate no-brainer dinner.

Preheat the oven to 180°C (350°F).

Are you ready? It's so simple. Basically, put all the ingredients in a bowl, toss them together and season really well (good seasoning is essential here). Then swap the bowl for a roasting tray and bake for 45–50 minutes. This smells divine and tastes even better.

PER PORTION

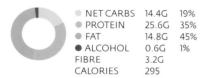

● NET CARBS	14.4G	19%
● PROTEIN	25.6G	35%
● FAT	14.8G	45%
● ALCOHOL	0.6G	1%
FIBRE	3.2G	
CALORIES	295	

Roast chicken bake

8 skinless, boneless chicken thighs (360g)

2 red onions, quartered (300g)

1 red pepper, deseeded and quartered (160g)

1 yellow pepper, deseeded and quartered (160g)

1 punnet (8.8 oz) cherry tomatoes (250g)

4 garlic cloves, crushed (12g)

Few springs of thyme, oregano or rosemary (4g)

100ml (⅜c) white wine (100g)

2 tbsp olive oil (26g)

2 tbsp balsamic vinegar (23g)

1 tsp smoked paprika (2g)

Salt and pepper (3g)

Serves 4

Balsamic roast chicken with arugula, roast tomatoes and Parmesan

4 chicken breasts, skin on (520g)

2 tbsp olive oil (26g)

Few tablespoons balsamic vinegar (22.8g)

1 tbsp Worcestershire sauce (18g)

Few cloves of peeled garlic (9g)

Some thyme or rosemary if you have it (5g)

Salt and pepper (3g)

1 pack (9 oz) cherry tomatoes, sliced in half (250g)

4 handfuls of arugula (90g)

Few chunky shavings of Parmesan or Pecorino (20g)

Serves 4

Pure ease.

Preheat the oven to 180°C (350°F).

Plop the chicken into a roasting tray (wash your hands!) and pour over the olive oil, balsamic vinegar and Worcestershire sauce. Add in some garlic and herbs and season well, then add the cherry tomatoes (or leave them out if you hate them).

Cover the roasting tray with a baking tray to form a lid (this just stops it drying out too much, but foil will do) and cook for about 10 minutes. Remove the lid/tin foil, turn the chicken pieces over and baste with the cooking juices. Give it another blast for another 5–10 minutes, until the chicken is fully cooked through. If you aren't sure or if your chicken breasts are ginormous, then just slice one in half lengthways and give it a few more minutes if it looks a little pink.

Arrange the arugula on four plates, top with chicken and some tomatoes and loads of the cooking juices (which is like a warm and simple vinaigrette). Top with some Parmesan shavings and serve.

PER PORTION

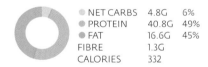

● NET CARBS	4.8G	6%
● PROTEIN	40.8G	49%
● FAT	16.6G	45%
FIBRE	1.3G	
CALORIES	332	

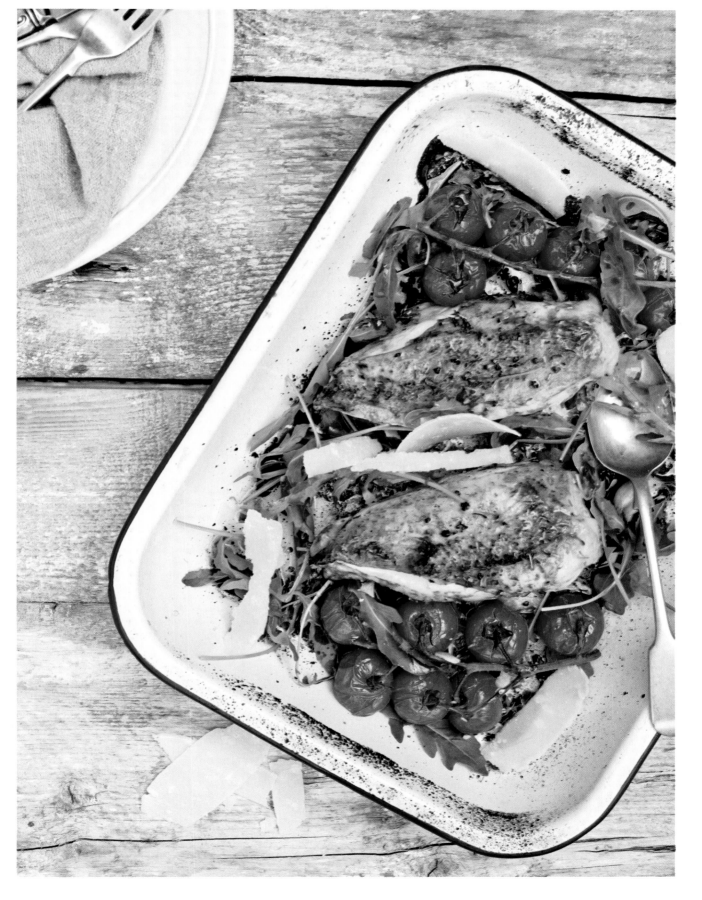

Grilled mint and chilli chicken

8 boneless chicken thighs (360g)
Large bunch of mint (12g)
2 chillies, deseeded and roughly
    chopped (40g)
3 garlic cloves, crushed (9g)
Zest and juice of 2 limes (4g + 40g)
1 tbsp olive oil (13g)
Good pinch of dried mint (1g)
½ tsp honey (4g)
Salt and pepper (3g)
Seeds of 1 pomegranate (120g seeds)
Chopped parsley, cilantro or mint (8g)

Serves 4

Mint and chilli, yum. If you want to use skinless thighs, do, and if you can only get thighs with the bone in them, then just be sure to cook them for 15 minutes longer.

Put the chicken thighs in a shallow dish that can go in the oven. Put the rest of the ingredients except the pomegranate seeds and parsley in your food processor and blitz. Pour over the marinade and try to leave for at least 1 hour to marinate or longer if you can, but it really doesn't need to be done overnight.

To cook, preheat your oven as hot as it will go and blast the thighs for 15 minutes. Sometimes they ooze out a lot of liquid. Turn them over, baste with the marinade, turn the oven down to 200°C (400°F) and cook for another 30–40 minutes, until cooked through. It's quite a wet marinade so they wont go uber-sticky, although you can help get this effect by sticking them under a hot grill. Garnish with pomegranate seeds and chopped parsley, cilantro or mint.

PER PORTION

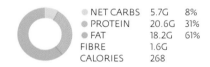

NET CARBS	5.7G	8%
PROTEIN	20.6G	31%
FAT	18.2G	61%
FIBRE	1.6G	
CALORIES	268	

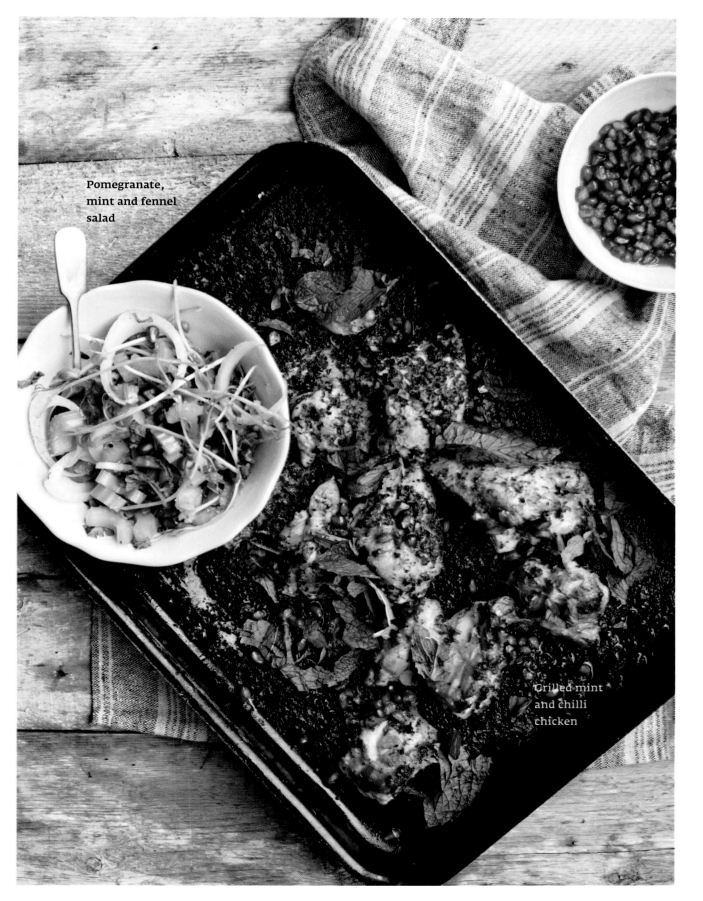

Pomegranate,
mint and fennel
salad

Grilled mint
and chilli
chicken

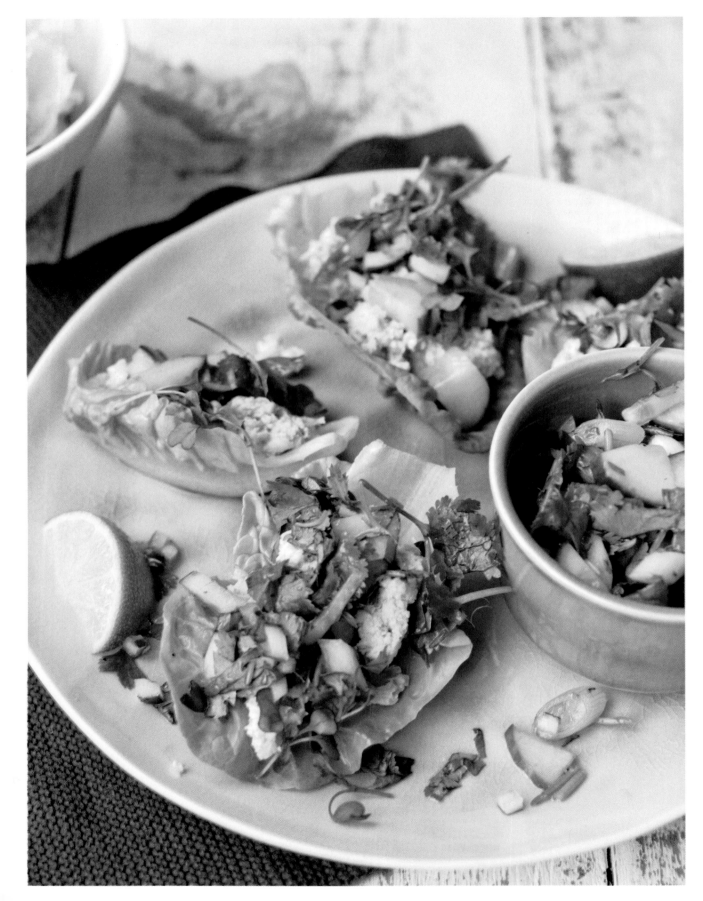

Fragrant, fresh and delicious.

In a food processor, pulse the chicken so that the meat becomes finely minced. If you don't have a food processor, then chop it finely.

Heat the water in a large saucepan along with the chilli, garlic, ginger and fish sauce. When it comes to the boil, add the chicken and bring it back to the boil, then reduce the heat to a simmer. Break up the chicken with a wooden spoon so that it doesn't form clumps. Cook for a few minutes, then turn the heat off and allow the chicken to cook gently in the residual heat for another 10 minutes with the lid on. Mix well and check to make sure the meat is thoroughly cooked, then allow to cool. Hopefully most of the liquid will have cooked off.

Meanwhile, chop the herbs and mix them with the cucumber, red onion, scallions, lime juice, olive oil, tamari and mirin and season with some salt and pepper. Check the seasoning.

When the chicken has cooled down, spoon some of the chicken mix into each baby gem leaf, top with the herb and cucumber salad sauce and serve with toasted pistachios on top.

PER PORTION

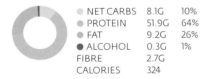

● NET CARBS	8.1G	10%
● PROTEIN	51.9G	64%
● FAT	9.2G	26%
● ALCOHOL	0.3G	1%
FIBRE	2.7G	
CALORIES	324	

Lime and mint chicken parcels

4–6 skinless chicken breasts, roughly chopped (600g)

500ml (2⅛c) water (500g)

1 chilli, deseeded and finely sliced (20g)

2 garlic cloves, finely sliced (6g)

Good knob of ginger, peeled and thinly chopped (10g)

2 tbsp fish sauce (36g)

Bunch of mint leaves (20g)

Bunch of cilantro (16g)

Bunch of basil leaves (15g)

1 cucumber, deseeded and finely sliced (360g)

1 small red onion, thinly sliced (60g)

Bunch of scallions, finely chopped (60g)

Juice of 4 limes (80g)

1 tbsp olive oil (13g)

2 tsp tamari (12g)

2 tsp mirin (11g)

Salt and pepper (3g)

2 baby gems, broken into individual leaves (300g)

2 tbsp pistachios, lightly toasted (14g)

Serves 4

Green Asian chicken salad

This is my ideal lunch if there is any leftover chicken from the roast on page 52. Unlikely, but that's why I will sometimes roast two chickens, so I have enough meat left over for one or two ace dishes, like this lovely salad.

Large bag of kale (170g)

Bunch of scallions, finely chopped (60g)

Leftover roast chicken – about 150g per person, chopped (300g)

1 ripe avocado, chopped (240g)

20g (0.7 oz) sesame seeds (20g)

Dressing:

1 garlic clove, crushed (3g)

1 tbsp chopped mint (4g)

1 tbsp sesame oil (12g)

1 tbsp fish sauce (18g)

1 tbsp honey or maple syrup (21g honey)

1 tbsp mirin (15.9g)

1 tbsp tamari (18g)

Serves 2

Raw kale can be too harsh for some folks because of its goitrogen load, so a quick steam or even just putting it in a colander and pouring boiling water over it will help. Just dry it as much as possible and proceed as normal.

Start by washing, destalking and drying the kale and shredding it into bite-sized shards about 8cm (3in) or so across. Patricia recommends steaming kale to help reduce the goitrogen load. I do and I don't. If you want to, I find the best way is to put it on a baking tray and let it wilt in a hot oven for about 5 minutes. Job done.

Next, make the dressing by mixing all the ingredients together in a large bowl. Add the raw kale and scallions and leave them to marinate for about 20 minutes or so, until the kale is wilted a little. Finally, add in the chopped chicken, avocado and sesame seeds, mix well and serve.

PER PORTION

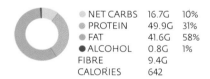

NET CARBS	16.7G	10%
PROTEIN	49.9G	31%
FAT	41.6G	58%
ALCOHOL	0.8G	1%
FIBRE	9.4G	
CALORIES	642	

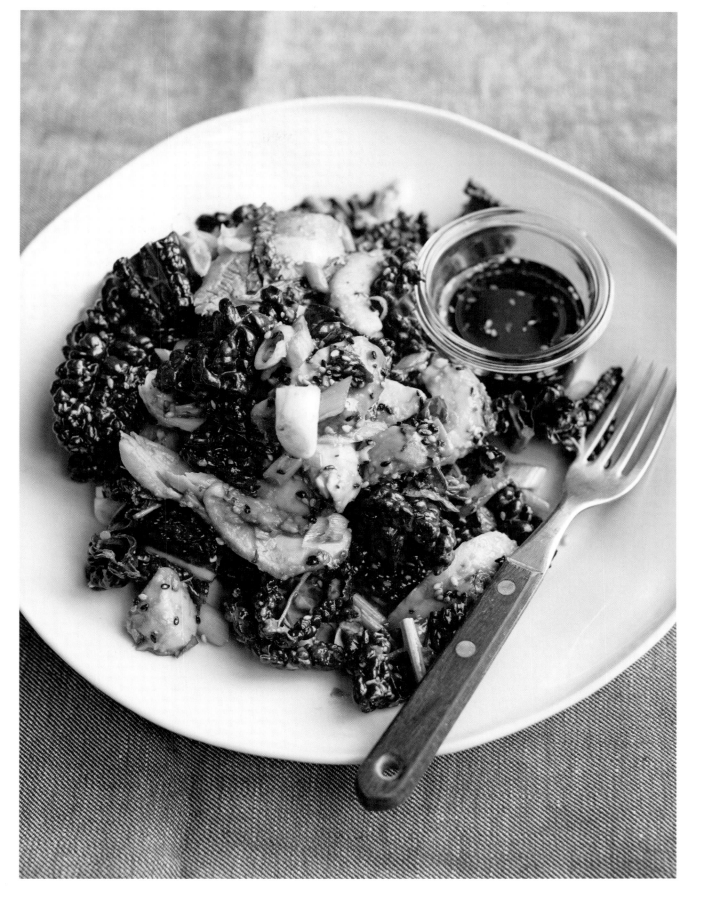

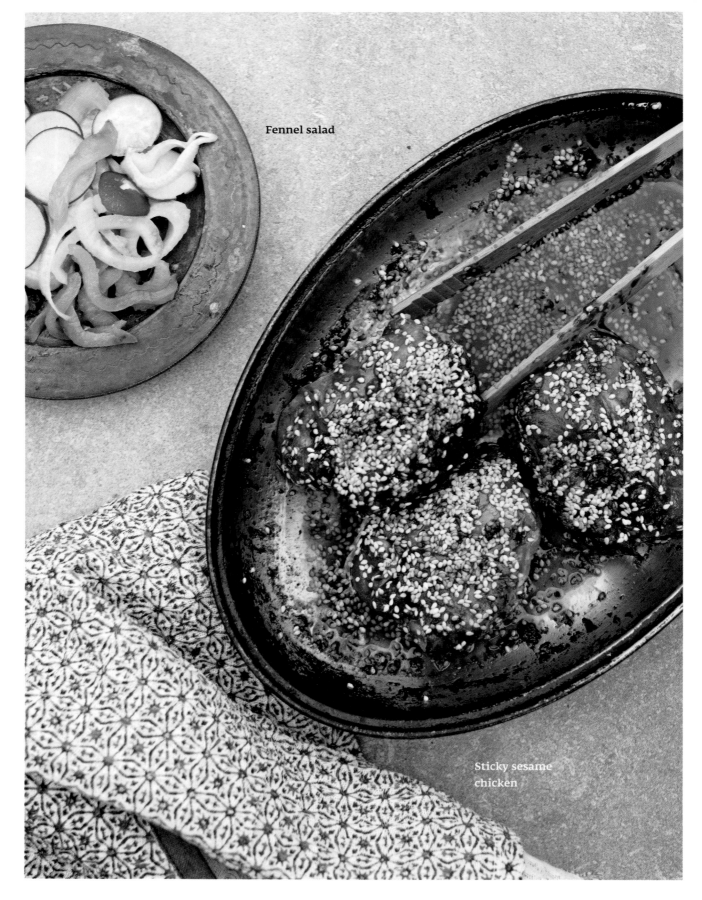

Fennel salad

Sticky sesame chicken

You can make this with drumsticks or chicken breasts, if you like. Allow two thighs per person. I used to make this with lots of brown sugar but have modified it to be better behaved, sugar wise. Grrr. It's a fun dish and very tasty, but the original is truly evil.

Preheat the oven to 200°C (400°F).

Heat the butter in a small saucepan and add the garlic, tamari, fish sauce, sesame seeds, sesame oil, honey and black pepper. Whisk well and pour the sauce over the chicken. It may seem like you don't have much sauce, but it will get quite liquid when it cooks.

Bake for about 40 minutes, until golden brown and sticky. You can turn the chicken pieces over about halfway through cooking and baste with the sauce. You could serve this with loads of chopped scallions and cilantro.

Sticky sesame chicken

50g (3½tbsp) butter (50g)
3 garlic cloves, sliced (9g)
3 tbsp tamari (54g)
3 tbsp fish sauce (54g)
2½ tbsp sesame seeds (27.5g)
1 tbsp sesame oil (12g)
1 tbsp honey or maple syrup (21g honey)
Black pepper (1g)
8 chicken thigh fillets, bone in and skin on (600g)

Serves 4

PER PORTION

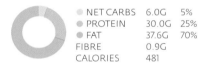

NET CARBS	6.0G	5%
PROTEIN	30.0G	25%
FAT	37.6G	70%
FIBRE	0.9G	
CALORIES	481	

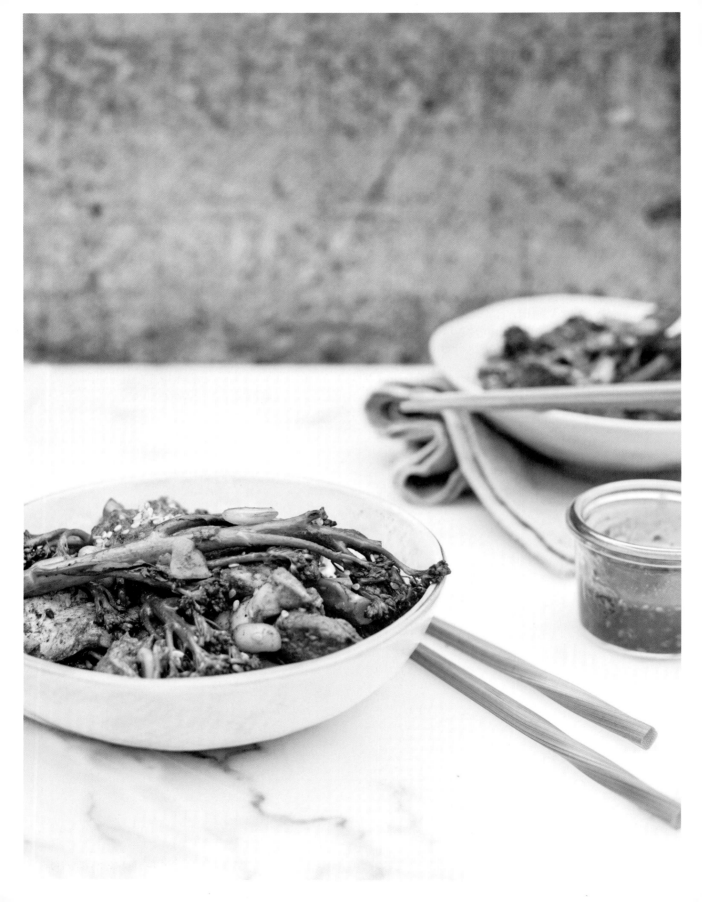

Just as time works its magic on a rich stew or slow roast, marinating does all the hard work for you. And marinating, for just a half hour or so, is all it takes to turn the chicken in this recipe into a tender, flavoursome and healthy supper. Oh, there's a few moments' steaming too, but again, this will hardly strain the muscles.

Start by marinating the chicken in the garlic, five spice and tamari about half an hour before you're ready to serve.

When you're ready to cook, heat the coconut oil in a frying pan and fry the chicken until it's coloured a little – about 3 minutes – before adding the broccoli stems and the water. Cover tightly with a lid, turn the heat down to medium and steam for about 5 minutes, until the chicken is cooked through and the stems are al dente. Remove the lid and check the seasoning (it shouldn't need salt) before adding the nuts and sesame seeds, tossing the whole lot together and serving on a bed of the broccoli rice on page 171.

Chicken, cashew and broccoli stir-fry

4 skinless chicken breasts, sliced into
   1.25cm (½in) strips (480g)
2 garlic cloves, sliced (6g)
1 tbsp five-spice powder (6g)
1 tbsp tamari (18g)
1 good tbsp coconut oil (27g)
400g (14.1 oz) broccoli stems (use
   the florets for the broccoli rice)
   (400g)
200ml (⅞c) water (200g)
2 tbsp cashews (20g)
1 tbsp sesame seeds (11g)

Serves 4

PER PORTION

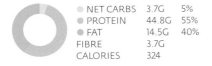

NET CARBS	3.7G	5%
PROTEIN	44.8G	55%
FAT	14.5G	40%
FIBRE	3.7G	
CALORIES	324	

Chicken with lemon and green olives

4–8 pieces of chicken (depending on size) with the skin on (520g)

1 tbsp butter (15g)

Salt and pepper (3g)

2 white onions, sliced (300g)

2 tsp ground coriander (4g)

1 tsp ground ginger (5g)

Good pinch of ground turmeric (1g)

Pinch of saffron (1g)

300ml (1¼c) chicken stock (300g)

100g (3.5 oz) green olives, stoned (100g)

2 lemons, fresh or preserved, sliced (260g)

Large bunch of flat-leaf parsley, chopped (20g)

Large bunch of cilantro, chopped (20g)

Serves 4

Whether a recipe calls for the zest, pulp, juice or even all three, lemons can lift a dish out of the ordinary into the realm of the sensational. And whether it's there to cut through fat or throw sweet flavours into sharp relief, lemons are something I could not imagine ever doing without.

Preheat the oven to 180°C (350°F).

You'll need a pot with a lid that will go from hob to oven for this. Start by browning the chicken pieces, skin side down, in the butter and season well. When they've got a good colour, set them aside.

Add the onions to the pot, turn the heat down to medium, put the lid on and sweat for 5 minutes. Add the spices, stirring well so all the flavours start coming together. Return the chicken to the pot and add the stock, olives and lemons. Bring to a simmer before transferring to the oven, lid on, for a further 40 minutes.

If you want to be fancy when serving it, lay the chicken pieces on a platter, then reduce the sauce to thicken it. Add the fresh herbs to the sauce and spoon it over the chicken.

PER PORTION

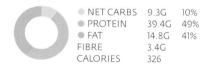

NET CARBS	9.3G	10%
PROTEIN	39.4G	49%
FAT	14.8G	41%
FIBRE	3.4G	
CALORIES	326	

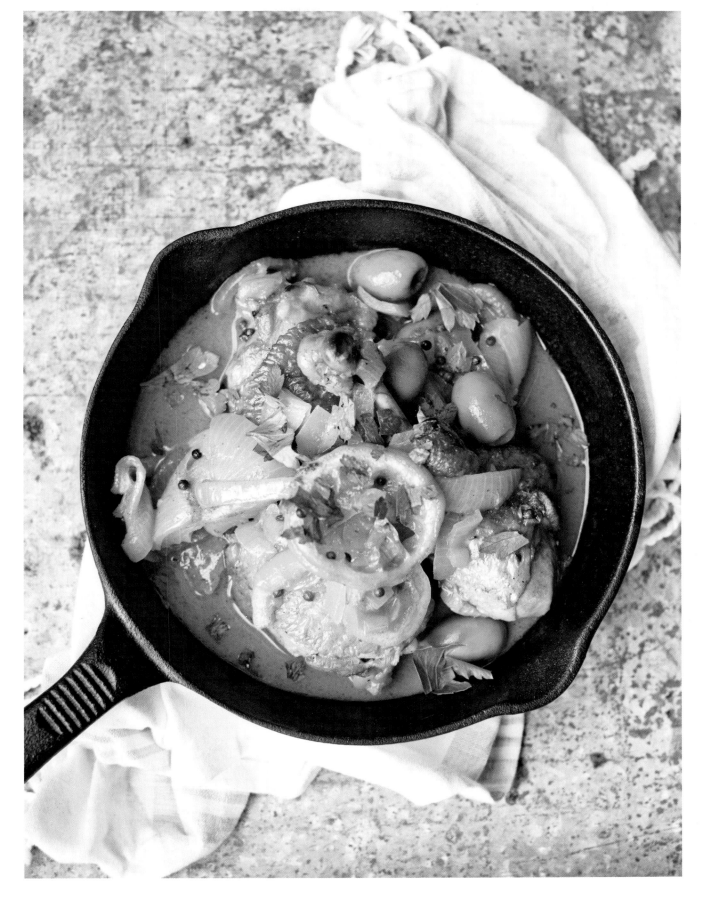

Pan-fried lemon chicken with celeriac remoulade

4 skinless chicken breasts (520g)
Knob of butter (15g)
1 tbsp olive oil (13g)
Squeeze of lemon juice (15g)
Few sprigs of thyme (4g)

Remoulade:

1 head of celery (540g)
1 medium celeriac (500g)
100ml (⅜c) crème fraîche or Greek
  yoghurt (100g)
Zest and juice of 1 lemon (2g + 40g)
1 tbsp Dijon mustard (24g)
1 tbsp wholegrain mustard (30g)
1 tbsp chopped capers (8.6g)
Handful of flat-leaf parsley,
  chopped (12g)
Salt and pepper (3g)

Serves 4

First make the remoulade. Slice the celery very thinly. Chop the top and bottom off the celeriac. It should sit still on your board. Cut the skin off using a knife, removing the skin from top to bottom, then cut the celeriac into thin slices and chop these into long, thin strips. Mix with the celery, crème fraîche, lemon zest and juice, both mustards and capers. Mix really well, add the parsley and season well. It will be fine for an hour or two.

Preheat the oven to 160°C (320°F).

Slice the chicken breasts in half horizontally. Place the pieces of breast, one at a time, onto a sheet of cling film and cover with another sheet of cling film. Bash the pieces of chicken flat with a rolling pin so that you end up with wide, flat, thin chicken breasts.

Heat the butter and olive oil in a large frying pan and brown the chicken pieces. Season them with plenty of black pepper, then transfer to a roasting pan or other serving dish. When all the breasts have been browned off, add a good splash of water and a squeeze of lemon juice to deglaze the frying pan.

Pour this over the chicken along with a few sprigs of thyme, cover loosely with tin foil and bake for 5–10 minutes, until fully cooked through. Serve with a big spoonful of the remoulade.

PER PORTION

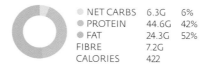

NET CARBS	6.3G	6%
PROTEIN	44.6G	42%
FAT	24.3G	52%
FIBRE	7.2G	
CALORIES	422	

The skin is left on, first to crisp up beautifully to a rich golden brown and then, over a lower heat, to render so it combines with the wine, garlic, herbs and lemon juice to form the most delicious sauce. This is how you make a creamy sauce without cream.

Heat the butter in a large heavy-based pan and brown the chicken on all sides for about 5 minutes, until golden brown. You might need to do this in batches. Make sure you get a good colour on it, then season well.

Next, add the garlic, wine, lemon juice and zest, thyme and bay leaves and mix thoroughly. Lower the heat to medium-low and cook with the lid on for 45 minutes. If your pan is a bit flimsy, then you may need to add a few splashes of water occasionally to stop it sticking (read burning). Sprinkle with fresh parsley before serving.

PER PORTION

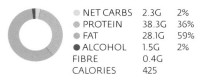

● NET CARBS	2.3G	2%
● PROTEIN	38.3G	36%
● FAT	28.1G	59%
● ALCOHOL	1.5G	2%
FIBRE	0.4G	
CALORIES	425	

Lemon and garlic poached chicken

Big knob of butter (25g)
Approx. 8 chicken pieces, on the
  bone and skin on (736g)
Salt and pepper (3g)
Approx. 10 garlic cloves (30g)
250ml (1c) white wine (250g)
Zest and juice of 2 lemons (4g + 80g)
Few sprigs of fresh thyme (4g)
2 bay leaves (2g)
Fresh parsley, chopped (8g)

Serves 4

Steeped chicken with scallion and ginger sauce

1 chicken (1.35kg)
Bunch of scallions (60g)
Few slices of fresh ginger (10g)
1 tbsp sea salt (15g)
Black pepper (1g)

Scallion and ginger sauce:
3 large bunches of scallions (180g)
3 garlic cloves, peeled (9g)
Good knob of ginger, peeled (10g)
100ml (⅜c) olive oil (100g)
2 tbsp tamari (26g)
1 tsp sesame oil (optional) (4g)

Serves 4

You can really play around with this sauce. Sometimes I use the soy sauce that's syrupy and sweet and sometimes I chuck in thinly sliced mushrooms or cilantro. Basically, anything goes!

Put the chicken in a large saucepan that you can fit a lid onto and cover it with water. Chuck in the rest of the ingredients and cook on a gentle heat until just simmering. Keep the lid on and simmer for 15–20 minutes, then take off the heat and keep covered with the lid for 1 hour.

Meanwhile, to make the scallion and ginger sauce, finely slice or chop the scallions, garlic and ginger and have them ready to go, sitting in a bowl. Heat the olive oil in a saucepan until it's hot but not smoking. Pour the hot oil over the scallions and mix well. The heat will cook the scallions, garlic and ginger just enough. Add the tamari and sesame oil, if using, and adjust the seasoning to your taste.

When the chicken is fully cooked, remove it from the saucepan, but be careful of hot water pouring out of the bird! Check it's cooked by slicing between the breast and the leg to make sure it's not pink, but if it is, dump it back in the water and heat it for another 10 minutes. Remove the skin and discard. Tear off the chicken and serve in chunks on a platter with a bowl of the scallion and ginger sauce.

PER PORTION OF THE CHICKEN

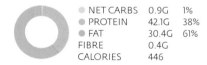

NET CARBS	0.9G	1%
PROTEIN	42.1G	38%
FAT	30.4G	61%
FIBRE	0.4G	
CALORIES	446	

PER PORTION OF THE SAUCE (¼ OF THE SAUCE RECIPE)

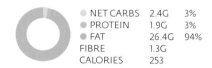

NET CARBS	2.4G	3%
PROTEIN	1.9G	3%
FAT	26.4G	94%
FIBRE	1.3G	
CALORIES	253	

This is my go-to recipe when I have chicken breast and nothing else, mainly because I always have full-fat or Greek yoghurt at home. You can mess with the spices in this one, but I really like the combo of coriander and fennel seeds, lemon and lots of black pepper.

I make this in minutes. Put the chicken strips or chunks into a gratin dish and pour on the yoghurt along with the lemon juice, oil, coriander and fennel seeds and seasoning. Mix it around – it doesn't need to be brilliant, but enough to smooth out the yoghurt and coat the chicken pieces.

Turn your grill to its highest setting and grill the heck out of it. After about 7 minutes it should be starting to char, at which point you turn the pieces over and rearrange them slightly to give the pale and anaemic bits a bit more charring. It should be cooked after 15 minutes of grilling on a high heat.

When it's cooked through, serve hot or warm. It's also delicious served cold in sandwiches the next day.

Coriander chicken

4 skinless chicken breasts, cut into
    strips or chunks (480g)
100g (3.5 oz) Greek yoghurt
    (½ big tub) (100g)
Juice of 1 lemon (40g)
1 tbsp olive oil (13g)
1 tsp coriander seeds (2g)
1 tsp fennel seeds (2g)
Salt and pepper (2g + 2.3g)

Serves 4

PER PORTION

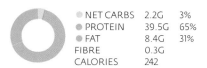

NET CARBS	2.2G	3%
PROTEIN	39.5G	65%
FAT	8.4G	31%
FIBRE	0.3G	
CALORIES	242	

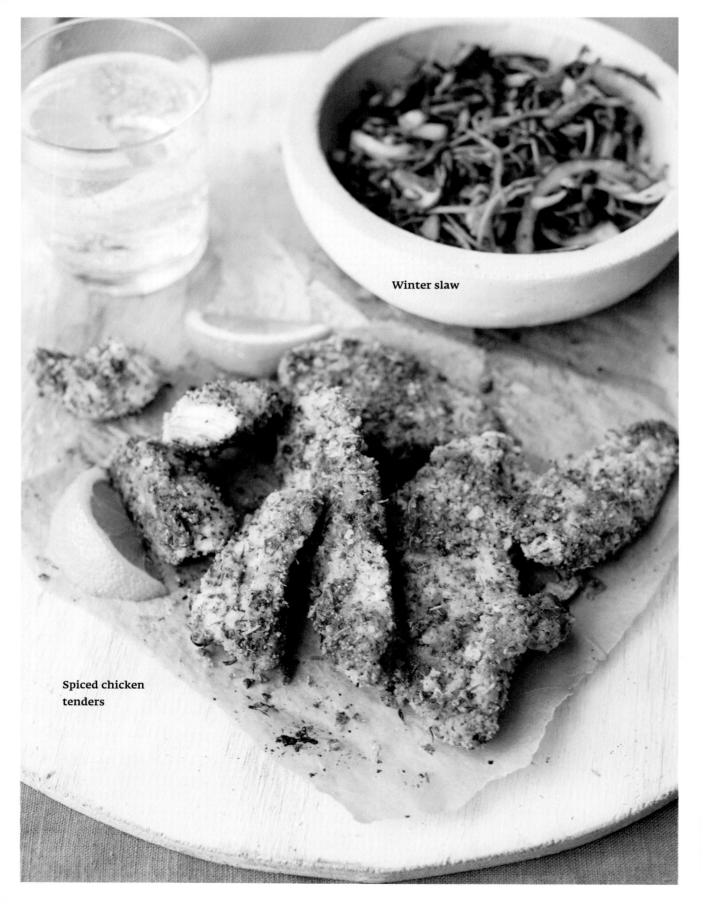

Winter slaw

Spiced chicken
tenders

Preheat the oven to 200°C (400°F).

Mix the coconut flour with all the dried ingredients and place in a shallow bowl or plate. Beat the eggs together in a large bowl. Drop the chicken strips into the egg wash and then plop them into the flour. Put the strips on an oiled non-stick baking tray or a tray lined with non-stick baking paper.

Drizzle with a bit more oil and cook in the hot oven until browned and crisp. This might take about 30 minutes in total, and halfway through cooking, it's a good idea to turn them over (gingerly) so they can brown on both sides.

PER PORTION

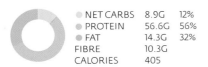

● NET CARBS	8.9G	12%
● PROTEIN	56.6G	56%
● FAT	14.3G	32%
FIBRE	10.3G	
CALORIES	405	

Spiced chicken tenders

100g (3.5 oz) coconut flour (100g)
1 tbsp dried oregano (5g)
1 tbsp dried thyme (3g)
1 tbsp dried rosemary (3g)
2 tsp ground white pepper (10.6g)
Good pinch of chilli flakes (2g)
Good pinch of sea salt (3g)
Loads of black pepper (2g)
2 eggs (114g)
4–6 skinless chicken breasts, cut into strips (600g)
1 tbsp olive oil (13g)

Serves 4

Tandoori chicken

6 garlic cloves, crushed (18g)

Good knob of ginger, peeled and finely chopped (10g)

2 tbsp olive oil (26g)

2 tbsp garam masala (12g)

2 tsp ground cumin (4g)

Good pinch of chilli flakes (2g)

200g (7 oz) plain or Greek yoghurt (200g)

Juice of 2 limes (40g)

2 tsp salt (10g)

4 skinless chicken breasts, cut into strips (480g)

Serves 4

This is a variation of the coriander chicken on page 73 for when you have more time.

Sweat the garlic and ginger in the olive oil, then add the spices after a few minutes. Cook for a few minutes to get the flavours going, then turn off the heat and cool down before mixing with the yoghurt, lime juice and salt.
Put the chicken strips in a gratin dish, pour on the tasty yoghurt and grill the heck out the chicken, as on page 73.

PER PORTION

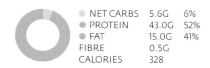

NET CARBS	5.6G	6%
PROTEIN	43.0G	52%
FAT	15.0G	41%
FIBRE	0.5G	
CALORIES	328	

'Medicine is a science of uncertainty and an art of probability.'
Sir William Osler

I use a whole chicken that I 'steep': I put it in a large saucepan, cover it with water and a bit of salt and pepper, bring it up to the boil, simmer it for couple of minutes and then turn it off and leave it for an hour to finish cooking. Then all you have to do is remove the skin, tear off bits of tender, juicy meat and when cool, dress it with your coronation sauce. Add the bones back to the leftover cooking stock, add some cider vinegar and make some more bone broth!

As mentioned above, put the chicken in a large pot, cover it with cold water, add some salt and pepper and bring up to the boil. Boil for few minutes, then reduce the heat and slosh out any scum with a large metal spoon. Simmer gently for at least 20 minutes, turn off the heat and leave the chicken to cook in the hot water for 1 hour. If your chicken is a giant, then simmer for 30 minutes before turning off the heat.

When the cooling-down hour has passed, carefully remove the bird from the water (hot water running out of the chicken will burn you if you're not careful), tear away the skin and discard, then tear the flesh off every nook and cranny and set aside. Chuck the carcass back into the stock and continue to cook for some bone broth (see page 423).

Meanwhile, make the coronation essence. Sweat the onion in the olive oil until soft. Add the curry powder and mix well. Turn up the heat and let it sizzle a bit, but sizzle doesn't mean burn. After a minute or so, add the tomato purée and mix well, then add the mango, wine, water, bay leaf and some seasoning. Mix well and allow it to reduce down until thick and a lovely rich, dark colour.

Allow it to cool and then mix with the mayo before adding the cooked chicken pieces and serving with crisp green leaves.

Coronation chicken

1 medium chicken (1.35kg)
Salt and pepper (3g)
1 onion, very finely chopped (150g)
2 tbsp olive oil (26g)
1 tbsp mild curry powder (6g)
Good squeeze of tomato purée (51g)
1 mango, peeled and finely diced
   (230g)
150ml (⅝c) red wine (150g)
120ml (½c) water (120g)
1 bay leaf (1g)
4 tbsp mayonnaise (88g)

Serves 4

PER PORTION

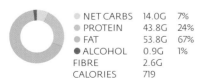

	NET CARBS	14.0G	7%
	PROTEIN	43.8G	24%
	FAT	53.8G	67%
	ALCOHOL	0.9G	1%
	FIBRE	2.6G	
	CALORIES	719	

Chicken with dried mushrooms

This chicken dish is pure comfort, rich and delicious. It's exactly what I crave in winter months and is lovely with dried morels, but any dried mushrooms will do nicely.

60g (2.1 oz) dried mushrooms (60g)
Big knob of butter (25g)
1 tbsp olive oil (13g)
8 chicken thighs or drumsticks (600g)
Salt and pepper (3g)
1 onion, very finely diced (150g)
1 glass of white wine (125g)
Few sprigs of thyme (4g)
200ml (⅞c) chicken stock (200g)
100ml (⅜c) cream (100g)

Feeds 4–6

Soak the mushrooms in warm water for 30 minutes, then drain and roughly chop. You don't need to keep the mushroom water, although you could use it as the 'stock' if you can strain it through some muslin, as the soaking liquid tends to be a bit gritty.

Preheat the oven to 170°C (340°F).

Heat the butter and olive oil in a heavy-based frying pan and fry the chicken (in batches, probably) on all sides over a high heat until golden brown. Season it very well. When the chicken is all well browned and well seasoned, transfer it to a suitable-sized casserole dish.

Sauté the onion in the leftover chicken fat until soft. Deglaze the pan with the white wine, then add the thyme, stock, cream and mushrooms and simmer gently for 10 minutes. Taste and season well.

Pour or spoon the hot creamy mixture over the chicken and bake for about 40 minutes. You may need to cover it with tin foil, but at 170°C (340°F), it's unlikely to burn.

PER PORTION (¼ OF THE RECIPE)

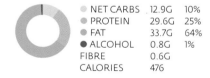

NET CARBS	12.9G	10%
PROTEIN	29.6G	25%
FAT	33.7G	64%
ALCOHOL	0.8G	1%
FIBRE	0.6G	
CALORIES	476	

The original recipe that inspired this dish was for rabbit legs braised with mustard in Anthony Demetre's book *Today's Special*. But perhaps because most butchers don't regularly stock legs from the cast of *Watership Down*, I've tweaked it to use chicken legs instead, which work just as well and eat beautifully. His recipe called for just one type of mustard (but I use two: Dijon and wholegrain) and interestingly had some smoked paprika in the dish, which I thought might be a little odd with all the mustard so I ended up using smoked sweet paprika. This was an incredibly tasty dish, and provided you have a good, heavy saucepan with a lid, it can be cooked on top of the stove or in the oven if you find that handier.

Melt the butter in a heavy-based saucepan. Season the chicken legs well and fry them over a high heat until they are an even golden brown on all sides. This will take a good 5–10 minutes. Take off the heat while you transfer the part-cooked chicken to a plate and then finish the sauce.

Add the vinegar to the saucepan and put it back on the heat. Make sure the fat isn't too hot, as it will sizzle and potentially catch fire – if in doubt, leave it to cool a little before adding the vinegar to the pan. Bring the vinegar to the boil and let it bubble away for about a minute, then add all the remaining ingredients, whisking so that it's well mixed, and bring up to the boil again. Taste and adjust the seasoning if necessary, then gently place the chicken legs back into the saucepan. Put the lid on and either cook on top of the stove over a low heat for about 25 minutes or cook in the oven at 160°C (320°F) for about 40 minutes. It should be bubbling away gently, but do keep an eye on it. Take off the heat or out of the oven, allow to cool for a bit and serve.

Chicken with mustard and smoked paprika

20g (1⅓tbsp) butter (20g)
4 chicken legs – use legs with the thigh still attached or else use about 6 drumsticks (540g drumsticks)
Salt and pepper (3g)
50ml (¼c) white wine vinegar (50g)
4 garlic cloves, crushed (12g)
Few sprigs of rosemary (12g)
2 bay leaves (2g)
300ml (1¼c) chicken stock (300g)
50ml (¼c) cream (50g)
2 tbsp Dijon mustard (48g)
1 tbsp wholegrain mustard (30g)
2 tsp dried oregano (7g)
½ tsp smoked sweet paprika (1g)

Serves 4

PER PORTION

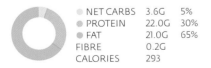

NET CARBS	3.6G	5%
PROTEIN	22.0G	30%
FAT	21.0G	65%
FIBRE	0.2G	
CALORIES	293	

Duck dal supper

4 cooked confit duck legs (1kg)
2 onions, finely chopped (300g)
4 garlic cloves, sliced (12g)
Knob of butter (15g)
1 tsp ground cumin (2g)
Pinch of chilli flakes (2g)
200g (7 oz) moong dal, rinsed well
   (200g)
400ml (1⅝c) vegetable stock (400g)
Rind of 2 lemons, chopped (4g of
   zest)
Salt and pepper (3g)
Big bunch of mint or cilantro,
   chopped (16g)

Serves 4 very generously

Everyone loves the buttery richness of this dish. I leave the chilli out if the rug rats are being fed, but play around with other spices. Even a little mild curry powder can get approval.

Preheat the oven to 180°C (350°F).

Heat up the duck legs according to the instructions on the pack.

Allow 40 minutes to cook the dal. Fry the onions and garlic in the butter in a large heavy-bottomed saucepan until they are just starting to colour, then add the cumin and chilli flakes. The butter gives it great richness, but if you want to leave it out, do. Add the rinsed dal and mix well so it gets coated with the flavours. Add the stock (or water plus extra salt), bring up to the boil and add the lemon zest. Stir well, then cover with the lid and cook for 40 minutes on a gentle heat. You may have to add some water. It will start to look like a mushy risotto or polenta. Season well.

Remove the duck from the oven, add some chopped mint or cilantro to the dal and serve with the duck.

PER PORTION

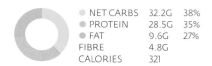

NET CARBS	32.2G	38%
PROTEIN	28.5G	35%
FAT	9.6G	27%
FIBRE	4.8G	
CALORIES	321	

Best brisket

What's the best cooking method for brisket? Well, it can be boiled, but I think oven-cooking coaxes out better flavour. For the beef in the chilli below, I took a 2kg (4.4lbs) joint of brisket, salted it a little and sat it in a shallow bath of stock, covered it with non-stick baking paper and baked it for hours until it was all nicely falling apart.

I used half of it for the chilli itself, while the other half got bagged up and stuck in the freezer for when the cupboard is bare. You can easily freeze this cut of meat, wrapped up in parchment paper and then put in freezer bags for easy access, allowing about 100g (3.5 oz) per adult and less for kids as something to add to a dish to make it a well-rounded dinner. All you have to do is take out a small portion of frozen meat the morning or day before and then use as required. The meat will be fully cooked, it will have thawed and therefore just needs to get hot again from being sautéed, heated in an oven or under the grill. This means that a stir-fry can be enlivened with a few shards of beautifully tender beef, or a salad that was looking kind of dull can be invigorated with some brisket that has been thawed and then grilled until crisp. A regular creamy onion soup can suddenly and easily become dinner with a few pieces of crisp grilled brisket on top. It also gets raided for an Asian-type salad with a sharp, salty dressing and plenty of raw or blanched veggies: lean, healthy and very, very tasty.

Preheat the oven to 160°C (320°F).

Pour about 2.5cm (1in) of stock or water into a deep roasting pan. Salt the meat by rubbing the salt in (this will help tenderise it) and then place the joint gently into its bath. Cover loosely with non-stick baking paper (you don't want it to brown) and bake for 6 hours, until it's falling apart; 6 hours should do it though. Leave to cool and then use for the chilli on page 84 or as the mood takes you (see the note above for ideas).

Chicken stock or water
1 tsp salt (3g)
2kg (4.4lbs) brisket (2kg)

PER 100G PORTION

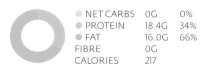

NET CARBS	0G	0%
PROTEIN	18.4G	34%
FAT	16.0G	66%
FIBRE	0G	
CALORIES	217	

Asian carpaccio

400g (14.1 oz) fillet of beef (400g)
400g (14.1 oz) snow peas (400g)
2 Portobello mushrooms, peeled
    and sliced (168g)
1 bunch of scallions, chopped (60g)
Few leaves of fresh basil, torn (3g)

Anything Asian dressing:
Knob of ginger, peeled and grated
    (5g)
1 garlic clove, crushed (3g)
25g (0.8 oz) sesame seeds (25g)
2 tbsp olive oil (26g)
2 tbsp tamari (36g)
1 tbsp mirin (16g)
2 tsp wasabi paste (20g)
2 tsp miso paste (20g)
1 tsp sesame oil (4g)
Splash of water (5g)

Serves 4

The secret to eating raw fish or meat is that it must be spanking fresh and of really good quality. It's easier to prepare and tastes better. Good sashimi is a wondrous thing – soft, silken slices that just melt in the mouth – but beef carpaccio is also tasty and very versatile. It's just as delicious with some Parmesan, arugula and truffle oil as it is in this salad recipe, where it revels in an Asian dressing that brings some umami oomph to the finely sliced, raw fillet of beef. The dressing is also fantastic with an Asian salad full of napa cabbage along with a few shards of the beef brisket on page 81.

Make the dressing by whisking together all the ingredients in a bowl. Set aside.

Chill the beef in the freezer for 15 minutes or so to firm up, then slice as thinly as you can. Put slices between sheets of cling film and bash until it's nice and thin. Lay out on a platter, cover loosely and refrigerate until required.

Blanch the snow peas in boiling water (you will need a rolling boil, not timid bubbles) for 1 minute, then refresh by running under cold water. This will keep their lovely colour and stop them overcooking.

In a bowl, mix the snow peas, mushrooms, scallions and basil with a spoonful or two of the dressing and spread it out on a platter or plate. Slice the beef thinly and carefully before layering it up on top of the salad, drizzling some more dressing on top and serving.

PER PORTION (WITH ¼ OF THE DRESSING)

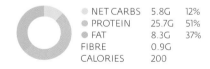

NET CARBS	5.8G	12%
PROTEIN	25.7G	51%
FAT	8.3G	37%
FIBRE	0.9G	
CALORIES	200	

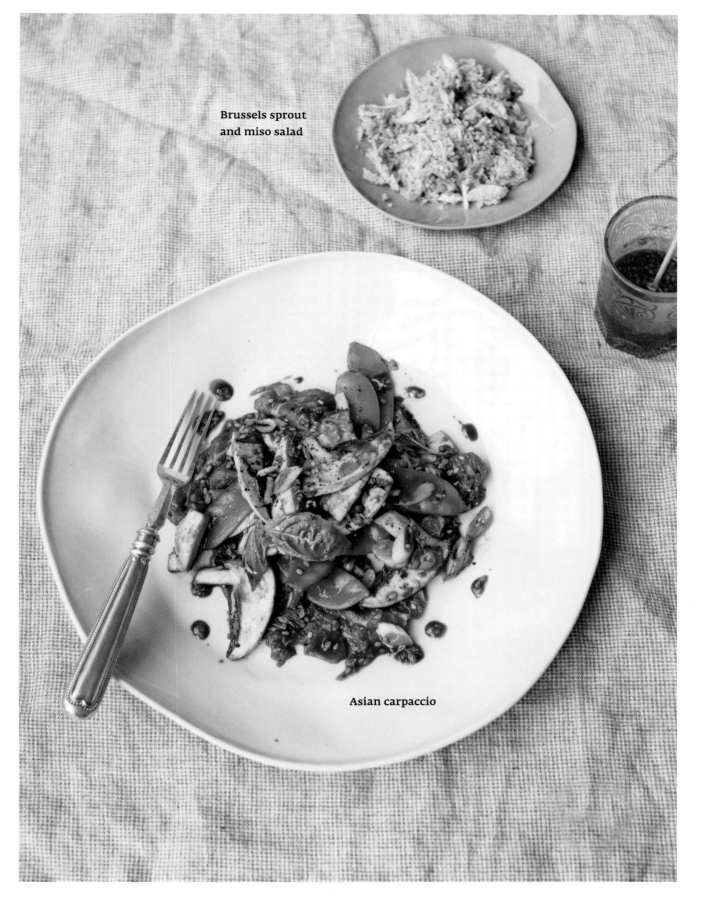

Brussels sprout
and miso salad

Asian carpaccio

Beef chilli

1 tbsp olive oil (13g)

1 large Spanish onion, chopped (240g)

2 tsp cumin seeds (4g)

1 tsp coriander seeds (2g)

1 tsp smoked paprika (2g)

1 tsp salt (3g)

Black pepper (1g)

800g–1kg (1.7–2.2lbs) cooked, chopped brisket (900g)

2 × 400g cans (28.2 oz) of chopped tomatoes (800g)

1 tbsp tamari (18g)

1 × 400g can (14.1 oz) of cooked kidney beans, drained and rinsed (240g)

50g (1.8 oz) dark chocolate (50g)

Serves 6–8

In a heavy saucepan, heat the olive oil and sweat the onion until soft – about 7 minutes. Add the spices, salt and pepper and stir for a minute or two, then add the meat, tomatoes and tamari. Cover and simmer for 10 minutes before removing the lid and cooking for a further 20 minutes.

Add the kidney beans 5 minutes before the end to heat them through, then the chocolate (believe me, it works) 2 minutes before the end so it melts but doesn't cook. Delicious on its own with a bit of grated cheese and maybe some chopped scallions.

PER PORTION (¹/₆ OF THE RECIPE)

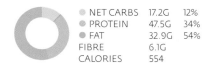

NET CARBS	17.2G	12%
PROTEIN	47.5G	34%
FAT	32.9G	54%
FIBRE	6.1G	
CALORIES	554	

'Fat gives things flavour.'
Julia Child

Venison stew

The venison stew is nutritionally sound because like most red meat, venison is a source of protein, zinc, iron and selenium, but is viewed as even more nutritious than red meat.

Heat the oil in a large saucepan and sweat the onions over a high heat until they are just starting to colour. Keep the heat up, add the bacon and let it brown. After 5 minutes, add the venison and thyme and season. Chuck in the mushrooms, then add the prunes, garlic and stock. Bring up to a simmer, cover with a lid and cook for 30 minutes. Add the artichokes, cover again, but only partially, and stew for at least another hour. Taste, season and serve once the venison is tender.

1 tbsp olive oil (13g)
2 onions, finely chopped (300g)
Few pieces of bacon, diced (40g)
1kg (2.2lbs) venison, diced (1kg)
Few sprigs of thyme (4g)
Salt and pepper (3g)
300g (10.5 oz) mushrooms, chopped (300g)
50g (1.8 oz) dried prunes (50g)
4 garlic cloves, sliced (12g)
500ml (2⅛c) vegetable stock or water (500g)
200g (7 oz) Jerusalem artichokes, peeled and cut in half (200g)

Serves 8

PER PORTION

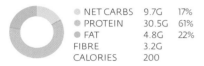

NET CARBS	9.7G	17%
PROTEIN	30.5G	61%
FAT	4.8G	22%
FIBRE	3.2G	
CALORIES	200	

'He is the best physician who is the most ingenious inspirer of hope.'
Samuel Taylor Coleridge

Roast shoulder of lamb

1 shoulder of lamb (1.5kg including bone)
1 tsp olive oil (4g)
1 tsp flaky sea salt, preferably Maldon (5g)
Black pepper (2g)
½ bottle of white wine (375g)
Handful of any fresh herbs: oregano, sage, thyme or rosemary (12g)
1 good tsp fennel seeds (3g)
1 good tsp coriander seeds (3g)
1 head of garlic, cloves peeled (30g)
½ tsp honey (4g)

Serves 4

The key is very slow roasting (after an initial blast in the oven) to create what has to be my favourite way of cooking lamb. Boiled spuds (but only one or two small ones if you're trying to stay low-carb) and a few peas make this complete along with a big spoonful of salsa verde (see page 192), which helps keep this roast meat summery.

Preheat the oven to 200°C (400°F) or higher.

Place the lamb shoulder, fatty skin side up, in a large roasting pan. Smear with olive oil and season generously with salt and pepper. Roast on a high heat for about 25 minutes, until some good caramelisation is taking place, then turn down the oven to about 140°C (280°F) and take the lamb out while you doctor it up.

Add the wine, herbs and spices and the whole peeled cloves of garlic. Wrap the roasting pan very securely with tin foil to seal it as much as possible while still giving you the ability to baste the lamb. Cook for another 2–3 hours, occasionally basting and checking to see that the roasting pan still has wine in it. If not, then you need to improve your tin foil roof. What I tend to do, though, is give it 2–2½ hours of slow cooking, then give it a final blast at about 160°C (320°F) without the foil and a drizzle of honey. The lamb should be a lovely dark brown and literally melting away.

It's fine to keep it warm, well wrapped up, for up to an hour after this. I also like to smear the very soft garlic cloves onto the skin halfway through before the final blast. Once you master this, it will become a firm favourite.

To carve, think about portioning the shoulder into rectangles rather than slices.

PER PORTION

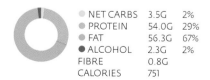

NET CARBS	3.5G	2%
PROTEIN	54.0G	29%
FAT	56.3G	67%
ALCOHOL	2.3G	2%
FIBRE	0.8G	
CALORIES	751	

To make this dish, the lamb is rubbed and covered with a thick paste made from onions, garlic and the classic North African spice blend ras el hanout, with its fragrant notes of cinnamon, cloves, cumin and a dozen other spices. The lamb then gets plonked on a bed of thickly sliced onions and the roasting dish is half-filled with water before being consigned to the oven for between 3 and 5 hours – just the right amount of time to read the papers of a Sunday.

And don't get cranky that I'm not being more specific. In autumn and winter, lamb can be awfully hard to figure out in the toughness stakes. Sometimes it's meltingly tender after 3 hours, other times it needs double the cooking time. Just keep topping up with water, keep it covered with foil and eventually it will feel as though with one little tug, it's all yours.

Preheat the oven to 200°C (400°F).

Blitz the chopped white onions, garlic and spice mix together in a food processor to form a sludgy paste, then season well. Cover the bottom of your roasting pan with the sliced red onions and place the lamb on top. Season it well, then smear the whole joint with the sloppy onion spice mix and fill the dish halfway up with water.

Roast for 1 hour to get some colour going before basting it, covering it with tin foil and returning it to the oven for another 3–5 hours at 170°C (340°F), until the meat is falling off the bone. Keep topping it up with water if it's drying out. Rest for half an hour before carving and eating.

Lamb shawarma

4 white onions, roughly chopped (600g)
8 garlic cloves, peeled (24g)
3 tbsp ras el hanout spice mix (18g)
Salt and pepper (3g)
4 red onions, cut into 1.25cm- (½in-) thick slices (600g)
1 shoulder of lamb or lamb on the bone (2kg)

Serves 6

PER PORTION

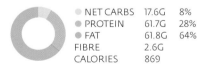

● NET CARBS	17.6G	8%
● PROTEIN	61.7G	28%
● FAT	61.8G	64%
FIBRE	2.6G	
CALORIES	869	

Piquant lamb stew

3 red onions, sliced (450g)

1 good tbsp liquid coconut or olive oil (27g coconut oil)

2 red chillies, deseeded and thinly sliced (40g)

3 garlic cloves, sliced (9g)

Good knob of ginger, peeled and chopped (10g)

1 tbsp Chinese five-spice powder (6g)

1.2kg (2.6lbs) diced lamb (1.2kg)

2 × 400g cans (28.2 oz) of chopped tomatoes (800g)

50g (1.8 oz) prunes, diced (50g)

1 litre (4¼c) chicken or vegetable stock (1kg)

50ml (¼c) fish sauce (50g)

50ml (¼c) tamari (50g)

1 tbsp miso (25g)

Big bunch of cilantro, chopped (20g)

Serves 6–8

Sauté the onions in the coconut oil in a heavy-based saucepan until they are just starting to colour. Add the chillies, garlic, ginger and Chinese five-spice powder. Turn up the heat and give it a good blast and mix well. This blast of heat gets some colour onto the base of your stew and gets the spices working their magic. Add the lamb and mix well so that it's well coated. Turn down the heat and add the tomatoes, prunes and stock.

Cook on a very gentle heat for about 1½ hours with a lid on or cook in the oven at 160°C (320°F) for about 2 hours. Add the fish sauce, tamari and miso and mix well. Adjust the seasoning and serve with lots of chopped cilantro.

PER PORTION (⅛ OF THE RECIPE)

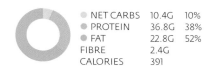

- NET CARBS   10.4G   10%
- PROTEIN   36.8G   38%
- FAT   22.8G   52%
- FIBRE   2.4G
- CALORIES   391

This tagine is ideal for a large group and is great with some rice, but only a little! The harissa gives it heat with body rather than outright fire, but feel free to add more.

Heat the olive oil in a large heavy-based saucepan and brown the lamb well on all sides. Season generously. When you've got a good colour on the meat after a solid 5 minutes of stirring and browning on a relatively high heat, add the onions, garlic and ginger and cook out for another minute or two, until the onions start to soften and caramelise. Add the harissa and spices and mix really well. Cook out for another few minutes so that the spices and harissa coat the meat.

Add the stock, cover with a lid, turn down the heat and simmer for at least 1 hour, stirring occasionally to make sure nothing is burning on the bottom of your saucepan. After the lamb has undergone the first hour of cooking, you can cool it down at this stage and leave it overnight for the flavours to develop, but allow for at least another hour of cooking time the next day. But if you want to make it all in one go, then add the tomatoes, prunes, olives and pistachios and cook, uncovered, for another hour. At this stage it should have reduced to a nice consistency and the flavours should be really good. The bottom line is that the lamb needs to cook for at least 2 hours in total, which can be done in one go or split over two days. Garnish with the cilantro.

Lamb and prune tagine

1 tbsp olive oil (13g)
1kg (2.2lbs) diced lamb (1kg)
Salt and pepper (3g)
2 onions, chopped (300g)
4 garlic cloves, chopped (12g)
Big knob of ginger, peeled and chopped (20g)
1 tbsp harissa (18g)
2 tsp ground cumin (4g)
1 tsp ground cinnamon (2g)
1 tsp fennel seeds (2g)
1 litre (4¼c) chicken stock (1kg)
4–6 large, ripe tomatoes, roughly chopped (1.2kg)
200g (7 oz) prunes (200g)
100g (3.5 oz) green olives, stoned (100g)
100g (3.5 oz) shelled pistachios (100g)
Bunch of cilantro, chopped (20g)

Serves 6

PER PORTION (WITHOUT RICE)

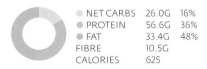

● NET CARBS	26.0G	16%
● PROTEIN	56.6G	36%
● FAT	33.4G	48%
FIBRE	10.5G	
CALORIES	625	

Lamb rendang

1 tbsp coriander seeds (6g)

2 tsp ground turmeric (4.4g)

1 tsp cumin seeds (2g)

1 cinnamon stick (2.3g)

4 cloves (1g)

Good pinch of dried chillies (2g)

1 good tbsp coconut oil (27g)

2 onions, chopped (300g)

Good knob of ginger, peeled and
  sliced (10g)

6 garlic cloves, sliced (12g)

2 sticks of lemongrass, finely
  chopped (4.8g)

1kg (2.2lbs) diced lamb (1kg)

Salt and pepper (3g)

1 × 400ml can (14.1 oz) of coconut
  milk (400g)

Bunch of cilantro, chopped (12g)

Serves 4 plus leftovers

Very easy-going flavours. Everyone from kids to grannies will eat this.

Put all the spices in a large saucepan and gently heat for a minute to dry roast them. Either grind them up in a pestle and mortar or pour into a cup and crush them with the end of a rolling pin.

Pour the crushed, dry-roasted spices back into the saucepan and add the coconut oil, then add the onions, ginger, garlic and lemongrass and sweat for a few minutes. Add the meat and mix so it's well coated in the spices, then season well with salt and pepper and add the coconut milk.

Cook for at least 2 hours on a very gentle heat. I don't keep a lid on it as I want it to reduce, but do give it the occasional stir, as it tends to burn on the bottom of the pan. Eventually the meat should be incredibly tender and the sauce should be nice and thick. If it has dried out too much, just add a few splashes of water and check the seasoning.

Adjust the seasoning and serve with loads of chopped cilantro and some boiled rice, but only a little! This is one of those dishes that also tastes very good the next day.

PER PORTION (1/6 OF THE RECIPE)

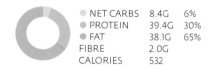

NET CARBS	8.4G	6%
PROTEIN	39.4G	30%
FAT	38.1G	65%
FIBRE	2.0G	
CALORIES	532	

Lamb can take big, robust flavours like garlic and rosemary, but it's also wonderful with subtle, warming, aromatic spices like coriander, fennel and cumin. The cannellini beans do a great job of soaking up much of the flavour and juices from the meat. They also mean you don't really need a carb-based accompaniment such as spuds or rice, but the 'smash' on page 96 makes a good accompaniment too.

Preheat the oven to 150°C (300°F).

In a large casserole dish (or a saucepan that transfers to the oven), fry the bacon in the knob of butter until it's done (i.e. brown and crisp) and then set aside.

Brown the shanks in the bacon fat over a high heat until they've got some good colour. Remove them from the pan and set the shanks aside with the bacon.

Add the olive oil to the pan – though you may not need it if there's enough fat remaining – and over a very gentle heat, sauté the carrots, onions and garlic. Next, deglaze the pan by adding all the white wine and simmering for a bit. Add the bacon, tomatoes, stock and herbs and mix thoroughly.

Nestle the shanks in well, cover the dish with a lid and cook in the oven for 3–4 hours, until the meat comes away easily from the bone. Now, I must stress that I ended up cooking mine for nearly 6 hours one day. The meat genuinely needs to be falling away from the bone. If it isn't, top it up with more water or stock and keep cooking. Add the cannellini beans about 40 minutes before the stew is done and serve with the 'smash' on page 94.

If you want to do this the day before and make it into more of a ragout, then simply allow it to cool a bit, tear the meat off the bones, discard the bones (or use them to make bone broth!), add the cannellini beans and cool it down, then simply reheat the next day.

Deliciously rich lamb shank and white bean stew

250g (8.8 oz) bacon (250g)
Knob of butter (15g)
4 lamb shanks (2.4kg)
50ml (¼c) olive oil (50g)
4 large carrots, peeled and chopped (480g)
2 onions, chopped (300g)
8 garlic cloves, sliced (24g)
½ bottle of white wine (375g)
1 × 400g can (14.1 oz) of cherry tomatoes (400g)
350ml (½c) chicken or vegetable stock (350g)
Few sprigs of thyme (4g)
1 bay leaf (1g)
1 × 400g can (14.1 oz) of cannellini beans, drained and rinsed (246g)

Serves 4

PER PORTION

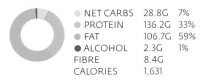

- NET CARBS   28.8G   7%
- PROTEIN   136.2G   33%
- FAT   106.7G   59%
- ALCOHOL   2.3G   1%
- FIBRE   8.4G
- CALORIES   1,631

Lamb skewers with pistachio aioli

500g (1.1lbs) minced lamb (500g)

2 garlic cloves, crushed (6g)

Salt and pepper (3g)

4–6 rosemary stalks or wooden skewers (soaked) or metal ones

1 tbsp olive oil in a bowl or saucer (13g)

Pistachio aioli:

110g (3.9 oz) shelled pistachios (110g)

Big bunch of parsley (20g)

2 tbsp capers (9g)

2 tsp olive oil (8g)

1 egg yolk, at room temperature (18g)

3 garlic cloves, crushed (9g)

100ml (⅜c) olive oil (100g)

Juice of 1 lemon (40g)

½ tsp sherry vinegar (2g)

½ tsp honey (4g)

Salt and pepper (3g)

50ml (¼c) olive oil or water (50g)

Serves 4 as a starter or as part of a large buffet

These lamb skewers are very easy – don't feel any pressure to use rosemary skewers. The only reason I did is that the ones that had survived the winter in my garden were so stalky and tough, I decided to give them a final hurrah in the frying pan.

The pistachio aioli is wonderful. It's so good, in fact, that I urge you to slather it on all sorts of fish and chicken, or even just keep it to blob on some cooked broccoli. The colour is gorgeous and even though minced lamb can sometimes be too 'lamby', this recipe is delicious. The aioli will make more than you need for this recipe, but it becomes a tad addictive after a while, so embrace the extra quantity for use for the rest of the week.

First make the pistachio aioli. On pulse mode, whizz the pistachios and parsley in a food processor until they form a coarse and slightly chunky crumb. You may need to give them a shove with a spatula so that you blitz them in an even fashion. Add the capers and the 2 teaspoons of olive oil, give it one final blitz and once you have an even crumb, leave it in the food processor.

Whisk the egg yolk with the garlic in a bowl, then start adding the 100ml (⅜c) of olive oil very slowly until you can feel it emulsifying. Then you can add this a bit more steadily. Once you are at the halfway point of adding the oil, mix in the lemon juice and continue with the rest of the oil. Add this to the ground-up pistachios along with the splash of sherry vinegar, squeeze of honey and some salt and pepper. Pulse to process, then you can add either another 50ml (3⅓tbsp) of olive oil or water, depending on how loose or rich you want it to be. Do this until you get your desired consistency, but taste and adjust the seasoning. You may need to add more lemon juice, sherry vinegar or salt. Refrigerate until ready to use.

Mix together the lamb, garlic, salt and pepper, then mould an equal amount of meat on the skewers or stalks using your hands (dip your hands into the oil so that the meat doesn't stick to them). Put them all on a plate and chill, covered, in the fridge until you're ready to cook.

When you're ready to cook, heat a bit more olive oil in a large frying pan. When it's nearly smoking, fry the skewers on each side until they're good and brown. You want them to form a good, dark crust so that they will stay fixed onto the skewers. Turn them over in the pan and shake them gently. You don't want to manhandle them, but rather coax them into cooking on all sides. Put on a large platter or individual plates with a blob of the aioli and some mixed leaves.

PER PORTION (WITH ⅛ OF THE AIOLI)

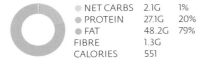

NET CARBS	2.1G	1%
PROTEIN	27.1G	20%
FAT	48.2G	79%
FIBRE	1.3G	
CALORIES	551	

'The idea that dietary carbohydrate, sugars and starches have some unique power to make people fat is pretty old.'
Dr Richard Feinman

Spiced lamb patties with cucumber salad

500g (1.1lbs) minced lamb (500g)

50g (1.8 oz) sesame seeds (50g)

2 garlic cloves, crushed (6g)

1 tbsp black mustard seeds (6g)

2 tsp garam masala (4g)

Salt and pepper (3g)

1 good tbsp coconut oil or ghee, for
    frying (27g)

Cucumber salad:

2 cucumbers, diced (1.2kg)

Small bunch of mint, chopped (20g)

1 garlic clove, crushed (3g)

4 tbsp yoghurt (160g)

½ tsp white wine vinegar (2g)

Salt and pepper (3g)

Serves 4

It's fair to say we are rather too fond of over-charring our beef and lamb – who isn't? But all that charred, caramelised, crisp deliciousness can produce carcinogens once it hits your digestive system. Now don't get me wrong, I shall still eat the occasional BBQ and am always fond of charred bits of anything, but for midweek goodness, I try to behave a little better. These spiced lamb patties avoid charring or heavy frying and instead opt for a gentler, oven-cooked approach, which still produces some fine flavour. Accompanying it is a cooling, rehydrating relish-cum-salad of cucumber in yoghurt. Lovely as a midweek supper or lunch.

Preheat the oven to 180°C (350°F).

To make the patties, simply mix together all the ingredients except the oil with your hands in a large bowl and shape into eight patties about 8–10cm (3–4in) across. Fry gently in a little coconut oil to brown, then transfer to a baking tray and cook in the oven for about 15 minutes, until cooked through.

To make the salad, again, simply place all the ingredients in a large bowl and mix well. Season thoroughly before serving.

PER PORTION

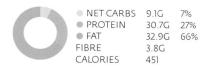

NET CARBS	9.1G	7%
PROTEIN	30.7G	27%
FAT	32.9G	66%
FIBRE	3.8G	
CALORIES	451	

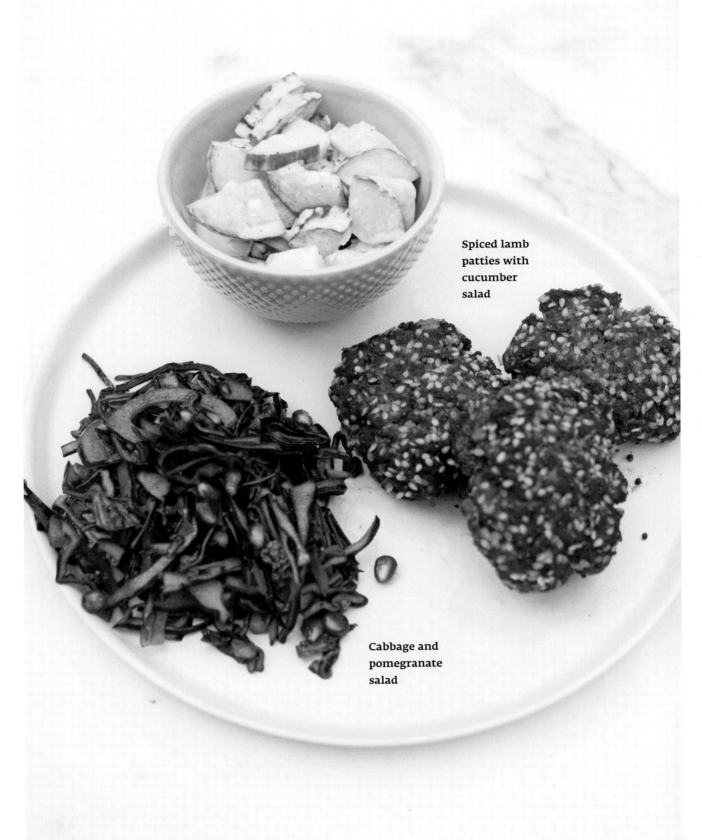

Spiced lamb patties with cucumber salad

Cabbage and pomegranate salad

Spiced lamb with eggplant and chickpea smash

1 tbsp olive oil (13g)

2 onions, finely chopped (300g)

500g (1.1lbs) lamb mince (500g)

Good splash of verjus or wine (12g/ 1 tbsp wine)

1½ tsp Worcestershire sauce (8g)

1 tsp ground cumin (2g)

1 tsp ground coriander or coriander seeds (2g)

1 tsp fennel seeds (2g)

Salt and pepper (3g)

100ml (⅜c) hot water (100g)

50g (1.8 oz) raisins or barberries (or both!) (50g)

4 garlic cloves, crushed (12g)

50g (1.8 oz) shelled pistachios (50g)

Eggplant and chickpea smash:

1 large eggplant (400g)

1 × 400g can (14.1 oz) of chickpeas, drained and rinsed (230g)

2 garlic cloves, crushed (6g)

Juice of 2 lemons (80g)

2–3 tbsp olive oil (32g)

1 tbsp light or dark tahini (18g)

Lots of chopped parsley, to garnish (16g)

Salt and pepper (3g)

Serves 4

Lamb can be a bit, how shall I say it . . . lamby. When looking to add a bit of sharpness to this spiced mince dish, I got to offload some barberries that were sitting idle in the store cupboard. 'Barberries?' I hear you say. Well, I bought mine from one of the best little food stores, Roy Fox's in Donnybrook, about a million years ago and they have been goading me to put them to good use ever since. But needless to say they hovered in the back of the press, along with unused bottles of hot sauce bought on some holiday, and a few more jars of foodie tat that you usually end up collecting at Christmastime. But back to the dried barberries. They are rich in vitamin C, quite tart and used a lot in Iranian cooking. They seem to have a host of health benefits: anti-inflammatory and good for digestion. But as for the flavour, when you want tart and sharp (as opposed to the sweetness of raisins or dried cherries), then these are for you. They work well here to cut through all the creamy richness of blitzed eggplants and chickpeas and to give the lamb that touch of piquancy that I like. But if you can't get them, add some raisins or currants and an extra squeeze of lemon juice. Sweeter, but still sharp.

Preheat the oven to 180°C (350°F).

To make the smash, pierce the eggplant all over with a fork, place on a baking tray and bake whole, with the skin on, for 30 minutes. Set aside to cool.

Meanwhile, to prepare the lamb, heat the olive oil in a medium-sized saucepan and sauté the onions for a good 5 minutes over a medium heat, till they're translucent, before adding the mince and letting it brown. Add the wine, Worcestershire sauce and spices, stirring well to get all those caramelised bits off the bottom of the saucepan, then season and add in about 100ml (⅜c) of hot water. Reduce the sauce till it's drier but not dry. This will give you a chance to break up all the mince and make it into a wetter sauce before letting the heat work its magic and dry it up a bit. Add the raisins and garlic and season well before finishing off by stirring in the pistachios.

When the eggplant is cool, simply cut the top off, peel
it like a giant banana and discard the skin. Put it in
a food processor with the chickpeas and all the other
ingredients except the parsley. Blitz until smooth. Add
more olive oil if you need to make it less pappy. Season
well to taste. Garnish generously with parsley and a good
dribble of your best olive oil and serve with the lamb.

PER PORTION OF LAMB

●	NET CARBS	17.2G	15%
●	PROTEIN	28.1G	26%
●	FAT	27.7G	58%
	FIBRE	3.6G	
	CALORIES	427	

PER PORTION OF EGGPLANT SMASH

●	NET CARBS	12.3G	25%
●	PROTEIN	6.2G	13%
●	FAT	12.6G	62%
	FIBRE	5.6G	
	CALORIES	184	

'Perhaps the hardest thing
to deal with is the idea that
the whole field of professional
nutrition is fundamentally
flawed.'
Dr Richard Feinman

Asian lamb stir-fry

400g (14.1 oz) snow peas (400g)

2 Portobello mushrooms, peeled and sliced (168g)

1 bunch of scallions, chopped (60g)

Few basil leaves, torn (2.5g)

400g (14.1 oz) lamb steak, sliced (400g)

1 tbsp olive oil (13g)

Salt and pepper (3g)

Dressing:

25g (0.9 oz) sesame seeds (25g)

Good knob of ginger, peeled and grated (10g)

1 garlic clove, crushed (3g)

2 tbsp olive oil (26g)

2 tbsp tamari (36g)

1 tbsp mirin (16g)

2 tsp wasabi paste (20g)

2 tsp miso paste (20g)

1 tsp sesame oil (4g)

Splash of water (7g)

Serves 4

Make the dressing by whisking all the ingredients together. Set aside.

Blanch the snow peas really briefly, then refresh. Mix with the mushrooms, scallions, basil and a tablespoon or two of the dressing, then lay out on a platter.

Stir-fry the lamb in a hot pan with some olive oil and a little salt and pepper. Cook to your liking and then plate up, drizzle some more dressing on top and serve.

PER PORTION

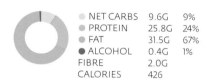

NET CARBS	9.6G	9%
PROTEIN	25.8G	24%
FAT	31.5G	67%
ALCOHOL	0.4G	1%
FIBRE	2.0G	
CALORIES	426	

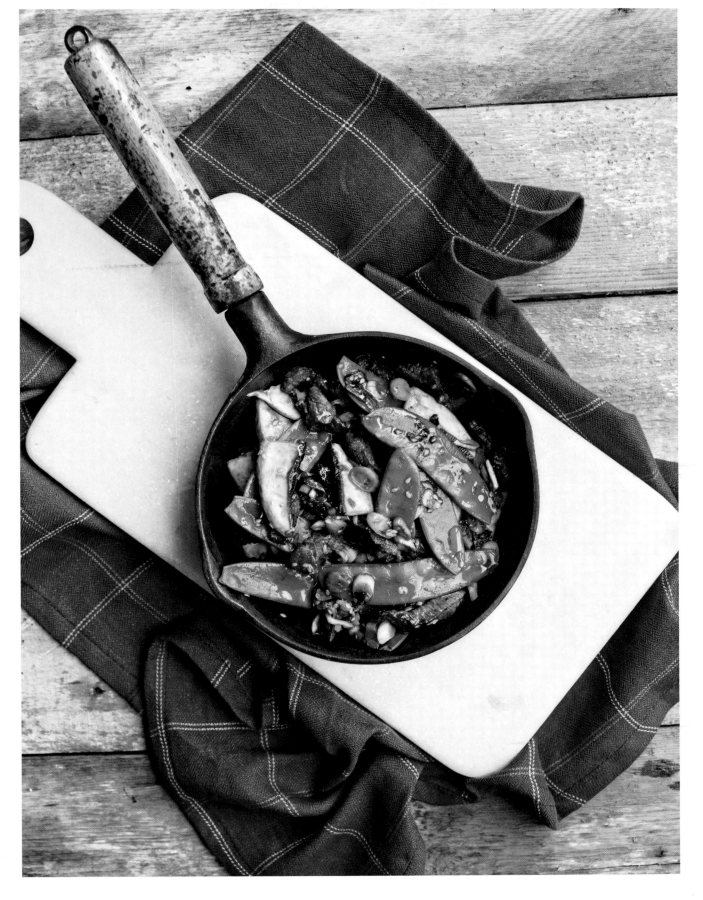

Shepherd's light pie

2 onions, diced (300g)

2 tbsp olive oil (26g)

3 garlic cloves, chopped (9g)

1 red chilli, deseeded and very thinly sliced (20g)

Good big knob of ginger, peeled and finely chopped (10g)

½ tsp ground coriander (1g)

½ tsp ground cumin (1g)

Salt and pepper (3g)

500g (1.1lbs) minced lamb (500g)

1 × 130g tube (½c) tomato purée (130g)

200ml (⅞c) water or vegetable or chicken stock (200g)

Good few shakes of Worcestershire sauce (6g)

Topping:

1kg (2.2lbs) celeriac, peeled and chopped into chunks (1kg)

50g (1.8 oz) Parmesan, finely grated (50g)

50ml (¼c) cream (50g)

Few dots of butter (5g)

Serves 4 plus leftovers

This shepherd's pie certainly offers a few twists on the classic number. First up, there's the sauce. It's got an Asian vibe going on, with spices, ginger and chilli, which are great to add to anything. Then there's the topping, which swaps spuds for a sweeter, less carby celeriac mash made rich by a small amount of cream and Parmesan, and I do mean small. It might sound as if it shouldn't work, but it's really, really moreish.

Preheat the oven to 180°C (350°F).

To make the meat bit, sweat the onions in the olive oil until soft. Turn up the heat and add the garlic, chilli, ginger, coriander and cumin. Let the onions start to brown and season them just a little. Add the minced meat, break it up with the spoon and mix it well so the spices and flavours get hold of the meat. Add the tomato purée and mix well, and when it's cooked out, add the stock or water (which is better if it's hot) along with the Worcestershire sauce. Cook over a moderate heat, letting it bubble, simmer and reduce but giving it a stir occasionally.

Meanwhile, get the topping on the go. Cook the celeriac in boiling water until very tender. Drain and put back in the saucepan over a very low heat with a tea towel on top to absorb the heat and help keep it warm. Add the cheese and cream, season very well and set aside.

When the mince is cooked out and very tasty, pour or spoon it into a 25cm × 33cm (9in × 13in) gratin dish. Cover with the celeriac topping and dot with butter. Bake straight away for about 30 minutes, until bubbling and golden brown. If you want to do this in advance, let the mince and celeriac cool separately (because they will cool down faster that way) and then layer them up, and when they hit room temperature, refrigerate for a couple of days. Bake for 40 minutes but be careful it doesn't burn – you may have to cover the topping with foil.

PER PORTION (¹/₆ OF THE RECIPE)

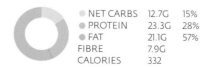

NET CARBS	12.7G	15%
PROTEIN	23.3G	28%
FAT	21.1G	57%
FIBRE	7.9G	
CALORIES	332	

There is increasing evidence that not just omega-3s, but also folic acid and polyphenols all do fantastic work on improving the brain and its braininess. The more we can eat directly from natural foods, the better it is for us in the long run. Surely a varied diet with plenty of raw foods and natural snacks, like nuts rather than crisps, has to be better for us than poor diets full of processed foods and supplemented with a handful of pills? I am lazy about eating mackerel and need to do better.

Mix the crème fraîche with the dill and mustard and set aside.

In a small saucepan, heat the vinegar with the chilli and bay leaf. Bring to the boil, then strain the liquid and allow it to cool. Chuck the bay leaf.

If you want to be good, you should salt the cucumber to remove excess liquid. I never bother, so just peel the cucumber, slice it thinly and mix with the grated apple, the onion, chopped chives and the chilli and vinegar syrup. Season to taste.

Turn up your grill to high and dot the mackerel skin with some butter or a drizzle of olive oil and season with some salt and pepper. Grill, skin side up, until the skin starts to bubble, blister and char. It really does cook very quickly, maybe 2–3 minutes.

Serve the mackerel with a spoonful of the mustard crème fraîche and marinated cucumber.

PER PORTION

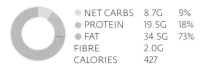

● NET CARBS	8.7G	9%
● PROTEIN	19.5G	18%
● FAT	34.5G	73%
FIBRE	2.0G	
CALORIES	427	

Grilled mackerel with marinated cucumber and mustard crème fraîche

4 mackerel fillets (320g)
1 tbsp butter or splash of olive oil (15g)
Salt and pepper (3g)

Marinated cucumber:
100ml (⅜c) white wine vinegar (100g)
1 chilli, finely chopped, with or without seeds (20g)
1 bay leaf (if you have one) (1g)
1 big cucumber (650g)
1 apple, grated (100g)
1 small onion or a couple of shallots, finely chopped (60g)
Bunch of chives, finely chopped (3g)
Salt and pepper (3g)

Mustard crème fraîche:
1 small tub (6 oz) of crème fraîche (170g)
Small bunch of dill, finely chopped (8g)
1 tbsp Dijon or wholegrain mustard (24g)

Serves 4

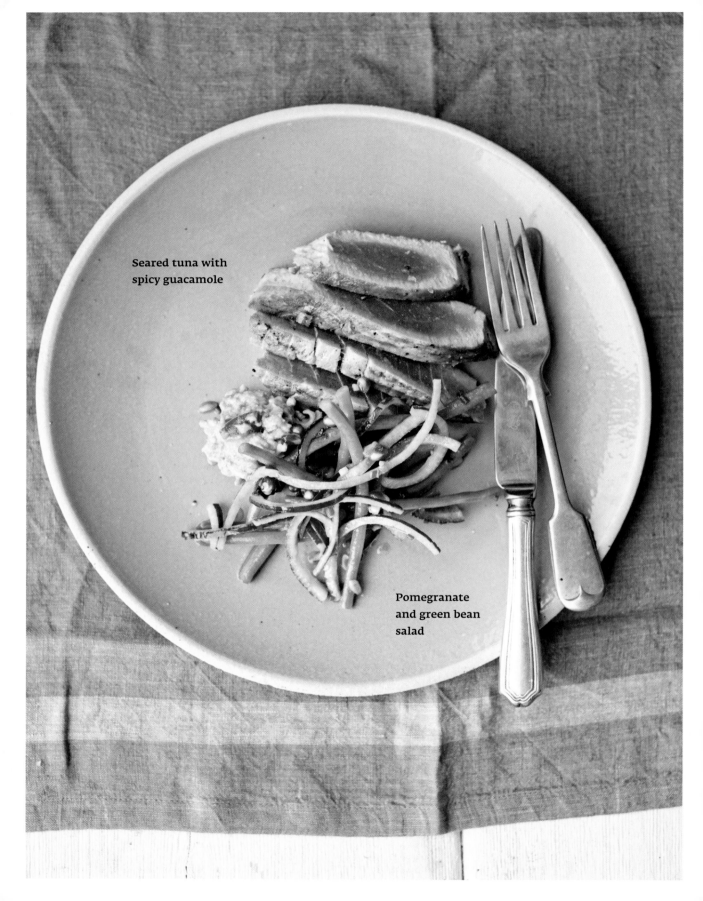

Seared tuna with
spicy guacamole

Pomegranate
and green bean
salad

I love tuna, but no matter how hot my pan gets at home, I always seem to overcook it. Having the tuna very cold helps. I sometimes stick it in my freezer for 15 minutes so that the inside stays rare, but it doesn't always work.

Some of the little tricks food companies get up to make me laugh. I recently picked up a jar of green goo that was supposed to be some sort of guacamole dip. Do you know, it didn't contain one ounce of real avocado but was flavoured with avocado powder. It was the most oxymoronic product I have seen in a long time. Imagine buying an avocado dip that doesn't contain any avocados. Mental. You could make this dip in the same amount of time it would take you to read the label. Tuna and guacamole go perfectly together.

To make the guacamole, cut the avocadoes in half, remove the stone and scoop out the flesh. Mash with a fork, then mix with the tomatoes, garlic and lime juice. Season well, including a few chilli flakes if you like, and cover with a thin layer of extra lime juice and cling film pressed down directly on the surface, unless you are going to serve it straight away.

Heat the olive oil until the oil is just about smoking. Season the tuna, going heavy with the black pepper, and cook for 10 seconds on each sides. It will take this long, provided your pan is hot enough. As soon as you have some colour on the outside, remove from the heat onto a plate to stop it from overcooking.

Seared tuna with spicy guacamole

1 tbsp olive oil (13g)
400g (14 oz) tuna, probably 2 × 200g
  (7 oz) tuna loin steaks (400g)

Spicy guacamole:
2 avocados (360g)
1 ripe tomato, finely chopped (130g)
2 big garlic cloves, crushed (7g)
Juice of 2 limes (40g)
Salt and pepper (3g)
A few chilli flakes (optional) (1g)

Serves 2

PER PORTION

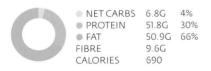

NET CARBS	6.8G	4%
PROTEIN	51.8G	30%
FAT	50.9G	66%
FIBRE	9.6G	
CALORIES	690	

Crab salad in baby gem parcels

Approx. 450g (1lb) pack of fresh or
    frozen cooked crab meat (450g)
100g (3.5 oz) crème fraîche (100g)
2 scallions, finely sliced (20g)
Small bunch of cilantro,
    chopped (8g)
Juice of 1 lemon (40g)
Good splash of olive oil (15g)
3–4 drops of hot sauce (no sugar) (5g)
1–2 tsp anchovy sauce (3g)
Salt and pepper (3g)
2 packs of baby gem (600g)

Avocado cream:
2 avocados (360g)
Juice of 2 limes (40g)
Salt and pepper (3g)
2 shakes of hot sauce (no sugar) (5g)

Serves 6

Mixing crab salad with some crème fraîche and a little splash of anchovy sauce (my new secret ingredient for mega-umami hits) and hot sauce is really delicious. This was a great dish to have instead of a starter, as friends just grabbed one along with a napkin and wolfed in. It's also extremely quick and handy, as you can easily buy frozen crab meat in plenty of fishmongers and supermarkets. Just thaw it out, wash your hands really well and have a little search and rescue for any excess shell. It's not entirely necessary (unless you run a professional kitchen and are in the restaurant business), but every now and then you will find a teeny tiny bit of shell that is never that nice to crunch down onto. After that, you just have to mix it with a flurry of ingredients and chill it, and once your avocado cream is made, all that's left is just a little last-minute assembly for a delicious bit of zingy crab salad. This dip is also lovely with cucumber sticks.

Pick through the crab meat with very clean hands, then mix with all the ingredients except the baby gems. Season with plenty of black pepper, but go easy on the salt because the anchovy sauce (and the crab itself) are quite salty. Chill until ready to serve.

Either mash or blend the avocados until super smooth with the lime juice, salt, pepper and hot sauce, which you can leave out of the crab too if kids are about or you have sensitive souls.

When ready to serve, cut the stalky bit off the baby gems to separate the leaves. Lay out the leaves and spoon some avocado cream onto each one, then top with a generous spoonful of crab. Serve on a big platter with some extra lemon wedges if necessary and a glass of something white and very well chilled.

PER PORTION (¹/₆ OF THE RECIPE)

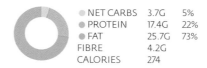

NET CARBS	3.7G	5%
PROTEIN	17.4G	22%
FAT	25.7G	73%
FIBRE	4.2G	
CALORIES	274	

If this sounds like a lot of work, feel free to ditch the haddock, just make the celeriac purée and serve with a poached egg and a handful of greens for a comfort dinner at its best.

Peel and roughly chop the celeriac. Place it in a large saucepan of cold water, add the thyme and a good pinch of salt, then bring to the boil. Reduce the heat and simmer for about 15 minutes, until the celeriac chunks are soft. Drain and ditch the thyme.

Get a blender or food processor out and add the celeriac, crème fraîche, mustard and a knob of butter. Whizz until smooth, but pulse it often rather than turn it into baby food. You're making a purée, not a smoothie. Put it back in a small saucepan and add another knob of butter, check the seasoning and reheat when you're about to serve.

Now poach your eggs. If I was doing this in a large batch, then I would just plop them in without worrying too much about swirling the water and so on, so just get on with it. Get a frying pan and fill it with water. Bring it up to the boil and add the white wine vinegar, then reduce the heat so that it's barely bubbling. Crack the eggs into the water, keeping the water simmering very gently. After 1½–2 minutes, lift the eggs out of the saucepan with a slotted spoon and pat them dry with some kitchen paper.

Bring some water and a splash of milk to the boil in a frying pan. Add the haddock fillets and barely simmer for 5–10 minutes. Drain and serve with a big spoonful of the celeriac purée and a poached egg on top. Garnish with watercress or baby spinach.

Poached haddock and egg with celeriac purée

1kg (2.2lbs) celeriac (1kg)
Few sprigs of thyme (4g)
Salt and pepper (3g)
2 good tbsp crème fraîche or Greek
   yoghurt (100g crème fraîche)
1 tbsp Dijon mustard (24g)
Few knobs of butter (25g)
Splash of white wine vinegar (2g)
4 very fresh eggs (228g)
Splash of milk (15g)
4 × 150g (5.3 oz) smoked haddock
   fillets (150g each)
20g (0.7 oz) watercress or baby
   spinach (20g)

Serves 4

PER PORTION (¼ OF THE RECIPE)

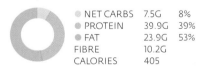

● NET CARBS	7.5G	8%
● PROTEIN	39.9G	39%
● FAT	23.9G	53%
FIBRE	10.2G	
CALORIES	405	

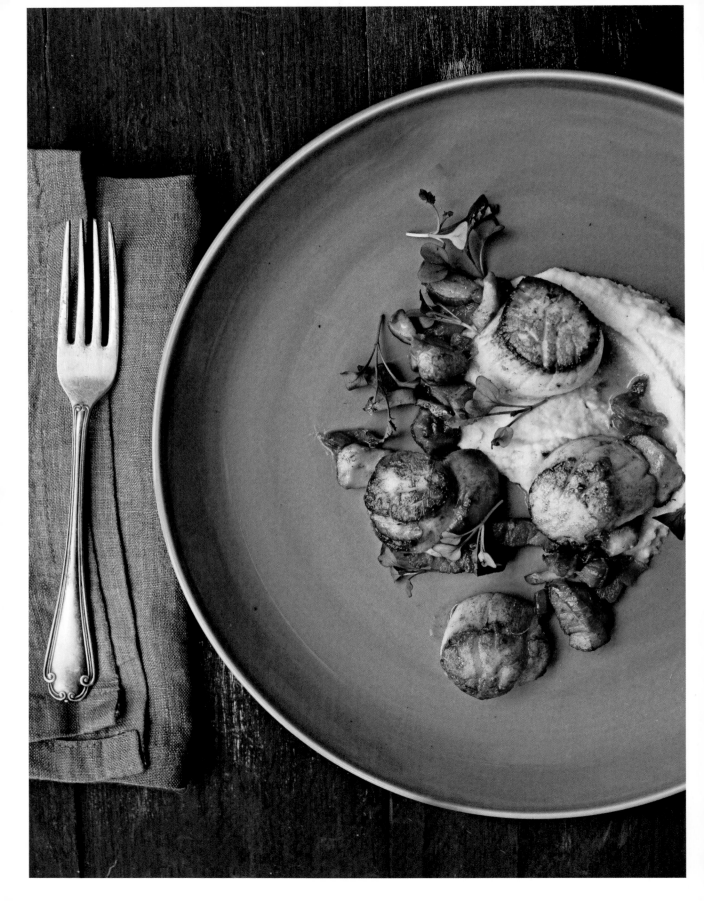

The strong flavour of cauliflower goes beautifully with scallops. When all these flavours are combined, you are going to feel like a Michelin-star chef on day release.

Preheat the oven to 160°C (320°F). Start by making the cauliflower cream. Break the cauliflower up into small florets, put them in a roasting tray, dot with half of the butter and a few splashes of water and cover with foil. Roast for about 30 minutes, until tender.

Process in a blender with a little of the olive oil and some salt and any juices left in the roasting pan. You may have to add a few tablespoons of water to get it to process, maybe even another knob of butter.

Next, make the mushroom and bacon mixture. Cook the lardons in a splash of olive oil until very crispy and caramelised. Transfer to a bowl and set aside. Using the same frying pan, heat 10g (2¼tsp) of butter and sweat the onion and garlic, then dice the mushrooms very finely and add to the soft onions. Add the wine, turn the heat up and reduce. Put in the chestnuts and add the bacon back in along with the thyme. Cook slowly and add a little water or more wine or even some stock, but cook it for about 30 minutes, until you have a delicious sort of mushroom compote. Season if necessary and set aside.

To cook the scallops, heat up the remaining 10g of butter until it's foaming, then place the scallops in the pan, flat side down, season lightly and let the heat and burning butter solids caramelise the outside of them. Turn them over and briefly cook on the other side. This should only take a couple of minutes on each side if they are pretty chunky.

Ideally the mushroom mix and cauliflower cream should be nice and hot. Plate up by making a nice bed of mushroom mix. Spoon a few arty blobs of the cauliflower cream onto each plate, plonk the lovely seared scallops onto each plate and serve.

Scallops with chestnuts, bacon and cauliflower cream

1 small head of cauliflower (500g)

40g (2¾tbsp) butter (40g)

2 tbsp olive oil (26g)

Salt (2g)

150g (5.3 oz) bacon lardons (150g)

1 small onion, very finely diced (60g)

2 garlic cloves, crushed (6g)

150g (5.3 oz) ceps or any fancy mushroom mix (150g)

150ml (⅝c) white wine (150g)

12 cooked, peeled chestnuts, roughly chopped or crumbled (120g)

Few sprigs of thyme (4g)

Black pepper (1g)

16 scallops, roe removed (160g)

Serves 4

PER PORTION

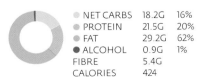

NET CARBS	18.2G	16%
PROTEIN	21.5G	20%
FAT	29.2G	62%
ALCOHOL	0.9G	1%
FIBRE	5.4G	
CALORIES	424	

Poached scallops and Asian salad

1 red onion, chopped (150g)

50g (1.8 oz) ginger, peeled and finely sliced (50g)

1 green or red chilli, deseeded and finely chopped (20g)

2 garlic cloves, chopped (6g)

1 good tbsp coconut oil (27g)

1 × 400ml can (14.1 oz) of coconut milk (400g)

Juice of 2 limes (40g)

1 tbsp fish sauce (18g)

16 scallops (160g)

300g (10.6 oz) snow peas (300g)

300g (10.6 oz) beansprouts (300g)

Salt and pepper (3g)

Big bunch of cilantro, chopped (30g)

Serves 4

In a large pot over a medium heat, sweat the onion, ginger, chilli and garlic in the coconut oil for a few minutes before adding the coconut milk, lime juice and fish sauce to make a tasty sauce. Let it cook for about 25 minutes or so on a gentle heat to let the flavours really develop.

Add the scallops and cook over a medium heat for about 2 minutes before adding the snow peas and beansprouts and cooking for a further 2 minutes. Season well and serve in bowls with lots of chopped cilantro.

PER PORTION

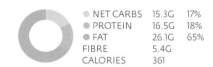

NET CARBS	15.3G	17%
PROTEIN	16.5G	18%
FAT	26.1G	65%
FIBRE	5.4G	
CALORIES	361	

In short, most of us are not eating nearly enough fish. Which is a shame, because fish, when fresh, is delicious and has the benefit of being a genuine 15-minute supper. It cooks fast, it's full of goodness and it's also very versatile. And though it's always tempting just to grill or fry it and serve it up with a bit of lemon and butter – nothing wrong with that – there are other ways of making it much more tempting, which helps if you're trying to feed a family. But what about heading west of Asia for spicy inspiration – what about a tagine? Recently I decided to try one. Firm, succulent salmon was a natural choice, but I also used hake and monkfish, as they're 'meaty' enough to take the cooking. The flavours are gentle but aromatic and the whole thing works surprisingly well.

In a large saucepan, sweat the onions and garlic in the olive oil over a medium heat until soft. Add the green peppers, tahini, cumin seeds and nigella seeds and cook for a further 5 minutes, until the peppers are just starting to soften. Add the diced fish, tomatoes and lemon juice and cook for 10 minutes over a gentle heat, until the fish is opaque. Don't overdo it, though; remember that fish will continue cooking once it's off the heat. Gently spoon the chopped herbs through the fish before serving.

Fish tagine

2 onions, chopped (300g)

4 garlic cloves, crushed (12g)

1 tbsp olive oil (13g)

2 green peppers, deseeded and diced (320g)

2 tbsp tahini (30g)

2 tsp cumin seeds (4g)

1 tsp nigella seeds (4g)

600g (1.3lbs) salmon fillets, diced generously into 5cm (2in) pieces (600g)

200g (7 oz) firm white fish, diced (cod, hake, pollack, monkfish) (200g)

1 punnet (8.8 oz) cherry tomatoes, halved (250g)

Juice of 3 lemons (120g)

Big bunch of parsley, chopped (15g)

Big bunch of cilantro, chopped (15g)

Serves 4

PER PORTION

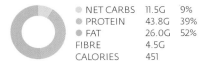

NET CARBS	11.5G	9%
PROTEIN	43.8G	39%
FAT	26.0G	52%
FIBRE	4.5G	
CALORIES	451	

Scallop and avocado ceviche

½ cucumber, deseeded, peeled and
 very finely diced (150g)
½ red onion, diced (75g)
1 small chilli, deseeded and diced
 (20g)
Juice of 2 limes (40g)
Salt and pepper (3g)
300g (10.6 oz) scallops (300g)
2 avocados, diced (360g)
1 tbsp olive oil (13g)
Bunch of cilantro, very finely
 chopped (20g)

Serves 4

Any good raw fish can be substituted for the scallops – salmon, monkish and sea bass work nicely when 'cold-cooked'.

Mix together the cucumber, red onion, chilli and lime juice to make a salsa and season very well.

Remove the little muscle that is attached to the roe and discard the roe along with this little gristly bit. Very finely slice or dice the scallops and mix with the cucumber and red onion salsa. Chill down and marinate for about 30 minutes. This is fine for a few hours in the fridge but it will probably need more salt, as when chilled it will taste blander than at room temperature.

Add the diced avocado and olive oil just before serving along with some chopped cilantro.

PER PORTION

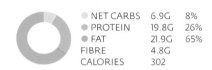

NET CARBS	6.9G	8%
PROTEIN	19.8G	26%
FAT	21.9G	65%
FIBRE	4.8G	
CALORIES	302	

I love this kind of one-pot wonder, as it's easy to make, can be bumped up to easily feed 12 or 18 and works well with chicken, prawns or the monkfish as per the recipe below, or it could even stay veggie by using hunks of zucchini and more eggplant in place of the fish.

In a large heavy-based saucepan, sauté the onion in the olive oil for a few minutes, until it's starting to soften a bit. Keep moving it around so it doesn't burn. Sprinkle the curry powder on top and add the garlic, lemongrass, chilli and ginger. Mix this around and season. It should start to smell really great after a few minutes, but if you feel it's going to start burning in patches, add a splash of water to deglaze the pan to allow you to keep cooking it out.

Add the eggplants to the pot and stir them around to get them well coated. Season again, then add the coconut milk and stock. If you use water, you'll just have to season it more. Add the star anise, lime leaves and desiccated coconut. Cook on a gentle simmer for about 20 minutes, until the eggplants are getting tender.

At this stage you can leave it to cool down fully and then reheat it and add in the fish to cook for about 10 minutes, or just add the fish about 10 minutes before you want to serve. It should be gently bubbling and simmering so the fish will cook quickly, but you need to taste it and adjust the seasoning. You should also remove the star anise. If you feel it's a bit bland, some lime juice, fish sauce or salt will help. Serve with limes wedges and chopped cilantro.

PER PORTION

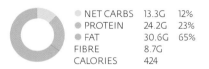

● NET CARBS	13.3G	12%
● PROTEIN	24.2G	23%
● FAT	30.6G	65%
FIBRE	8.7G	
CALORIES	424	

Monkfish, eggplant, lemongrass and coconut curry

1 onion, sliced (150g)

1 tbsp olive oil (13g)

1 small tbsp mild curry powder (5g)

2 garlic cloves, crushed (6g)

1–2 stalks of lemongrass, finely sliced (6g)

½ chilli, deseeded and sliced (optional) (10g)

Good knob of ginger, peeled and very finely sliced (10g)

Salt and pepper (3g)

2 eggplants, cut into chunks (600g)

1 × 400ml can (14.1 oz) of coconut milk (400g)

250ml (1c) vegetable stock or water (250g)

3 star anise

3–4 dried lime leaves (1g)

50g (1.8 oz) desiccated coconut (50g)

Approx. 500g (1.1lbs) diced monkfish (500g)

2 limes, cut into wedges (144g)

Bunch of cilantro, finely chopped (20g)

Serves 4

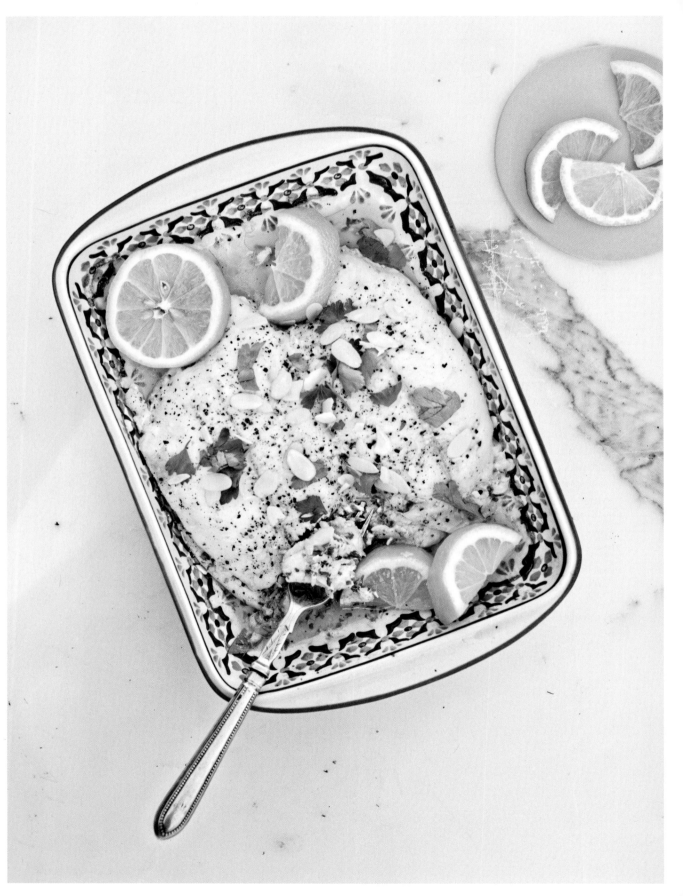

This is the kind of dish that feels like it doesn't even need a recipe, it's so 'throw it all together', but I'd forget to make something like this without a little reminder. This is fast food at its very best. Flaked almonds are a great store cupboard ingredient that give a nice crunch to savoury dishes without taking over, like some nuts do (yes, we're talking about you, Mr Walnut). A big bunch of flat-leaf parsley works a treat to keep it green and meaningful, and once you have skinned the fillets, this recipe takes just minutes to prepare and about 15 minutes in the oven. Simple, light and delicious.

Preheat the oven to 180°C (350°F).

Lightly oil the base of a medium-sized gratin dish and place four fillets on the bottom of the dish.

Mix together the parsley, lemon juice, capers, almonds and soft butter. Season with pepper and mix so that it forms a really rough sort of salsa. Spoon some of this on top of each fish fillet in the dish, then top with the remaining four fillets and press down, then spoon some more butter on top. Season the outside of the fish.

Bake, uncovered, for 10–15 minutes, depending on the size of your fillets and how cold your ingredients were to begin with. My oven is pretty ferocious, so these were done after 10 minutes. Let them rest for a minute before transferring onto a plate. Some purple sprouting broccoli would be magic with this.

Lemon sole parcels

½ tsp olive oil to grease the gratin dish
8 small skinless lemon sole or plaice fillets (960g)
Big bunch of flat-leaf parsley, finely chopped (20g)
Juice of 2 lemons (80g)
2 tbsp capers (17g)
80g (2.8 oz) flaked almonds (80g)
80g (5½tbsp) butter, very soft (80g)
Salt and pepper (3g)

Serves 4

PER PORTION

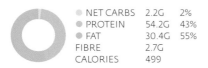

NET CARBS	2.2G	2%
PROTEIN	54.2G	43%
FAT	30.4G	55%
FIBRE	2.7G	
CALORIES	499	

Herb and curry crusted fish fillets

4 × 150–200g (5.3–7 oz) white fish
  fillets (700g)
1 tbsp olive oil (13g)
Salt and pepper (3g)
Approx. 3 tablespoons mayonnaise
  (42g)
1 garlic clove, crushed (3g)
1 tsp mild curry powder (2g)
Zest and juice of 1 lemon (2g + 40g)
100g (3.5 oz) flaked almonds (100g)
Bunch of flat-leaf parsley or cilantro,
  chopped (20g)

Serves 4

This dish and the lemon sole parcels on page 113 remind me of something that could come out of the microwave in the sense that they are both incredibly instant. I would normally be a bit snobby about using mayonnaise to embellish home cooking, but after reading Ferran Adrià's tip for making gazpacho extra silky by putting a good spoonful of mayonnaise into the soup before blitzing, I figured if it's good enough for Mr El Bulli, then it's certainly good enough for me. For a 'ready meal' type dish that's full of flavour and is Speedy Gonzales to make, then it's fine to cheat once in a while with something from a jar. This is one of those dishes that kids will particularly love, and although you can ditch the curry powder, I find a lot of them like it. It's good to expand taste buds in this way, but tweak to suit your own household. It's a straightforward, user-friendly dish that will be a bit of a crowd pleaser – not dinner party nosh, but perfect for when you have barely 30 minutes to get dinner on the table.

Preheat the oven to 200°C (400°F).

Place the fish in a shallow gratin dish, drizzle with a little olive oil and season lightly.

Mix together the mayonnaise, garlic, mild curry powder and lemon juice. Spread a layer over each piece of fish. Mix the almonds with the lemon zest, the parsley or cilantro and some salt and pepper. This is easier to do in a food processor, but if you're too lazy to wash it up, just chop the parsley like crazy and give it a good mix with the almonds and a couple glugs of olive oil.

Sprinkle this generously on top of the mayonnaise topping, then bake for about 15 minutes. The fish should be well cooked through and the almond crumbs should just be starting to brown in parts. If they are browning too quickly, just cover the dish with some foil.

PER PORTION

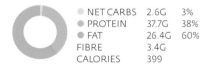

	NET CARBS	2.6G	3%
	PROTEIN	37.7G	38%
	FAT	26.4G	60%
	FIBRE	3.4G	
	CALORIES	399	

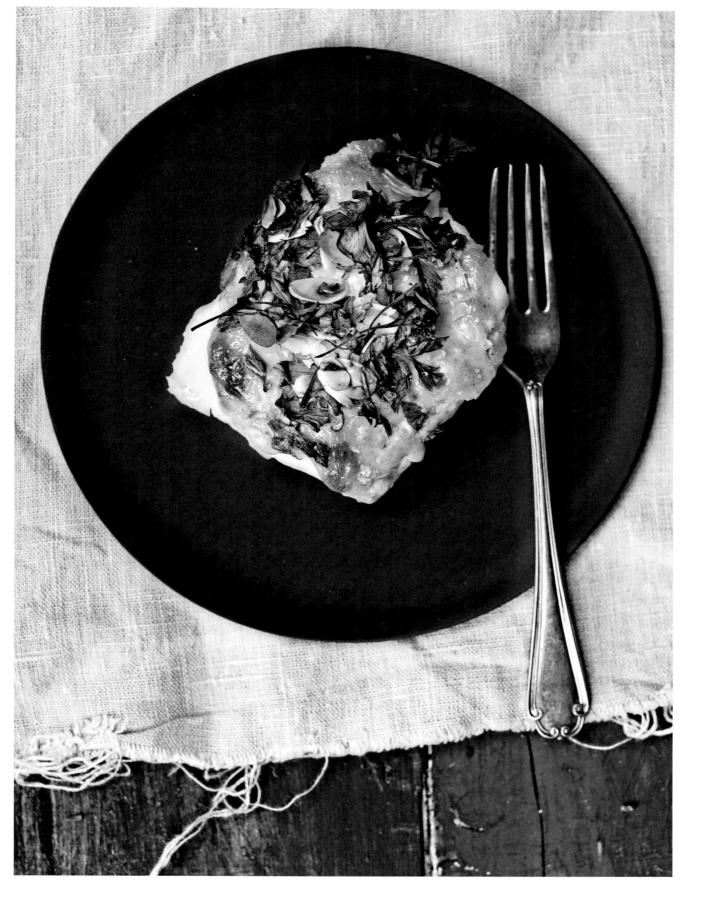

Baked fish supper with fennel and celery

4 × 150g (5.3 oz) fillets of firm white
    fish (600g)
1 head of celery – you'll be using just
    the inside stems (120g)
1 fennel bulb, cut into 0.5cm- (⅛in-)
    thick slices (87g)
About 8 small anchovies, drained
    and chopped (24g)
2 garlic cloves, chopped (6g)
4 tsp capers (11g)
½ tsp chilli flakes (1g)
Good knob butter or olive oil (20g
    butter)

Serves 4

Preheat the oven to 180°C (350°F).

Line a roasting pan with enough non-stick baking paper
to create a large parcel for the fish. Next, chop the celery
and mix well with all the other ingredients except for
the butter.

Place the fish fillets on the paper, pile the celery mixture
over each fillet, dot generously with butter or olive oil,
wrap up well and bake for 20 minutes.

To serve, remove each fillet from the wrapper with
enough topping for a portion each. But when opening
the paper, beware as steam may come out and burn you,
so open up with caution.

PER PORTION

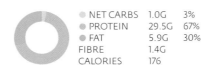

● NET CARBS	1.0G	3%
● PROTEIN	29.5G	67%
● FAT	5.9G	30%
FIBRE	1.4G	
CALORIES	176	

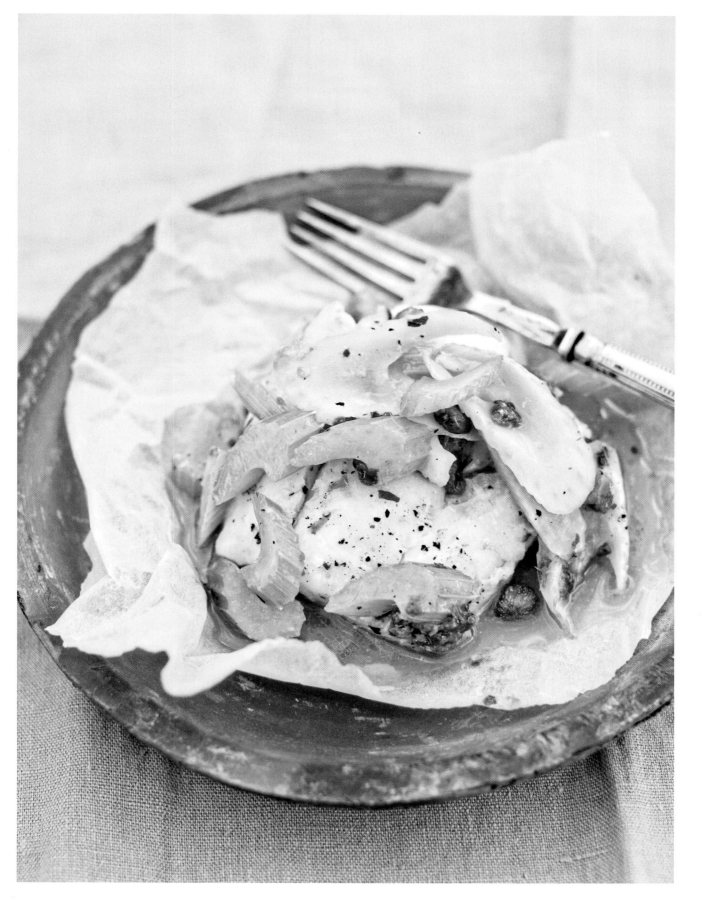

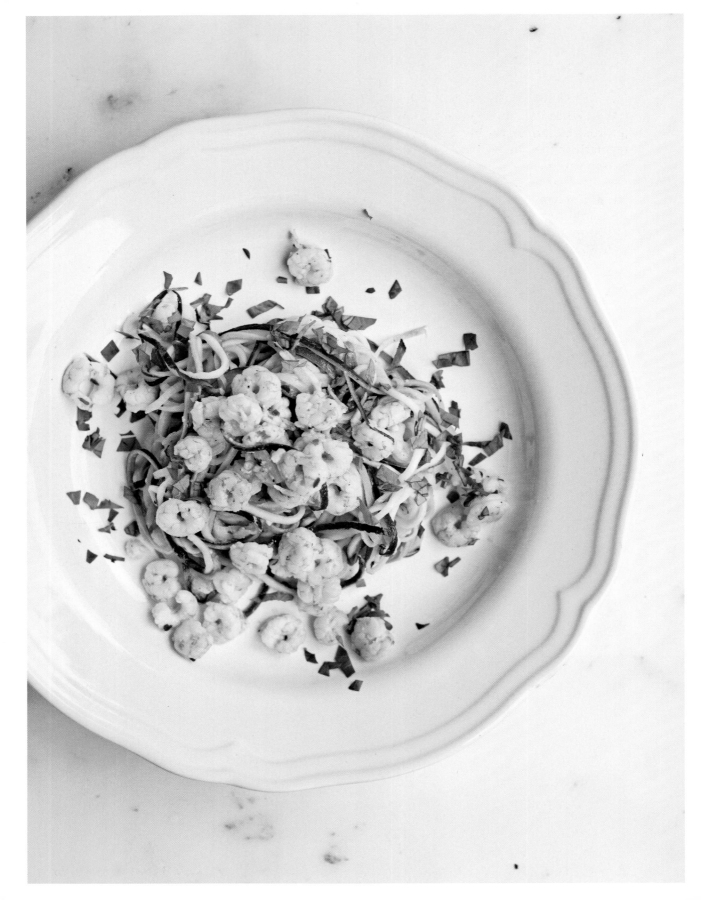

I love this gutsy-flavoured dish.

Melt half or all of the butter and add the garlic and chilli flakes. When hot (but don't let the garlic burn), add the prawns and turn up the heat. Cook them out, tossing regularly so they are well coated in butter and garlic. Season with plenty of black pepper and just a little salt. Add the chopped parsley, the lemon juice, the remaining butter if you didn't use it all before and finally the zucchinis. Mix well and when it's heated through and the prawns are fully cooked, spoon onto plates. Eat immediately.

PER PORTION

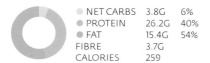

● NET CARBS	3.8G	6%
● PROTEIN	26.2G	40%
● FAT	15.4G	54%
FIBRE	3.7G	
CALORIES	259	

Prawns with garlic, chilli and zucchini spaghetti

40g (2½tbsp) butter (40g)

6 garlic cloves, crushed (18g)

Good pinch of chilli flakes (2g)

500g (1.1lbs) frozen prawns (500g)

Salt and pepper (3g)

Bunch of flat-leaf parsley, finely chopped (12g)

Juice of 2 lemons (80g)

2 zucchinis, grated or spiralised (482g)

Serves 4

Ridiculously tasty prawns

8 garlic cloves (24g)

50ml (¼c) olive oil (50g)

Few sprigs of thyme (if you have it) (4g)

Salt and pepper (3g)

Knob of butter (15g)

400g (14.1 oz) raw or frozen prawns, whatever you can get (400g)

Splash of white wine (15g)

25g (0.9 oz) flat-leaf parsley, chopped (25g)

Serves 4

I recently snatched up some raw prawns on some sort of dodgy supermarket offer and shoved them in the freezer for a 'bad mommy' day. That's a day when there is nothing left in the house to eat except a bit of old bread in the freezer, a few cloves of garlic and a can of beans. 'Not to worry,' I yelled, 'dinner will be ready in a jiffy!'

The family sat around the table, confirming they weren't eating porridge at night or any 'beans and prawns' combo. For a moment I thought I may have been on to a thrifty version of surf 'n' turf, but luckily, common sense prevailed. This dish ended up as gourmet 'prawns on toast' as I put it on some nice brown bread for them, which was truly delicious and repaired my damaged reputation . . . somewhat. I bulked out my dinner with extra broccoli, which is delicious as a side dish, especially with all those garlicky, buttery juices.

Don't peel the garlic cloves – leave the skin on. Heat the olive oil in a small saucepan and cook the whole garlic cloves very gently for 3–4 minutes. Cover with a lid to stop any oil splattering. Add the thyme and season lightly. If the oil gets too hot, the garlic will burn and become bitter. If that happens, start again with new cloves of garlic.

Stick a knife into one of the cloves – if it's soft, remove the cloves from the oil (keep the oil) and drain on kitchen paper. Leave them until they are cool enough to manhandle safely.

Heat up the knob of butter and an extra splash of olive oil (leftover from the confit garlic) in a large saucepan. Fry the prawns on a high heat until they start to get a good colour and caramelise in parts. Squeeze the garlic from its skins and add to the prawns along with the wine and plenty of black pepper. Squish the garlic with a wooden spoon and mix well, sautéing the prawns until cooked through (which should only take a couple of minutes). Garnish with the parsley.

PER PORTION (¼ OF THE RECIPE)

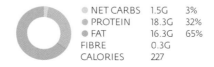

● NET CARBS	1.5G	3%
● PROTEIN	18.3G	32%
● FAT	16.3G	65%
FIBRE	0.3G	
CALORIES	227	

I apologise for calling these parcels 'fragrant'. It sounds more than a little poncey, but there's something about basil that really does make everything quite fragrant, so I feel the OTT adjective is just about permissible.

These can be wrapped up and left for a few hours before baking. They don't take long but I would bring them to room temperature before cooking, so leave them out of the fridge for 30 minutes before plonking in the oven.

Put each salmon fillet onto a larger rectangle of non-stick baking paper. The salmon pieces I had were all long and skinny, so I was able to sandwich or fold them over, stuffed with a couple of basil leaves, some cilantro and a slice of lime. Splash with a bit of lime juice and a few generous drops of olive oil and season well. Wrap up and secure loosely with string. These will be grand for a few hours in the fridge.

When ready to cook, take them out so they get to room temperature and place in a roasting pan. Preheat the oven to 190°C (375°F).

Splash the parcels randomly with some water (3–4 tablespoons) and bake for 10–15 minutes. I was happy with mine after about 10 minutes, mainly because I liked the fact that they were not fully cooked in the middle. But please, this is up to you, so open one up, pull it slightly apart and you'll know quite quickly how well done they are. But remember that if they are nearly done, they will keep on cooking in their parcels. Either way they'll remain moist, so even if you cook them to Timbuktu, they will still be delicious.

Fragrant salmon parcels

4 × 200g (7 oz) skinned pieces of
   salmon (800g)
4–8 basil leaves (3g)
4 small bunches of cilantro (16g)
1 lime, sliced (72g)
1 lime, juiced (20g)
1 tbsp olive oil (13g)
Salt and pepper (3g)

Serves 4

PER PORTION (¼ OF THE RECIPE)

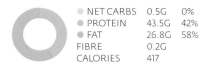

● NET CARBS	0.5G	0%
● PROTEIN	43.5G	42%
● FAT	26.8G	58%
FIBRE	0.2G	
CALORIES	417	

Prawn korma

Glug of olive oil (10g)

1 large white onion, finely sliced
    (240g)

3 garlic cloves, sliced (9g)

1 tbsp mild curry powder (6g)

¼ tsp turmeric (1g)

Good pinch of chilli flakes (2g)

Handful of button mushrooms
    (optional) (65g)

1 eggplant (optional) (250g)

Salt and pepper (3g)

1 × 400ml can (14.1 oz) coconut milk
    (400g)

400–500g (14 oz–1lb) prawns (450g)

1 tbsp lime juice (15g)

Big bunch of cilantro, chopped (30g)

Serves 4–6

If you're in the mood to feed a gang, then I'd be happy with this recipe purely for ease and flavour, based on Sarah Raven's recipe in her lovely book *Food for Friends and Family*. If you want to bulk the dish out, you could add some mushrooms when sweating off the onions, or even some diced eggplant. Any frozen prawns would do, cooked or uncooked. You would obviously just need to cook the raw ones for longer, but in reality they cook so fast that either are fine. Fresh ones are even better to use, but frozen ones are so handy. Serve with your favourite type of rice – mine is the cauliflower rice on page 180.

Heat the olive oil in a large heavy-based saucepan and sweat the onion until it's soft but not coloured. Do this slowly – allow about 7 minutes. Turn up the heat, add the garlic and spices, mix well and if using, add the button mushrooms (which you can cut in half) and the eggplant (which you should cut into small dice). Keep the heat up high and cook out the mushrooms and eggplant, which may go a bit soggy, so keep them on the move so they don't burn, but don't keep at them with a wooden spoon or they won't dry out. If you need to add another glug of the olive oil, do, as the eggplant and mushrooms will soak up the fat. Season them well and taste them at this stage. If they are tasty and well seasoned then it's okay to add the coconut milk. If not, keep cooking and season them some more (as well as adding some more spices) till they develop some flavour.

When you're nearly ready to serve, add the prawns and lime juice. Let the prawns cook until they change from translucent to pinky orange and are hot through. Bring the curry up to a simmer and check the seasoning. You can serve it straight away, or if you want to make this in advance, don't add the prawns or cilantro until you're ready to serve. Instead, bring it to the stage of adding the coconut milk and lime juice and cook for a few minutes, then cool to room temperature and refrigerate overnight. You can reheat it gently and when it's hot and simmering, add the prawns and cilantro. Cook fully and serve with rice in big bowls.

PER PORTION (¼ OF THE RECIPE)

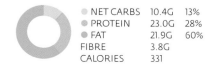

NET CARBS	10.4G	13%
PROTEIN	23.0G	28%
FAT	21.9G	60%
FIBRE	3.8G	
CALORIES	331	

Sometimes you need a no-nonsense kind of dish that is good for a Sunday lunch or dinner and ticks some nutritional boxes and another that shows you have a bit of dazzle up your sleeve. This salmon and leek bake is a dish that screams 'I am a grown-up' and can be rustled up in a jiffy. It shows a streak of sensible and will please slightly fussy types that like things piping hot and quite plain. It is one of those dishes, though, that looks really lovely before it cooks but then loses its sleek green lustre once it has baked in the oven.

Preheat the oven to 200°C (400°F).

Mix together the leeks and frozen peas in a bowl along with the cream. Season lightly, then pour this mixture on the bottom of a gratin dish. Place the salmon fillets on top, then top the salmon with a good glug of olive oil, the lemon juice and herbs. Season and loosely cover with foil.

Bake for 20–30 minutes. Be careful when you peel back the foil, as you can get a nasty burn from the steam. It won't look as appetising as when you started, colour wise, but it's a lovely dish that is incredibly easy to prepare.

Salmon and leek bake

2 leeks, thinly sliced (300g)
50g (1.8 oz) frozen peas (50g)
30ml (2tbsp) cream (30g)
Salt and pepper (3g)
2 × 150g (5.3 oz) salmon fillets, skinned (300g each)
1 tbsp olive oil (13g)
Juice of 1 lemon (40g)
Fresh tarragon or dill, chopped (8g)

Serves 2

PER PORTION

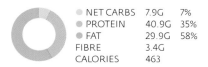

- NET CARBS 7.9G 7%
- PROTEIN 40.9G 35%
- FAT 29.9G 58%
FIBRE 3.4G
CALORIES 463

Baked salmon and horseradish mash

4 fresh medium beetroot, trimmed
   and peeled (320g)
4 × 150g (5.3 oz) salmon fillets
   (600g)
Juice of 1 lemon (40g)
2 tbsp horseradish sauce (more if
   you want it) or some fresh grated
   horseradish (48g)
Knob of butter (15g)
Salt and pepper (3g)

Serves 4

Beetroot is packed with goodness – it guards against coronary artery disease and stroke, for example, and lowers cholesterol levels – but its sweet, earthy flavour is not everyone's cup of tea. So to make it a regular feature on the menu, you need to be clever. Pair sweet roasted beetroot with nuts and salty cheeses like feta or Roquefort to make a substantial salad. Or serve it with salmon. Salmon is one fish that even fish-haters will eat. It's familiar and very good for you too. Beetroot and salmon work surprisingly well together, but good seasoning is crucial. In this recipe, baked fillets are partnered with a rich beetroot mash that gets its kick from a good dose of horseradish that balances out all that sweetness, which is enhanced by a knob of butter. But for younger mouths, feel free to leave the horseradish out.

Preheat the oven to 180°C (350°F).

Boil the beetroot until it's soft when poked with a knife. It took about 40 minutes for me one day and less the next, so give it plenty of time or even do it the day before.

Meanwhile, wrap each fillet of salmon in non-stick baking paper, sprinkling over some lemon juice before you seal the paper, and bake in the oven for 20 minutes, until cooked through.

Drain the beetroot and mash them well with the horseradish sauce and butter – this can be done with a masher or even in a food processor. Season well and serve with the salmon.

PER PORTION

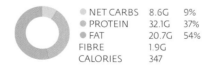

● NET CARBS	8.6G	9%
● PROTEIN	32.1G	37%
● FAT	20.7G	54%
FIBRE	1.9G	
CALORIES	347	

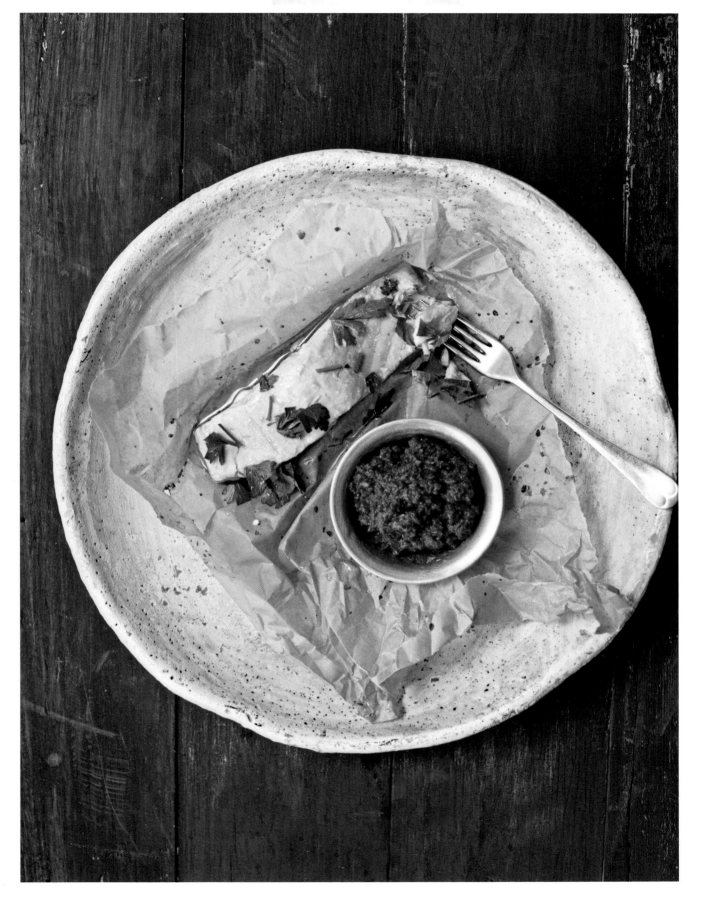

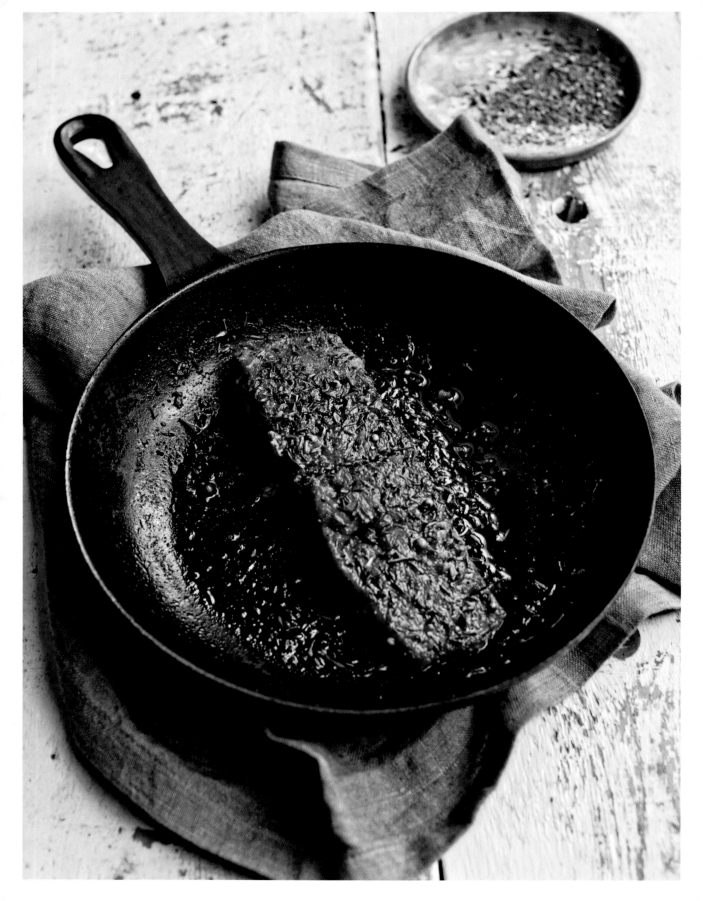

The spice blend for the salmon would also be delicious with monkfish or chicken. If you're doing it with chicken breasts, be sure to finish it off in the oven after cooking on both sides. Fish cooks so much quicker than chicken breasts, so about 4 or 5 minutes in a frying pan will do for the fish, but the chicken will need a good frying on both sides and then 7–10 minutes in an oven at 180°C (350°F) to ensure it's cooked all the way through. You could fry the fish in a little butter instead of the olive oil, which will blacken it even more as the milk solids in butter brown quite quickly. Serve the salmon with some diced cucumber mixed with yoghurt, mint, garlic, lemon juice, salt and pepper.

Grind the coriander seeds in a pestle and mortar or crush them in a cup with a rolling pin. Mix with all the other herbs and spices and the salt.

Place the salmon fillets on a baking tray and sprinkle with half of the spice mix. (Keep the other half for use another night.) Press the spice mix into both sides of the salmon and leave out for 20 minutes or so before frying.

Heat a good glug of olive oil in a large frying pan. When it's nearly smoking, fry the salmon on each side for about 4 minutes in total, longer if you like it well done. You may need to do this in two batches, especially if the heat on your hob isn't great. You need a good strong heat to get colour on the fish and to cook the spices, which is why you don't need to dry-roast the spices before frying.

'Blackened' salmon

1 tbsp coriander seeds (6g)
2 tbsp smoked paprika (14g)
1 tbsp ground cumin (6g)
1 tbsp garlic powder (10g)
1 tbsp ground black pepper (7g)
1 tbsp dried thyme (3g)
1 tbsp dried oregano (5g)
1 tsp flaky sea salt (preferably Maldon) or a few pinches of fine sea salt (3g)
4 × 100g (3.5 oz) salmon fillets, skinned (400g)
1 tbsp olive oil (13g)

Serves 4
Makes enough spice rub for at least 8 portions

PER PORTION (WITH ⅛ OF THE RUB)

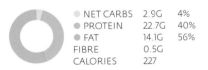

● NET CARBS	2.9G	4%
● PROTEIN	22.7G	40%
● FAT	14.1G	56%
FIBRE	0.5G	
CALORIES	227	

Cured salmon with avocado and wasabi purée

Zest of 1 lime (2g)

Zest of 1 lemon (2g)

Zest of 1 orange (2g)

3 large tsp flaky sea salt (preferably Maldon) (15g)

Lots of black pepper (2g)

800g (1.75lbs) salmon fillets (800g)

2 tsp maple syrup (13g)

Baby leaves (36g)

Avocado purée:

2 avocados (360g)

Juice of 2 limes (40g)

1 tsp wasabi paste (3g)

Salt and pepper (3g)

Sauce:

50ml (¼c) tamari (50g)

Good knob of ginger, peeled and grated (10g)

1 tsp honey (7g)

Serves 4–6

The avocado purée takes seconds to make and the tamari is sweetened, and therefore softened, with some honey. The salmon has an excellent flavour after being cured so you don't want to go overboard on the tamari, but I find that its flavour is gentler than soy sauce.

Mix together the zest, salt and pepper and scatter onto a baking tray or gratin dish. The salmon needs to be skinned and pin bones need to be removed. Then you need to chop the salmon into bite-sized pieces and pour on a splash of maple syrup. This should leave you with about 600g (1.3lbs). Plop the salmon pieces onto the zest mixture and turn them so they are well coated. Wrap the tray or dish really well with cling film, so well that you can give the salmon a good shake around the place and scatter and coat it without having to open it up, move it about with a fork and wrap it in cling film again. Place in the fridge and allow the salmon to cure for at least 8 hours or overnight.

When you are nearly ready to serve, rinse off the salmon pieces and pat them dry on a clean tea towel or kitchen paper, but be careful as the salmon can stick to the kitchen paper (in which case, just rinse it off and use a clean tea towel). Chill until ready to plate up.

Purée the avocados with the lime juice, wasabi and salt and pepper, then spread onto a nice platter.

Mix the tamari with the ginger and honey. Scatter some baby leaves on the avocado. Top with the salmon, then drizzle with some of the sauce. Serve on a big platter and let people help themselves.

PER PORTION (¹/₆ OF THE RECIPE)

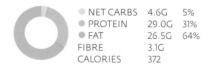

NET CARBS	4.6G	5%
PROTEIN	29.0G	31%
FAT	26.5G	64%
FIBRE	3.1G	
CALORIES	372	

This poached salmon recipe is a real favourite and we cook a fancier version of it when catering for large buffet parties. Even though salmon is relatively fatty in comparison to something like cod, you would think that poaching it in olive oil would be too rich, but in fact it's bang on. It really is a great dish to do for large numbers and is grand served cold the next day or lukewarm, when it takes on an almost custard-like texture.

Don't fret if you don't have pink peppercorns or tarragon. What is important here is the slow, gentle cooking of the fish in a salty, olive oil-based broth. You could always use green peppercorns or a few sprigs of rosemary instead.

Put the olive oil, tarragon, peppercorns and salt in a smallish saucepan with the water and heat until the salt dissolves. Carefully place the salmon fillets in the saucepan – don't worry if they are all squashed together. There should be enough liquid to half-submerge them. Gently bring to the boil, then reduce the heat so that it barely simmers for about 5 minutes. Turn off the heat and leave the salmon in the hot liquid for about 30 minutes, uncovered, turning the salmon once or twice so that it cooks evenly. You can then serve it lukewarm or else cool it entirely and then refrigerate in its poaching liquid and serve cold the next day. This works really well if served with a homemade mayonnaise and some watercress salad.

Olive oil poached salmon with tarragon and pink peppercorns

100ml (⅜c) olive oil (100g)
Small bunch of tarragon (10g)
1 tbsp pink peppercorns (5g)
2 tsp salt (10g)
400ml (1⅝c) water (400g)
4 × 200g (7 oz) salmon fillets with
   the skin on (800g)

Serves 4

PER PORTION

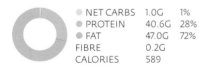

NET CARBS	1.0G	1%
PROTEIN	40.6G	28%
FAT	47.0G	72%
FIBRE	0.2G	
CALORIES	589	

Green tea poached salmon with roasted broccoli and tahini lime dressing

Clean and light with an air of frugality about it. The green tea imparts an interesting taste and ensures a feeling of virtue. This dressing will be enough to do you for a couple of days, but it's a pain to make in smaller batches, so spoon some on stir-fries or anything that needs some oomph.

Preheat the oven to 200°C (400°F).

Cut the broccoli into florets, rinse and put into a roasting pan. Toss with the olive oil and some salt and pepper and roast for 20–30 minutes, until slightly charred.

Meanwhile, to make the dressing, whisk together all the ingredients and set aside.

Heat up the 250ml (1c) water in a shallow saucepan that can hold the four pieces of salmon. Put the tea bags in a cup and add boiling water, then let them steep while the water in the saucepan is heating up. Add the green tea water (don't add the tea bags, as they are likely to burst) to the saucepan along with the green peppercorns and the mirin. Season the water well with salt.

Carefully slide the fish into the water, cover the pan and bring back up to a gentle simmer. Cook for a couple of minutes, then turn the heat off and leave it to sit for 7–10 minutes. If you like it well done, then simmer it for longer. You can always peek into the middle of the fish by gently parting each end of one fillet to see how pink or poached it looks.

Give it a light pat dry before putting on a plate with some broccoli and the dipping sauce to share. It's also good served with the wild rice salad on page 179.

Salmon and broccoli:
2 small heads of broccoli (350g)
2 tbsp olive oil (26g)
Salt and pepper (3g)
250ml (1c) water (250g)
3 green tea bags
1 tbsp green peppercorns (21g)
120ml (½c) mirin or white wine (120g)
4 × 200g (7 oz) salmon fillets (800g)

Tahini lime dressing:
Good knob of ginger, peeled and grated (10g)
2 garlic cloves, crushed (6g)
Zest and juice of 1 lime (1g + 20g)
3 tbsp tamari (54g)
2 tbsp olive oil (26g)
2 tbsp honey (42g)
1 tbsp toasted sesame oil (12g)
1 tbsp tahini (18g)

Serves 4

PER PORTION (WITH ⅛ OF THE DRESSING)

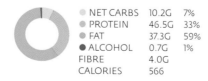

NET CARBS	10.2G	7%
PROTEIN	46.5G	33%
FAT	37.3G	59%
ALCOHOL	0.7G	1%
FIBRE	4.0G	
CALORIES	566	

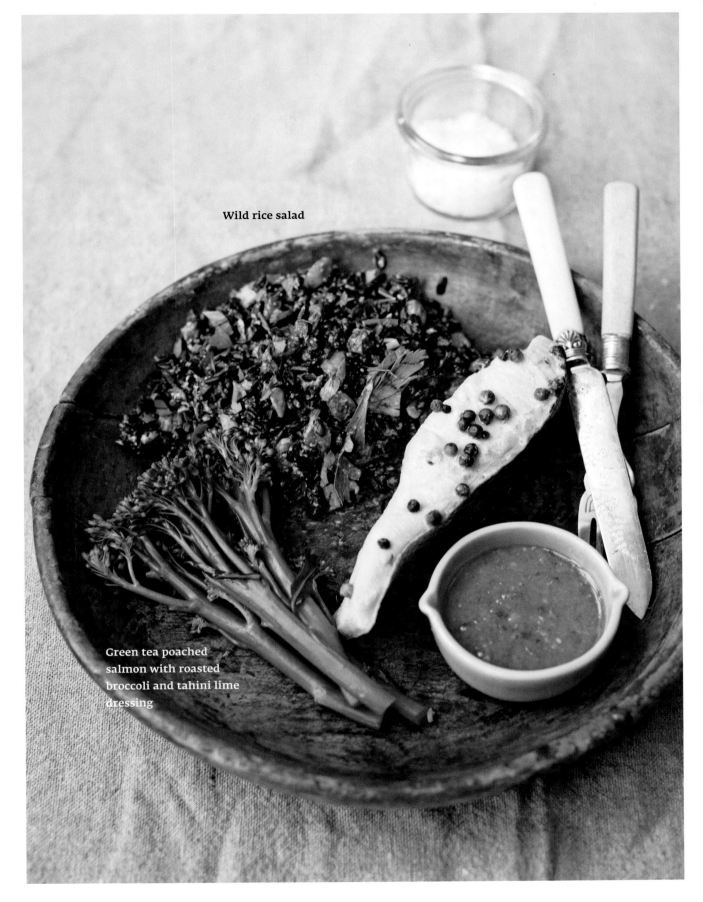

Wild rice salad

Green tea poached
salmon with roasted
broccoli and tahini lime
dressing

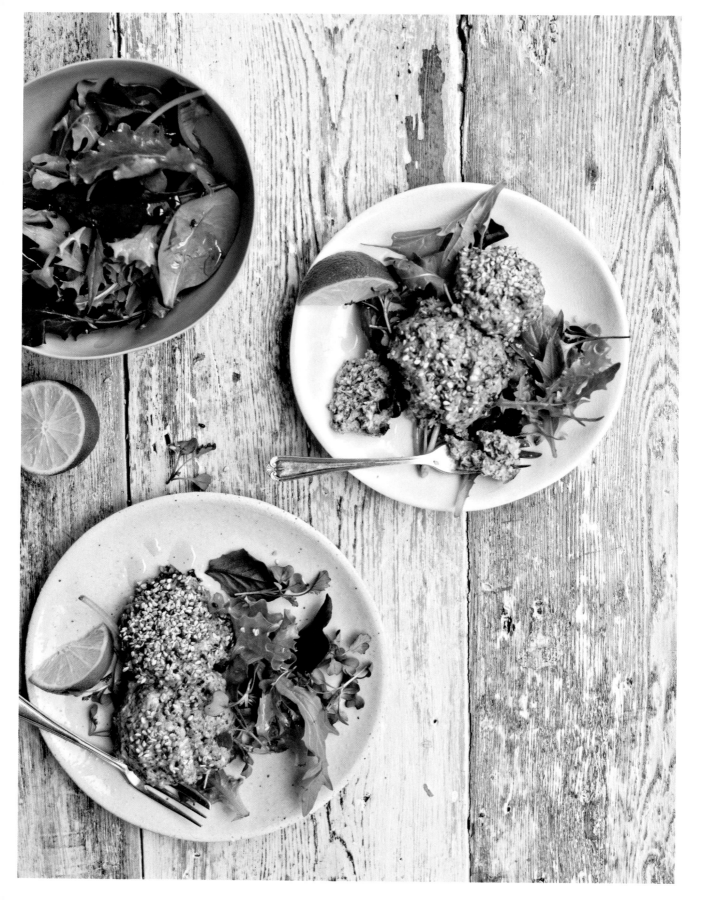

Low-carb fish cakes

There is something very addictive about crisp fishcakes with a panko crumb fried until golden brown and slathered in some delicious emulsion . . . STOP! To keep it low-carb, you have to ditch the flour, egg and crumb approach. These aren't bad!

Preheat the oven to 200°C (400°F). Line a baking tray with non-stick baking paper.

Whizz all the ingredients except the fish and sesame seeds together in a food processor until smooth. Add the fish and pulse so that it's processed but not total mushy baby food. Shape the fish into balls and place them on the lined baking tray. If you can, chill them for 10 minutes.

Sprinkle with sesame seeds, then bake for 10–12 minutes. If you can, gently turn them over halfway through so they can brown on both sides. They cook quite quickly and you may like to serve them a bit rare inside. Let them settle for a second before removing from the paper (they are quite delicate, as there is no egg to bind them). Serve with a good squeeze of lime juice.

2 red onions, diced (300g)
2 red chillies, deseeded and diced (40g)
Small bunch of cilantro (4g)
Small bunch of basil (4g)
Good knob of ginger, peeled (10g)
1 stalk of lemongrass (4g)
2 lime leaves (0.6g)
Juice of 2 limes (40g)
2 tbsp tamari (36g)
1 tsp fish sauce (6g)
1 tsp sesame oil (4g)
200g (7 oz) fresh salmon fillet, skinned and roughly chopped (200g)
200g (7 oz) fresh tuna fillet, skinned and roughly chopped (200g)
Handful of sesame seeds (22g)

Serves 4 as a starter, 2 as a main

PER PORTION (¼ OF THE RECIPE)

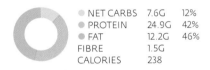

● NET CARBS	7.6G	12%
● PROTEIN	24.9G	42%
● FAT	12.2G	46%
FIBRE	1.5G	
CALORIES	238	

Thai fish cakes

1 onion, roughly chopped (150g)

Knob of ginger, peeled and roughly chopped (5g)

1 stalk of lemongrass, roughly chopped (5g)

Zest of 1 lime (2g)

½ tsp maple syrup (3g)

½ tsp fish sauce (3g)

1 bunch of scallions, very finely sliced (60g)

Approx. 600g (1.3lbs) skinned salmon, cut into chunks (600g)

Approx. 200g (7 oz) green beans (200g)

Salt and pepper (3g)

1 tbsp olive oil (13g)

Serves 4–6

Salmon (especially wild salmon if you can get it) is a great source of omega-3s, as are trout, mackerel and sardines. We often hear people saying our omega-3s and 6s are really important, but unfortunately, most Western diets tend to contain far too many omega-6s rather than 3s. When I can't remember which is which, I just keep thinking of that De La Soul song, 'Three is the magic number', because it really is.

Ask your fishmonger to skin and roughly chop about 700g (1.5lbs) of salmon for you so you end up with about 600g (1.3lbs) of skinned salmon chunks. You can also use trout or other fish in this. Also, my green beans come in a 165g pack, so don't get too hung up on the quantity. Use whatever is handy.

Preheat the oven to 180°C (350°F). Line a baking tray with non-stick baking paper.

Put the onion, ginger, lemongrass, lime zest, maple syrup and fish sauce in a food processor and whizz until it makes a finely chopped paste. Add the scallions and salmon and pulse until mixed well enough that you can form them into fish cakes. You don't want it to be total mush, but slightly chunkier than minced beef, if possible. Slice the green beans very finely then throw them in and season the whole mixture lightly.

Mix with a spoon and shape into eight decent-sized fish cakes. Place them on the lined baking tray. Drizzle each one with a little olive oil and brush or rub it in with your fingers.

Bake for 12–15 minutes. They may brown ever so slightly on top, but they do cook quite quickly. Serve with a squeeze of lime juice.

PER PORTION (¼ OF THE RECIPE)

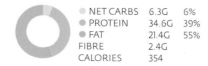

NET CARBS	6.3G	6%
PROTEIN	34.6G	39%
FAT	21.4G	55%
FIBRE	2.4G	
CALORIES	354	

Loosely based on a Diana Henry recipe.

To make the sauce, sweat the peppers, carrot, onion and chilli in the olive oil with a lid on for about 20 minutes, until soft. Add in everything else except the water and cook for another bit. After about 5 minutes, blitz in a blender until smooth by adding some water until it's as thick as you like it. Check the seasoning. Set aside and serve at room temperature. It will taste better once it has cooled down.

To make the fishcakes, preheat the oven to 180°C (350°F).

In a food processor, pulse all the ingredients for the fish cakes together except for the fish until well combined, then add the fish chunks and pulse until well combined again, but don't blend to a mush. If you can, shape into approx. 24 patties and chill on a baking tray. Bake for about 10 minutes. Try to get some colour on them and then carefully turn over and cook for another 5 minutes. Serve while warm with the red pepper sauce.

PER PORTION

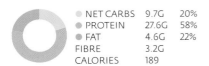

● NET CARBS	9.7G	20%
● PROTEIN	27.6G	58%
● FAT	4.6G	22%
FIBRE	3.2G	
CALORIES	189	

Spicy fish cakes with red pepper sauce

Bunch of scallions, finely chopped (60g)
Bunch of cilantro, finely chopped (20g)
1 garlic clove, crushed (3g)
1 egg, beaten (57g)
Zest and juice of 1 lemon (2g + 40g)
2 tsp ground coriander (4g)
1 tsp ground cumin (2g)
1 tsp fennel seeds (2g)
½ tsp chilli flakes (1g)
Salt and pepper (3g)
700g (1.5lbs) white fish, skinned and filleted (700g)

Red pepper sauce:
2 red peppers, deseeded and sliced (320g)
1 carrot, peeled and chopped (100g)
1 onion, chopped (150g)
1 chilli, deseeded and chopped (20g)
Glug of olive oil (10g)
2 ripe tomatoes, roughly chopped (260g)
50ml (¼c) white wine vinegar (50g)
½ tsp saffron (1g)
Salt (2g)
50–100ml (¼–⅜c) water (75g)

Serves 6 – should make 24 cakes

Vegetarian

I love vegetarian food and was a veggie for about seven years, a million years ago. I think meat is unbelievably nutritious, but I also worry that as a society, we don't view meat as the luxury it is. At home, we try to eat meat only a couple of times a week to give us the chance to get some fish into us at least once a week, then the rest of the time we eat a vegetarian diet. These are some of my favourite vegetarian recipes and most of them give you some leftovers, which is always a nice perk.

This zucchini and mint frittata takes a simple concept and makes it tastier and a lot more interesting to eat. I used to use more eggs and less veg, but have since changed the balance and I prefer it this way. Dried mint is brilliant for you and is definitely one to plunge into everything you can. And remember, don't feel obliged to use cheese in recipes. I put it in for flavour and taste, but if you can't eat dairy, just leave it out. Either way, this is delicious served cold for lunch.

Preheat the oven to 180°C (350°F). You'll need a large ovenproof frying pan.

Heat the olive oil and sweat the onions and leeks very gently with the mint and lemon zest. I often put a lid on them to really make them sweat. When they have wilted down, season well and add the zucchinis. Take off the heat, mix well and then pour in the eggs. You'll have to use a fork to help the eggs reach every corner, making tracks in the veg and then evening everything out.

Top with the cheese and then put in the oven for 20–30 minutes. Leave it to 'settle' for 10 minutes, then slice and serve. There are so many veg in this that I often just serve this with a few spoonfuls of avocados and chopped tomatoes for little people and a crisp green salad for me.

Leek, zucchini and mint frittata

50ml (¼c) olive oil (50g)
2 red onions, diced (300g)
3 leeks, sliced (510g)
3 good tsp dried mint (2g)
Zest of 1 lemon (2g)
Salt and pepper (3g)
6 zucchinis, grated (1.2kg)
6–8 eggs, beaten (7 eggs or 400g)
200g (7 oz) soft goats' cheese or halloumi, cut into chunks (200g goats' cheese)

Serves 8 for a light supper or lunch

PER PORTION

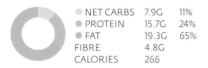

NET CARBS	7.9G	11%
PROTEIN	15.7G	24%
FAT	19.3G	65%
FIBRE	4.8G	
CALORIES	266	

Cauliflower, zucchini and goats' cheese pizza

Base:

1 head of cauliflower (1kg)

Approx. 200g (7 oz) soft goats' cheese (see note above) (200g)

1 egg (57g)

1 tsp dried thyme (1g)

Sauce:

1 tbsp olive oil (13g)

1 onion, diced (150g)

1 red pepper, cored and roughly chopped (160g)

4 garlic cloves, crushed (12g)

1 × 400g can (14.1 oz) of chopped tomatoes (400g)

2 bay leaves (2g)

1–2 tsp dried oregano (2g)

Pinch of smoked sweet paprika or cayenne pepper (1g)

Pinch of chilli flakes (1g)

Salt and pepper (3g)

Topping:

1 zucchini (200g)

1 tsp olive oil (4g)

Salt and pepper (3g)

Approx. 100g (3.5 oz) of your favourite goats' cheese (100g)

Serves 4–6

This cauliflower pizza is superb. I am a big, big fan of cauliflower but I tend to just roast it with curry powder, turmeric, olive oil and a little salt. In this recipe, the florets get blitzed to form cauliflower crumbs that then get bound up with some goats' cheese and an egg. When you spread it out and bake it, you end up with a fabulous golden brown base that is veggie, gluten-free and very good for you. A nice light sauce and some shavings of zucchini are my toppings of choice.

This would easily serve 4–6, but it's quite moreish and surprisingly filling. I think it's better when it cools down to room temperature. I use the Old MacDonnells Farm goats' cheese, though St Tola would also be soft enough to use.

To make the base, remove the green stalks from the cauliflower (these are good when you're roasting cauliflower, but they don't work here) and cut or break the florets into small pieces. Pulse in a food processor until you make white 'breadcrumbs' that look a little damp. Don't over process, but do make sure it's fully ground up.

Transfer the cauliflower crumbs to a large bowl and mix with the goats' cheese, egg and thyme. It's almost like beating sugar and butter together with no electric beater. I just did it with a spatula and it's easier if the cheese is soft and at room temperature. Eventually you will feel that everything is reasonably well distributed.

Line a baking tray or brownie pan with plenty of non-stick baking paper, then spread the 'dough' onto the paper and pat it down with the spatula. Put another sheet of baking paper over it and smooth out the cauliflower with your flat hands so that it spreads out until it's about 1.25cm (0.5in) thick. It's almost like pushing play dough into the corners. You can chill the base (even overnight) while the sauce is cooking away.

When you're ready, preheat the oven to 200°C (400°F) and cook the base on its own for about 20 minutes. It will start to look a little pale but golden on top. Lift up the paper to check that the bottom is okay. The edges may char a bit, but this is fine. Set aside to cool down.

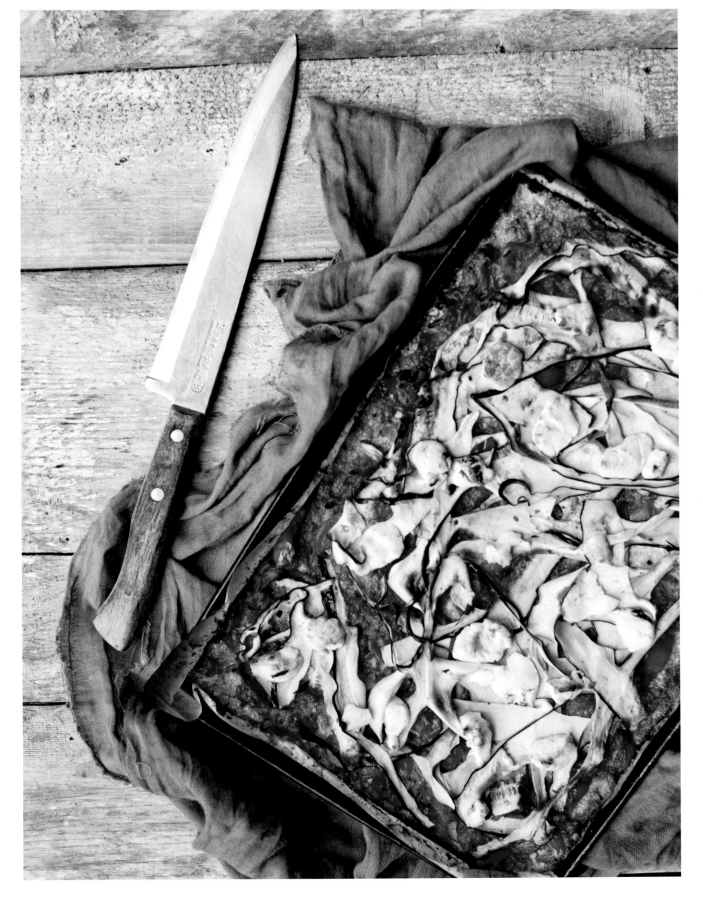

Heat the olive oil and sweat the onion, red pepper and garlic for a few minutes. Add the rest of the ingredients and simmer over a gentle heat for about 20 minutes. Remove the bay leaf and let the sauce cool down, then blitz until smooth in a blender. This will make too much sauce, but it can be frozen in batches so you have some ready to go the next time you want a homemade pizza sauce that's a bit fruitier than normal.

Cut the zucchini lengthways on a mandolin or very finely with a knife. Toss with the olive oil and salt and pepper.

When you're ready to do the final 10 minutes of cooking, spread a few tablespoons of sauce onto the pizza base, then top with slivers of the zucchinis and scatter some goats' cheese on top. Bake for 10 minutes, until the cheese is just starting to melt. Allow to cool and settle and serve. Just as good cold, if not better.

PER PORTION (¼ OF THE RECIPE)

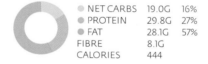

NET CARBS	19.0G	16%
PROTEIN	29.8G	27%
FAT	28.1G	57%
FIBRE	8.1G	
CALORIES	444	

This is a tart with a cauliflower base, a kind of veg 'pastry', that is loosely based on a Natasha Corrett recipe. I know it's annoying when you see 350g (12.3 oz) cauliflower (that's about three-quarters of a head of cauliflower), but roast the rest with some of your favourite spices and a lick of olive oil in a hot oven until it's starting to brown. The creamy filling of grated zucchini and goats' cheese is really nice. Thank goodness for food fashions! This one is a keeper.

Preheat the oven to 180°C (350°F). Grease a 27cm (11in) quiche pan.

To make the base, blitz the cauliflower in a blender until it forms 'breadcrumbs'. Add the almonds, egg and thyme, season well and blitz briefly again to form a wet dough/pastry. If you like, you can throw in a few other fresh herbs like oregano or marjoram; there are no rules here. Press the 'dough' into the greased quiche pan to form the base, bringing it up at the sides just as you would pastry, as you want to contain the filling. Bake the base in the oven for about 15 minutes, until it's just starting to colour at the edges.

While that's cooking, make the filling by simply whisking all the ingredients together in a bowl and seasoning well.

When the base is done, put the pan on a baking tray and pour in the filling. Return it to the oven and bake for 30–35 minutes, until golden and still a bit quivery, as the egg will continue to cook even out of the oven.

Cauliflower, almond and goats' cheese tart

Base:
350g (12.3 oz) cauliflower (350g)
75g (2.6 oz) ground almonds (75g)
1 egg (57g)
Few sprigs of fresh thyme, leaves chopped (1g)
Salt and pepper (3g)

Filling:
700g (1.5lbs) (approx. 3) zucchinis, grated (700g)
100g (3.5 oz) goats' cheese (100g)
4 eggs (228g)
200ml (⅞c) crème fraîche (200g)

Serves 6–8

PER PORTION (¹⁄₆ OF THE RECIPE)

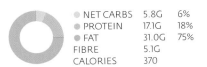

NET CARBS	5.8G	6%
PROTEIN	17.1G	18%
FAT	31.0G	75%
FIBRE	5.1G	
CALORIES	370	

Quinoa, cauliflower, raisin and feta cakes

200g (7 oz) quinoa (200g)
1 head of cauliflower (1kg)
1 large bunch of flat-leaf parsley
    (20g)
4 eggs, beaten (228g)
1 × 200g pack (7 oz) of feta cheese,
    crumbled (200g)
50g (1.8 oz) raisins, chopped (50g)
2 garlic cloves, crushed (6g)
Salt and pepper (3g)

Makes 12 cakes, which would easily serve 12

I loved my original version of these, and in an effort to be good I tried them without frying them – and they are still good. I've also added some more garlic (why not?) and used a whole head of cauliflower. They may be a little more fragile without that heat-sealing blast in the frying pan, but they are lighter and better for us. In every 100g (3.5 oz) oats, there are 70g carbs. You need 50–100g of carbohydrates a day to stay 'low-carb', although it depends very much on the type of person you are, what you do, how sedentary you are, etc. Anyway, the bottom line is that in the few recipes I have previously used oats in, I have subsequently replaced them with something else.

Cook the quinoa in boiling water for 15 minutes by simmering gently. Drain and let it cool down while it continues draining. You could also do this the day before, no prob.

Break the cauliflower into florets, then put the cauliflower in a food processor and pulse until it resembles fine breadcrumbs. You may have to do this in a few batches. Put the crumbs in a big bowl, then blitz the parsley and add it to the cauliflower crumbs.

Add the quinoa and the rest of the other ingredients to the cauliflower crumbs and mix really well. Shape into 12 patties and put on a baking tray or similar and chill in the fridge for at least 30 minutes or you could leave them overnight.

To cook, preheat the oven to 180°C (350°F). Line a baking tray with non-stick baking paper.

Transfer the patties to the lined tray and cook in the oven for about 30 minutes. If you can turn them over halfway through cooking, do, but if they look like they might fall apart, then don't.

They are delicious with the guacamole on page 103 or the quick olive salsa on page 196 and they are also good eaten cold.

PER CAKE:

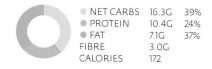

NET CARBS	16.3G	39%
PROTEIN	10.4G	24%
FAT	7.1G	37%
FIBRE	3.0G	
CALORIES	172	

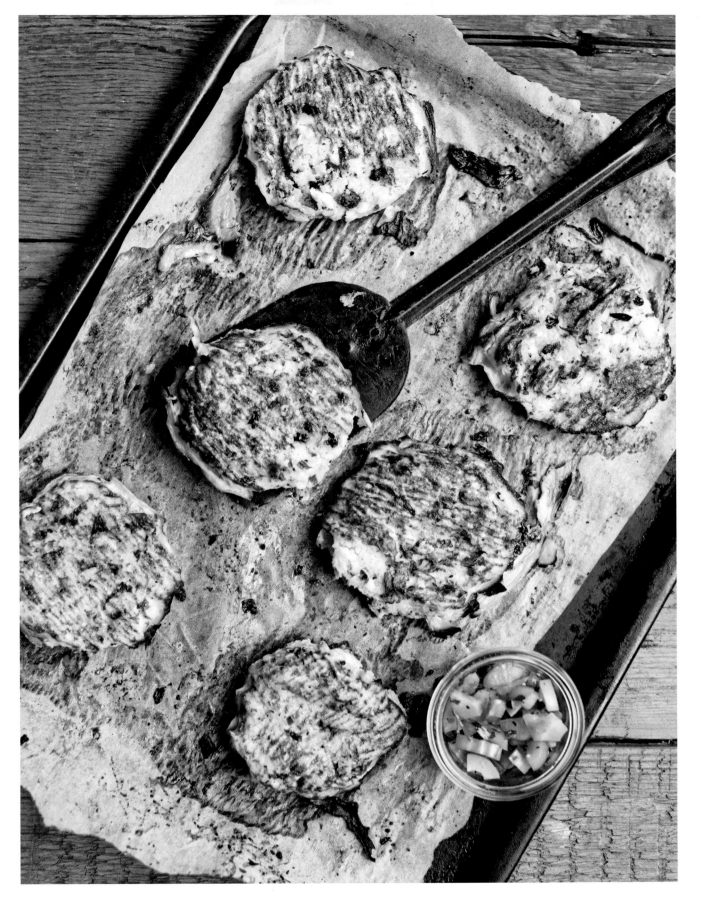

Roast tomato curry

2 onions, chopped (300g)

40g (2½tbsp) butter (40g)

1 green chilli, deseeded and chopped (20g)

2 garlic cloves, crushed (6g)

Good knob of ginger, peeled and finely chopped (10g)

1 tsp ground cumin (2g)

6–7 curry leaves (1g)

5 cardamom seeds (0.5g)

Approx. ½ × 400ml can (7 oz) of coconut milk (200g)

Salt and pepper (3g)

10 tomatoes, cut in half horizontally (1.3kg)

1 tbsp lime juice (15g)

Bunch of cilantro (16g)

Serves 4

This dish has a little fire in it, with vibrant colours that remind us we're due a good summer when tomatoes are in season. A handy recipe when you have a glut of tomatoes and little else!

Preheat the oven to 180°C (350°F).

Sweat the onions in the butter until soft, then add the chilli, garlic, ginger, cumin, curry leaves and cardamom. Cook over a gentle heat for about 5 minutes to help release all the lovely oils and aromas, then add the coconut milk, taste and season.

Place the tomatoes in a large gratin dish, skin side down. Spoon the sauce over the tomatoes and bake for 30 minutes, until bubbling. Allow to cool for a bit, then squeeze some lime juice on top and tear up some cilantro to garnish and serve.

PER PORTION (¼ OF THE RECIPE)

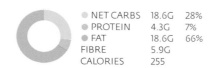

NET CARBS	18.6G	28%
PROTEIN	4.3G	7%
FAT	18.6G	66%
FIBRE	5.9G	
CALORIES	255	

Remember, you salt eggplants to force their air cells to collapse so that they don't absorb as much oil when cooking them. Thinking that you are removing the bitter juices is scientifically known as 'hooey'.

Put the tomatoes in a small saucepan along with the butter, garlic, herbs and seasoning. Bring up to a simmer and cook for about 20 minutes over a gentle heat until it's as thick as ketchup, stirring often with a wooden spoon as it can burn if you don't keep an eye on it.

Meanwhile, sprinkle the eggplants generously with salt and lay them out on a baking tray lined with kitchen paper.

In another saucepan, heat up the crème fraîche until simmering and reduced by a third. It will start to look like curdled yoghurt, but don't worry. Take it off the heat, mix in the Parmesan and set aside.

Taste both the tomato sauce and the crème fraîche and make sure you are happy with the seasoning. You can do both these stages the night before if that's handier and just leave them in your fridge until ready to assemble.

Preheat the oven to 180°C (350°F).

Wipe the salt off the eggplants and fry them in batches in olive oil until golden on both sides. Don't bother seasoning them except with pepper. Drain on kitchen paper and then layer up in a gratin dish once they have cooled down. Top with tomato sauce and then spoonfuls of the crème fraîche, which won't spread, so merely drop it on top of the tomato sauce with a spoon.

Bake for 25–30 minutes, until bubbling. Drizzle with more olive oil and let it rest for 10 minutes before serving with a green salad.

Baked eggplants with tomato, Parmesan and crème fraîche

1 × 400g can (14.1 oz) of chopped tomatoes (400g)
50g (3½tbsp) butter (50g)
4 garlic cloves, thinly sliced (12g)
Bunch of thyme or rosemary (16g)
Salt and pepper (3g)
2 eggplants, sliced into 2cm- (¾in-) thick rounds (600g)
1 × 250g tub (8.8 oz) of crème fraîche (250g)
50g (1.8 oz) Parmesan, finely grated (50g)
3 tbsp olive oil (39g)

Perfect supper for 2–3

PER PORTION (⅓ OF THE RECIPE)

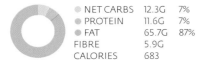

- NET CARBS 12.3G 7%
- PROTEIN 11.6G 7%
- FAT 65.7G 87%
- FIBRE 5.9G
- CALORIES 683

Eggplant dengaku

80g (2.8 oz) tahini (80g)

3 tbsp miso (90g)

1 tbsp mirin (16g)

1 tbsp rice wine vinegar (11g)

3 eggplants (900g)

3 tbsp olive oil (39g)

2 tbsp black and white sesame seeds (22g)

Serves 4

This eggplant dengaku is lovely served at room temperature. It does burn quite quickly, so do keep an eye on it. You want the filling to be nice and soft, but the topping should be caramelised rather than burnt. It's a vegetable that tastes quite meaty and can stand sitting out in the heat for an hour or so and still be vaguely edible.

Preheat the oven to 180°C (350°F).

Heat the tahini, miso, mirin and rice wine vinegar together and gradually whisk until it becomes a nice smooth paste, then take off the heat.

Cut the eggplants in half lengthways, then score the skin with a knife, like you'd do with fish, so the sauce sinks into the track lines. Put on a baking tray and drizzle generously with olive oil, then smear some of the (cooled down) paste on each surface and sprinkle with sesame seeds if you have them. Cook for 30–40 minutes. The eggplants should feel nice and soft and the tops should be caramelised. Allow to cool and settle and eat warm or even cold.

PER PORTION:

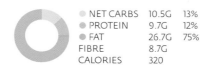

NET CARBS	10.5G	13%
PROTEIN	9.7G	12%
FAT	26.7G	75%
FIBRE	8.7G	
CALORIES	320	

Melt the coconut oil in a large heavy-based saucepan over a medium heat, then sweat the spices for a few minutes to release their aroma and flavour. Now this next bit takes some time. Add the diced eggplants and cook them slowly, stirring them every now and then, until they are golden all over and cooked through – this takes about 25 minutes. Add the tomatoes and halloumi and stir in until they are warmed through and slightly cooked/ melting. Just before serving, add the cilantro. Season well and serve.

PER PORTION

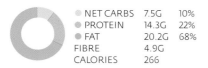

NET CARBS	7.5G	10%
PROTEIN	14.3G	22%
FAT	20.2G	68%
FIBRE	4.9G	
CALORIES	266	

Eggplant and halloumi mish-mash

1 good tbsp coconut oil (27g)

1 tbsp black mustard seeds (6g)

2 tsp garam masala (4g)

2 eggplants, diced (600g)

1 punnet (11.6 oz) cherry tomatoes, cut in half (330g)

1 × 200g pack (7 oz) of halloumi, diced (200g)

Bunch of fresh cilantro, chopped (16g)

Salt and pepper (3g)

Serves 4

'Cut out most of the carbs in your life and life is better.'
Dr Richard Feinman

Shakshuka

½ tsp cumin seeds (1g)

50ml (¼c) olive oil (50g)

2 onions, sliced (300g)

4 peppers (I use 2 red and 2 yellow), sliced (640g)

Good pinch of smoked sweet paprika (1g)

4–6 large, ripe tomatoes, roughly chopped (800g)

Few sprigs of thyme (2g)

Splash of hot sauce (no sugar) (3g)

Salt and pepper (3g)

4 eggs (228g)

Serves 2 people if you're starving, but you could increase the eggs to 6 and serve 3 people, but have slightly less sauce

Slow cooking is the key to the delicious red pepper and tomato base. I make it in a large frying pan with tall enough sides and one that a lid can fit on. It would be fair to say that this vegetarian dish has become a supper favourite instead of a breakfast one.

In a large, deep frying pan that you have a lid for, dry roast the cumin for a minute or so until you get the best smell, then add the oil and onions and slowly sweat for about 5 minutes, until soft but not coloured. Add the peppers and paprika after a minute, then after another minute or so add the tomatoes, thyme and hot sauce. The heat will start to break up the tomatoes. At this stage, put a lid on the pan, turn the heat down to low and cook for about 10 minutes, occasionally stirring, until it starts to turn into a lovely thick sauce. Taste and season well. You want the mix to taste fantastic!

You can either cool it down until the next day or else keep going by making a few wells in the sauce. Crack the eggs into the mixture and then leave them to poach on the surface of the tomato sauce. This will take a while, and I often find myself tipping the pan to try to get some of the tomato juices to run over the tops of the egg whites to get them to cook a tad more. Putting a lid on also helps the eggs to cook.

When ready to serve, carefully scoop out so the eggs stay intact. Delicious with some salad.

PER PORTION (½ OF THE RECIPE)

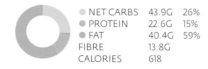

NET CARBS	43.9G	26%
PROTEIN	22.6G	15%
FAT	40.4G	59%
FIBRE	13.8G	
CALORIES	618	

If you're keen to eat more vegetables in new ways, the spiraliser or julienne peeler is for you. The nutritional benefits are considerable. Because the veg is raw or nearly raw, its nutrients remain largely intact. If your digestion is delicate, though, and too much raw food is a problem, up your intake gently. And the results are tasty, too. Kids like the noodles and you can easily mix up some carrots and zucchini if you feel like going crazy.

Following the spiraliser instructions or using a julienne peeler, spiralise the zucchinis into strips.

Heat the butter very gently in a large saucepan with the garlic, then add the zucchinis and warm through – just 2 minutes is all it takes; you don't want mush or browning of any kind. Squeeze over some lemon juice, season and serve straight away. You can toss the vi-coise sauce on page 190 through it and serve, or just sprinkle it on top.

Zucchini 'spaghetti'

4 zucchinis, rinsed and dried (800g)
Knob of butter (15g)
1 garlic clove, crushed (3g)
1 tbsp lemon juice (15g)
Salt and pepper (3g)
Vi-coise dip (page 190), to serve

Serves 4

PER PORTION (¼ OF THE RECIPE, WITHOUT THE DIP)

NET CARBS	4.0G	24%
PROTEIN	3.7G	23%
FAT	3.9G	53%
FIBRE	4.1G	
CALORIES	66	

Eat your greens . . . and everything in between

Spinach, kale, cabbage and everything in between, from broad beans to broccoli – greens are everywhere but can be a tough sell sometimes, particularly to children. Some experts believe this has to do with the fact that it's an in-built safety mechanism, still ingrained in their stubborn psyche, from when Mum and Dad were out hunting and gathering. We might have been left to inadvertently consume poisonous berries or leaves that no amount of juju could save us from.

This reluctance to eat unknown 'green things' may well have saved our junior predecessors, but now the pressure to eat our greens is hovering everywhere. And let's face it: processed food has been engineered to be as pleasing as possible to our palates. Vegetables, especially things like sprouts and cabbage, have to grow on you.

But a bit like Kermit, I'm always happy for green to take its place in the limelight. Green foods are overflowing with nutrients that protect your heart, nourish your digestion and give the kind of glow to your skin that only 20-year-olds bursting with collagen enjoy.

And don't forget the stems and extra green bits, especially of leeks and scallions. Although broccoli stems can seem 'woody', they are actually full of goodness. Eating lots of indigestible fibre is invaluable for good gut health!

Often the quickest and easiest way to cook vegetables like broccoli is to plunge the florets into boiling water and only cook for about 30 seconds or so before draining. While this is going on, I heat up a little olive oil or a small knob of butter, sauté some garlic and add the broccoli to the saucepan and let the heat cook out the garlic and finish off the broccoli. A bit of seasoning or a squeeze of lemon juice work wonders. This takes less than 5 minutes and is so, so good for you! Plus it's delicious, and making your vegetables taste wonderful is the best way to get everyone eating them. That might mean you rely on some dips and sauces initially to coax folks into eating their greens, but eventually you can go plainer because cooking three separate elements every night is a pain. So keep it simple: if you're cooking one of the meat or veggie main courses, then do something very quick and easy for your veg. But if you're eating leftovers, then take the time to put a bit more effort into your vegetable side dishes.

Once these basic rules are observed, you can loosen things up a bit because it's nice to have a few recipes where the veg are the star of the show.

These are very moreish, and if you can get the kids on board with these as a snack, you may even be able to wrangle the crisps away. They are also a nifty substitute when you're craving croutons in a salad.

Preheat the oven to 220°C (430°F).

Toss the chickpeas around a roasting pan with the rest of the ingredients. Get them well coated and then roast in the oven for 15 minutes or so, until golden, crunchy and well coated in the seasonings. Serve warm or cool (they do go a bit soggy when they cool down, but they're still very tasty) and stuff in sandwiches or eat as a snack.

PER PORTION (⅓ OF THE RECIPE)

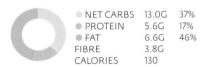

NET CARBS	13.0G	37%
PROTEIN	5.6G	17%
FAT	6.6G	46%
FIBRE	3.8G	
CALORIES	130	

Crunchy chickpeas

1 × 400g can (14.1 oz) of chickpeas, drained and rinsed (230g drained)
1 tbsp olive oil (13g)
Good pinch of dried rosemary or thyme (1g)
Good pinch of coriander seeds (1g)
Good pinch of smoked sweet paprika (1g)
Good pinch of ground turmeric (1g)
Salt and pepper (3g)

Serves 2–3 depending on what you do with them

Greek-ish salad

1 green pepper (160g)

2 tsp cumin seeds (4g)

2 tsp dried oregano (4g)

Juice of 2 lemons (80g)

120ml (½c) olive oil (120g)

Salt and pepper (3g)

Approx. 150g (5.3 oz) mixed leaves
(150g)

120g (4.2 oz) good black olives
(approx. 12–15 stoned olives) (120g)

100g (3.5 oz) feta, crumbled (100g)

1 cucumber, sliced (600g)

1 red onion, cut in half and very finely
sliced (150g)

1 punnet (11.6 oz) cherry tomatoes,
sliced in half (330g)

Bunch of mint, roughly chopped
(16g)

Serves 4

I love Greek salad, but I really love the way this one is a bit more robust with the cumin in it. Red wine vinegar also works instead of the lemon juice.

If you have a gas hob, stick the green pepper over a flame and char the skin. Alternatively, you can rub the skin with a little oil and grill it under a hot grill. Either way, remove the skin or be lazy and leave it on. Slice the pepper finely.

Toast the cumin seeds in a frying pan for a minute or two until you start to get a good roasted smell from them. Allow them to cool slightly, then whisk together the cumin, oregano, lemon juice and olive oil. Season well.

Toss the salad leaves with a little dressing, then layer up the other salad ingredients. Drizzle some more dressing on top and serve straight away.

PER PORTION (¼ OF THE SALAD)

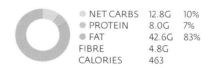

	NET CARBS	12.8G	10%
	PROTEIN	8.0G	7%
	FAT	42.6G	83%
	FIBRE	4.8G	
	CALORIES	463	

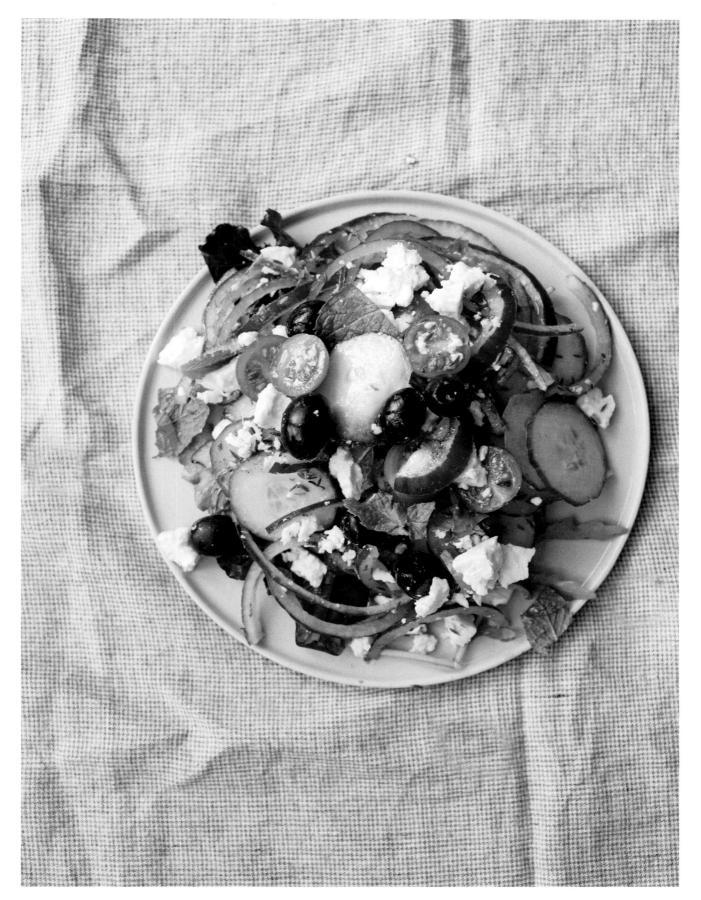

Braised baby gems

4 heads of baby gem (360g)
Large knob of butter (50g)
1 tbsp olive oil (13g)
100ml (⅜c) water (100g)
2 garlic cloves, crushed (6g)
Few sprigs of thyme (4g)
Salt and pepper (3g)

Serves 4

I know what you're thinking: 'Cooked lettuce? Are you mad?' But give it a go. Sometimes the leaves of the little baby gems are so tight that they seem reluctant to be made into a Caesar salad, so I teach them a lesson and cook the hell out of 'em for kicks (as well as for a tasty side dish that even the childer like). This dish only takes a few minutes to cook.

Slice the baby gems in half lengthways. If some outer leaves fall off, so be it: don't bother cooking them. Heat the butter and olive oil until foaming and fry the baby gems, flat side down, for about a minute, until just starting to colour in parts. Add about 100ml (⅜c) water, the garlic and thyme and season very well. Cook on a high heat for about another minute, then baste the lettuces or gently turn them over and serve with a small bit of the garlicky, buttery cooking liquid.

PER PORTION

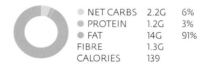

NET CARBS	2.2G	6%
PROTEIN	1.2G	3%
FAT	14G	91%
FIBRE	1.3G	
CALORIES	139	

Fennel salad

Have everything ready to be sliced and mixed together, as the fennel and radish can start to look a little grim if they don't get mixed with some acid (which comes from the lemon juice). Once it's mixed it will look fine for a few hours, but like all salads, it's better made closer to the time of consumption rather than sitting around gradually getting soggy and discoloured.

If you have a gas hob, stick the peppers over a flame and char the skin. Alternatively, you can rub the skin with a little oil and grill them under a hot grill. Either way, remove the skin or be lazy and leave it on, then finely slice the peppers.

Chuck everything into a bowl, mix well and season. If you find the salad too sharp and lemony, remove some of the juices, add 1 teaspoon of honey, mix well and pour back onto the salad.

2 yellow peppers (320g)
4 fennel bulbs, thinly sliced (348g)
½ head of celery, chopped (200g)
100g (3.5 oz) radishes, thinly sliced (100g)
Juice of 1 orange (55g)
Juice of 1 lemon (40g)
4 tbsp olive oil (52g)
Small bunch of chives or scallions, roughly chopped (20g)
Salt and pepper (3g)

Serves 4–6

PER PORTION (¹/₆ OF THE SALAD)

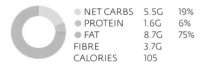

NET CARBS	5.5G	19%
PROTEIN	1.6G	6%
FAT	8.7G	75%
FIBRE	3.7G	
CALORIES	105	

Pomegranate, mint and fennel salad

50ml (¼c) olive oil (50g)

Juice 1 lemon (40g)

Juice and seeds of 1 pomegranate (190g whole)

2 fennel bulbs, finely sliced across the width of the bulb (174g)

1 head of celery, chopped (400g)

Handful of sprouted beans (any kind will do) (75g sprouted chickpeas)

1 bunch of mint leaves, chopped (16g)

Handful of tarragon leaves, chopped (20g)

Salt and pepper (3g)

Serves 4

This is a ridiculously crisp, crunchy salad of fennel, celery and pomegranate that just screams summer-is-round-the-corner freshness. This is one of those salads where you can practically feel the goodness going into your body. For starters it's rich in vitamin C, but there is also manganese and potassium in the fennel, and the sprouted beans that are the final flourish are alive with powerful enzymes as well as even more vitamin C. Not bad for one little salad, eh?

In a large bowl, gently whisk together the oil, lemon juice and pomegranate juice before adding in the pomegranate seeds, fennel and celery and tossing well. Sprinkle with the sprouted beans and chopped herbs, season well and mix gently before serving.

PER PORTION

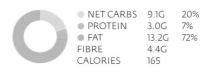

NET CARBS	9.1G	20%
PROTEIN	3.0G	7%
FAT	13.2G	72%
FIBRE	4.4G	
CALORIES	165	

Cabbage and pomegranate salad

1 red cabbage, sliced or grated (1kg)

½ tsp salt (3g)

Juice of ½ lemon (20g)

3 tbsp olive oil (39g)

2 pomegranates, seeds removed (380g whole)

1 red onion, finely diced (150g)

Big bunch of chopped mint (20g)

Black pepper (1g)

Serves 6

I'm trying to make this cabbage salad at least once a week, as cabbage will apparently protect you from every possible health goblin. But cabbage juice, which apparently is even better for you, is just a step too far.

Slice or grate the cabbage in a food processor. Season well with salt and leave to wilt for at least 10 minutes. When that's done, dress the salad with lemon juice and olive oil to your taste (some like it sharper than others) before tossing with the pomegranate seeds, diced onion, fresh mint and some freshly ground black pepper. Serve with the spiced lamb patties on page 94.

PER PORTION

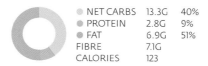

NET CARBS	13.3G	40%
PROTEIN	2.8G	9%
FAT	6.9G	51%
FIBRE	7.1G	
CALORIES	123	

Dead easy, dead handy.

Blanch the beans, scoop out the pomegranate seeds, make the dressing and toss the whole lot together.

PER PORTION (¹/₆ OF THE SALAD AND DRESSING)

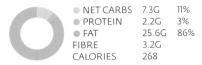

NET CARBS	7.3G	11%
PROTEIN	2.2G	3%
FAT	25.6G	86%
FIBRE	3.2G	
CALORIES	268	

Pomegranate and green bean salad

450g (1lb) green beans (450g)
1 pomegranate (190g when whole)
1 red onion, thinly sliced (150g)
Small bunch of flat-leaf parsley, roughly chopped (10g)
Small bunch of mint, roughly chopped (10g)

Dressing:
150ml (⅝c) olive oil (150g)
50ml (¼c) white wine vinegar (50g)
1 garlic clove, chopped (3g)
1 tsp Dijon mustard (8g)
Salt and pepper (3g)

Serves 4–6

Winter slaw

4 carrots, peeled and grated (400g)
2 Belgian endive, thinly sliced (170g)
1 red cabbage, thinly sliced (1kg)
1 red onion, thinly sliced (150g)
200g (7 oz) baby spinach leaves (200g)
100g (3.5 oz) pumpkin seeds (100g)

Green dressing:
Massive handful of parsley (25g)
Massive handful of mint (25g)
Massive handful of cilantro (25g)
6 garlic cloves, peeled (18g)
Good knob of ginger, peeled (10g)
Juice of 2 lemons (80g)
100ml (⅜c) olive oil (100g)
1 tbsp red wine vinegar (11g)
1 tbsp capers (9g)
Salt and pepper (3g)

Makes plenty for 6–8

The best part of this is the dressing, which is fragrant and fresh and would also be very tasty served with roast lamb.

Whizz all the dressing ingredients together, season and use as required. It does lose some of its lovely green colour if you keep it too long in the fridge, so it's best to make it only a few hours before you need it.

Mix all the salad ingredients together, add the green dressing and season. Chill until ready to serve.

PER PORTION (⅛ OF THE SALAD PLUS DRESSING)

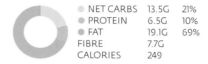

NET CARBS	13.5G	21%
PROTEIN	6.5G	10%
FAT	19.1G	69%
FIBRE	7.7G	
CALORIES	249	

Celery and cucumber salad

1 cucumber (600g)
1 head of celery (400g)
Salt and pepper (3g)
1 tbsp Dijon mustard (24g)
1 tsp English mustard (8g)
Juice of 1 lemon (40g)
80ml (5½tbsp) olive oil (80g)
Flat-leaf parsley (16g)

Feeds 6 as a side

This celery salad is quick and easy and good for outdoorsy parties as it stay pretty crunchy. It also lasts for ages, so it won't turn into silage if left out for a few hours.

Peel and chop the cucumber and toss into a bowl. Chop the celery as finely as possible, add to the cucumber and season well.

In a small bowl, mix the mustards with the lemon juice and slowly whisk in the olive oil. Season well and pour onto the salad. Add lots of chopped parsley and taste. Season as necessary, but this lasts well for a few hours.

PER PORTION

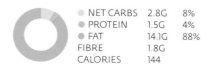

NET CARBS	2.8G	8%
PROTEIN	1.5G	4%
FAT	14.1G	88%
FIBRE	1.8G	
CALORIES	144	

One of my favourite salads. Delicious with some crumbled blue cheese in it too.

Preheat the oven to 190°C (375°F).

Cut the cauliflower into small florets and plonk them in a roasting pan. Pour a good glug or three of olive oil over them. Sprinkle with seasoning and the curry powder. Scoop them around so they get evenly coated in the spiced olive oil and are well seasoned. Roast for about 20 minutes, until tender and starting to brown (this may take longer). Taste them and make sure they are well seasoned.

Marinate the red onions and raisins in the red wine vinegar. Season well. Drain and rinse the chickpeas.

When you are ready to serve, mix the cauliflower with the red onions, raisins and chives, then add the chicory and the olives, if using. Taste and add some more olive oil and seasoning if necessary.

Roast cauliflower salad

1 head of cauliflower (1kg)
2 tbsp olive oil (26g)
Salt and pepper (3g)
2 tsp mild curry powder (4g)
2 red onions, sliced (300g)
50g (1.8 oz) golden raisins (50g)
1 tbsp red wine vinegar (11g)
1 × 400g can (14.1 oz) of chickpeas (230g drained)
1 bunch of chives, finely chopped (10g)
2 heads of chicory, sliced (200g)
50g (1.8 oz) black olives, stoned (optional) (50g)

Serves 6

PER PORTION

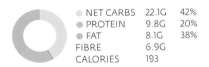

● NET CARBS	22.1G	42%
● PROTEIN	9.8G	20%
● FAT	8.1G	38%
FIBRE	6.9G	
CALORIES	193	

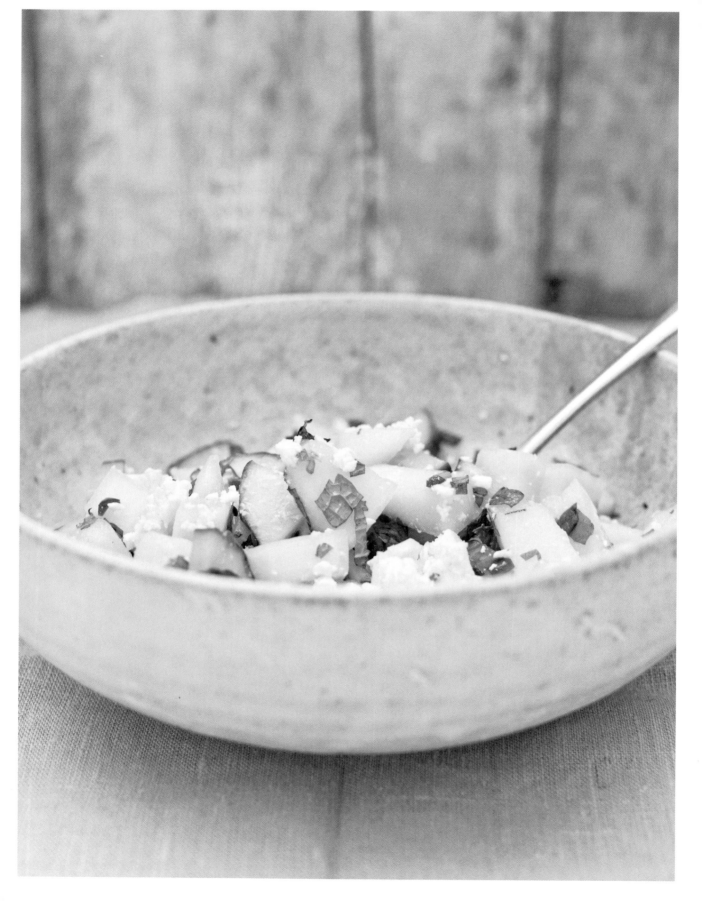

This melon and cucumber salad is a real hit, and although I use dried chilli flakes here, you could also use fresh ones and green ones would probably be even nicer. Chilli flakes are great, but if you get one stuck in the back of your throat, be warned – they sure are fiery.

Cut the melon into slices, remove the seeds, scoop out the flesh and chop it, then place in a large bowl. Wash the cucumber well and cut it in half lengthways, then cut it again so you have long quartered pieces that you can chop into decent-sized chunks before adding to the bowl with the melon. Chop the mint and add it in along with the lemon juice, olive oil and some salt and pepper. Add the chilli flakes and mix well, adjust the seasoning and then crumble in some feta.

PER PORTION

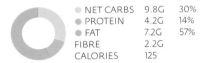

● NET CARBS	9.8G	30%
● PROTEIN	4.2G	14%
● FAT	7.2G	57%
FIBRE	2.2G	
CALORIES	125	

Melon, cucumber, chilli, mint and feta salad

1 honeydew melon (1.1kg whole)
1 large cucumber (600g)
25g (0.8 oz) mint (25g)
Juice of 1 lemon (40g)
2 tbsp olive oil (26g)
Salt and pepper (3g)
½ tsp chilli flakes (1g)
100g (3.5 oz) feta (100g)

Serves 6 – it's hard to eat too much of it

Quinoa, pea and scallion salad

200g (7 oz) quinoa (200g)
200g (7 oz) peas (200g)
1 bunch of scallions (60g)
2 tbsp olive oil (26g)
Salt and pepper (3g)
1 red onion, sliced (150g)
Juice of 2 lemons (80g)
1 avocado (180g)

Serves 6

I've noticed recently that scallions are having a bit of a pulled pork moment – they are on every fancy menu I have seen recently and are this year's foam or pea shoot as far as garnishes are concerned. I added them in not just because they are inevitably swimming around my subconscious as a de rigueur ingredient, but also because they are absolutely divine with a lick of olive oil and a generous amount of seasoning, swiftly grilled until wilted and delicious.

Cook the quinoa as per the instructions on the packet. Drain and allow to cool fully. You can also do this the day before so it really is well and truly cold.

Cook the peas in boiling water for 20–30 seconds, then drain and refresh in cold water. Make sure they, too, are really cold. Set aside.

Heat up your chargrill pan. Cut the scallions in half through the root to flatten them out, then rub with a little oil and char them on the pan. This will only take a minute or so. Season well and set them aside.

Marinate the red onion in the lemon juice and some salt. Cut the avocado into slices.

Mix the quinoa with the peas, then add some olive oil and the red onions and lemon juice. Season generously, then add the scallions and avocado. Taste, season and serve when you're ready. You can also add in some chopped herbs, but to be honest, it's delicious just as it is.

PER PORTION

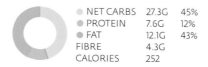

NET CARBS	27.3G	45%
PROTEIN	7.6G	12%
FAT	12.1G	43%
FIBRE	4.3G	
CALORIES	252	

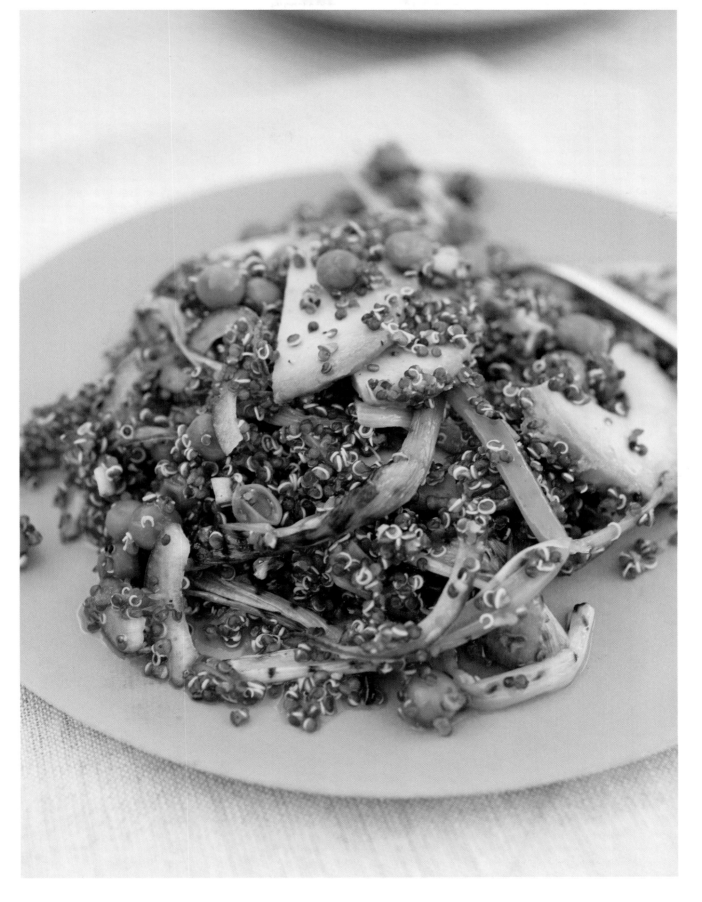

Super quick zucchini salad

4 zucchini (800g)
50ml (¼c) olive oil (50g)
Juice of 1–2 lemons (60g)
1 good tsp Dijon mustard (10g)
Squeeze of honey (3g)
Salt and pepper (3g)
Some chopped fresh dill (16g)

Serves 4

Feel free to change the herb: mint, basil, chives or scallions are also delicious with this. The main thing is that the lemons 'cold cook' the zucchini, making them soft and zingy, so there's no need to cook them.

Slice the zucchinis very thinly. Mix together the olive oil, lemon juice, mustard and honey. Season and taste. It should be lemony, but if you find it too sharp, add a splash more olive oil and honey. Pour some dressing over the zucchinis, toss and leave to marinate for 10 minutes. Toss again, add the dill, season if necessary and serve straight away.

PER PORTION (¼ OF THE SALAD)

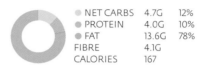

NET CARBS	4.7G	12%
PROTEIN	4.0G	10%
FAT	13.6G	78%
FIBRE	4.1G	
CALORIES	167	

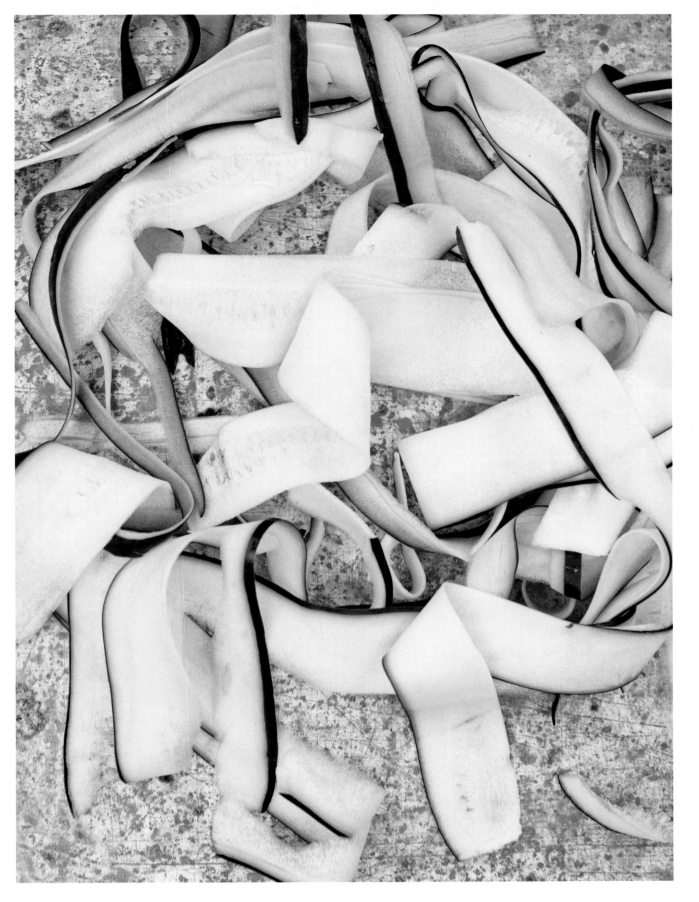

Broccoli salad with avocado and chilli dressing

1 head of broccoli, cut into florets (500g)

200g (7 oz) peas, boiled and blanched (200g)

100g (3.5 oz) flaked almonds (100g)

1 × 400g can (14.1 oz) of chickpeas, drained and rinsed (230g drained)

100g (3.5 oz) feta or firm goats' cheese, crumbled (100g)

Small bunch of scallions, finely chopped (40g)

1 bag of mixed baby leaves, such as spinach and mesclun (80g)

4 tbsp mixed seeds (linseeds, pumpkin, sunflower, etc.) (60g)

2 tbsp sprouted beans, to garnish (2 tbsp)

Avocado and chilli dressing:

1 very ripe avocado (180g)

1 green chilli, deseeded (20g)

Bunch of mint (16g)

75ml (⅓c) Greek yoghurt (75g)

Juice of 1 lime (20g)

1 tbsp olive oil (13g)

Salt and pepper (3g)

Serves 4 as a side

The broccoli recipe here is the perfect winter salad: filling, tasty and nutritious, and with its creamy avocado dressing, just that little bit luxurious. The mint adds zing and the chickpeas and toasted almonds add crunch and flavour. This is lovely on its own, but I've also had it with leftover shoulder of lamb and they complemented each other very nicely, thank you.

Blanch the broccoli for 1 minute in boiling water, then refresh (to stop it cooking) by running it under cold water until it's cooled down. Do the same with the peas, boiling them for just 30 seconds before refreshing. Drain them both really well so you're not making a salad out of waterlogged vegetables.

Toast the almonds in the oven or in a frying pan over a medium heat, then toss all the ingredients together to assemble the salad.

To make the dressing, place the ingredients in a blender and whizz until smooth. Season well.

To serve, spoon some salad onto plates and add a dollop of the creamy dressing, and for added goodness, a few sprouted beans.

PER PORTION (¼ OF THE RECIPE)

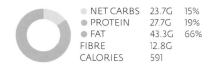

NET CARBS	23.7G	15%
PROTEIN	27.7G	19%
FAT	43.3G	66%
FIBRE	12.8G	
CALORIES	591	

A lovely, simple dish.

Melt the butter over a gentle heat. Roughly chop the hazelnuts, then add them to the butter and turn up the heat. When they are just starting to brown, add the lemon zest and juice and season well. Beware of splashes of hot fat. Keep the sauce warm.

Trim any stalky bits off the broccoli. Blanch in boiling water for a minute, drain and serve immediately with the hazelnut butter spooned over.

PER PORTION

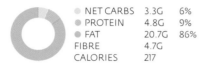

● NET CARBS	3.3G	6%
● PROTEIN	4.8G	9%
● FAT	20.7G	86%
FIBRE	4.7G	
CALORIES	217	

Purple sprouting broccoli with lemon and hazelnuts

80g (5tbsp) butter (80g)
2 tbsp hazelnuts (20g)
Juice and zest of 1 lemon (40g + 2g)
Salt and pepper (3g)
Approx. 400g (14.1 oz) purple
    sprouting broccoli (400g)

Serves 4 as a side dish

'The best diet is the one that works.'
Dr Richard Feinman

Broccoli and sugar snap peas with tahini dressing

200g (7 oz) broccoli (200g)

Approx. 1 × 180g (6 oz) pack of green beans (180g)

Approx. 100g (3.5 oz) sugar snap peas (100g)

3 tbsp sesame seeds (33g)

Knob of butter (14g)

Tahini dressing:

2 garlic cloves, crushed (6g)

Juice of 1 lime (20g)

2 tbsp tahini (36g)

2 tbsp tamari (36g)

2 tbsp rice vinegar or sherry vinegar (23g)

2 tbsp hot water (36g)

1 tsp honey (7g)

Salt and pepper (3g)

Serves at least 4 as a side dish

This is one of those dishes that stretches out a few leftover bits of green veg you may have lurking in your fridge. The vegetable weights below are approximate.

The trick to making the broccoli manageable and a bit more interesting is to trim it into tiny florets. Trim the green beans too. Cook the broccoli in boiling salted water for about 2 minutes. When it's 30 seconds away from being cooked, dunk in the green beans and follow with the sugar snap peas, which only need about 20 seconds. Drain and rinse really well until they are cold. Set them aside until you're ready to serve, or even refrigerate overnight.

Preheat the oven to 180°C (350°F).

Toast the sesame seeds in the hot oven for about 10 minutes, but do shake them around a bit. Keep an eye on them, as they may toast up in 5 minutes.

Mix all the ingredients for the dressing together and season to taste.

When you're ready to serve, heat the knob of butter in a large saucepan along with a splash of boiling water. Heat up the blanched vegetables, throwing them around so they get coated in some butter. When hot, plonk them on a platter and serve with the tahini dressing and toasted sesame seeds drizzled over them.

PER PORTION

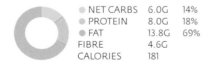

NET CARBS	6.0G	14%
PROTEIN	8.0G	18%
FAT	13.8G	69%
FIBRE	4.6G	
CALORIES	181	

The fact that kids will happily munch through a pile of florets if they are able to dip vegetables into something yummy makes this worth making.

Chuck all the ingredients for the dipping sauce into a food processor and whizz until smooth. Taste and adjust the seasoning if necessary. This will last in your fridge for a few days.

Trim the broccoli and chop up into florets. Blanch in boiling water for a couple of minutes until just tender. Drain and serve while still warm with the sesame seeds sprinkled on top and the dipping sauce on the side.

PER PORTION (¼ OF THE RECIPE)

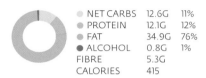

NET CARBS	12.6G	11%
PROTEIN	12.1G	12%
FAT	34.9G	76%
ALCOHOL	0.8G	1%
FIBRE	5.3G	
CALORIES	415	

Broccoli with sesame seeds and dipping sauce

2 small heads of broccoli (350g)
1 tbsp toasted sesame seeds, to garnish (11g)

Dipping sauce:
2 garlic cloves, crushed (6g)
Knob of ginger, peeled and grated (5g)
Juice of 1 lime (20g)
4 tbsp olive oil (52g)
3 tbsp tamari (54g)
2 tbsp tahini (36g)
2 tbsp crunchy peanut or almond butter (96g peanut butter)
2 tbsp mirin (32g)
1 tbsp honey (21g)

Serves 4–6 as a good side dish

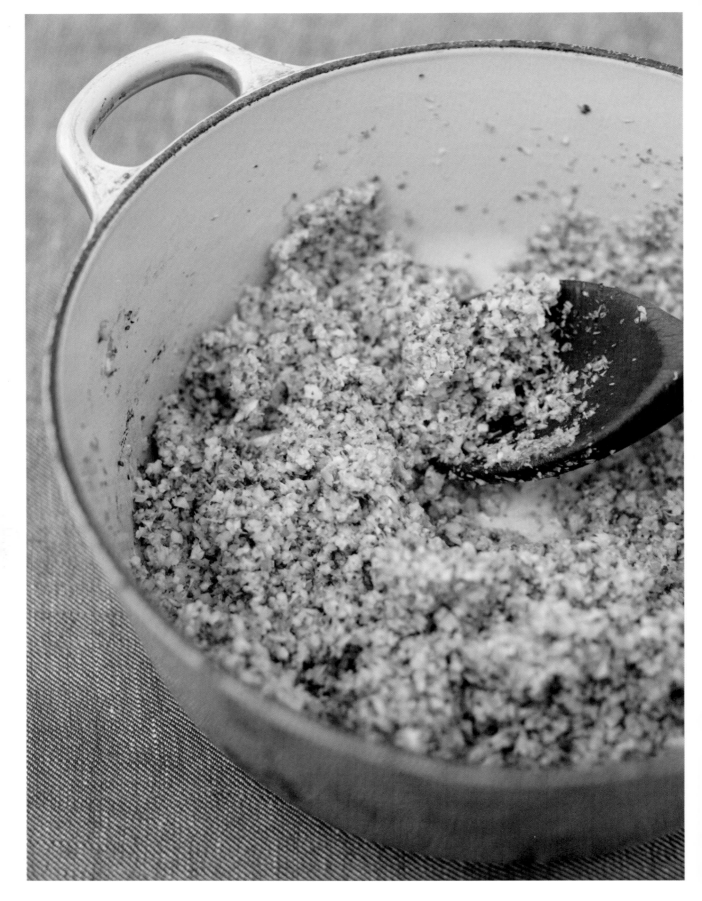

Working well with curries, stir-fries and anything saucy, this 'rice' is a versatile option and can also be made with cauliflower. In the last few years, an exciting movement has emerged that is doing all kinds of new and tempting things with vegetables, and this dish is just one example of it.

Blitz the broccoli florets in a food processor until they resemble fine crumbs.

Melt the butter or coconut oil in a saucepan before adding the water and the broccoli crumbs. Cook gently for 3 minutes over a medium to high heat, stirring regularly to help the water evaporate. Season well before serving and if you like, add another knob of butter.

Broccoli 'rice'

1 head of broccoli, broken into florets (500g)
Knob of butter or coconut oil (10g butter)
100ml (⅜c) water (100g)
Salt and pepper (3g)

Serves 4

PER PORTION (¼ OF THE RECIPE)

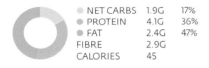

NET CARBS	1.9G	17%
PROTEIN	4.1G	36%
FAT	2.4G	47%
FIBRE	2.9G	
CALORIES	45	

Roast Brussels sprouts

500g (1.1lbs) Brussels sprouts (500g)
50ml (¼c) olive oil (50g)
Salt and pepper (3g)
Bunch of thyme (16g)
1 tsp honey (7g)

Serves 4

I tried these with frozen Brussels sprouts and they were okay, if a bit soggy. Frozen Brussels sprouts aren't great, although they will suffice if you're desperate.

Preheat the oven to 190°C (375°F).

Toss the Brussels sprouts in the olive oil and season really well. Put them in a roasting pan and blast them for 25 minutes. Add the thyme and honey, shuffle them about and give them a final blast.

PER PORTION

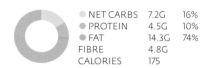

NET CARBS	7.2G	16%
PROTEIN	4.5G	10%
FAT	14.3G	74%
FIBRE	4.8G	
CALORIES	175	

Brussels sprout and miso salad

Juice of 2 limes (40g)
1 garlic clove, crushed (3g)
2 tbsp miso paste (any kind will do) (60g)
2 tbsp olive oil (26g)
1 tbsp sesame oil (12g)
1 tbsp mirin (16g)
500g (1.1lbs) Brussels sprouts, washed and shredded in a food processor (500g)

Serves 6

Making unpopular but nutritious foods more appealing can be an uphill struggle, and it can take longer with some veggies (and some people) than others. You just have to persevere. Take Brussels sprouts, for example. To echo a certain popular saying about pets, Brussels sprouts, despite what some (like many teenagers) might think, are not just for Christmas.

A member of the brassica family, which also includes cabbages and kale, Brussels sprouts are what nutritionists call 'nutrient dense'. Some even call them super. But let's not start that fight again.

In a large bowl, thoroughly mix all the ingredients together except the shredded sprouts, then add the sprouts and toss well before marinating for at least 30 minutes before serving. This keeps well for at least a day in the fridge.

PER PORTION

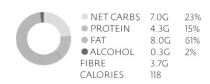

NET CARBS	7.0G	23%
PROTEIN	4.3G	15%
FAT	8.0G	61%
ALCOHOL	0.3G	2%
FIBRE	3.7G	
CALORIES	118	

Preheat the oven to 180°C (350°F).

Place the eggplants on a baking tray and toss in the olive oil. Cook in the oven for 30 minutes or so, until golden brown. Make sure they are cooked, as raw eggplant is not pleasant.

While they are cooking, you can assemble the rest of the salad by mixing all the other ingredients together in a large bowl. Season well before adding in the cooked roasted eggplant.

PER PORTION

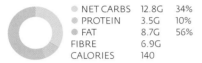

NET CARBS	12.8G	34%
PROTEIN	3.5G	10%
FAT	8.7G	56%
FIBRE	6.9G	
CALORIES	140	

Eggplant salad

2 eggplants, diced (600g)
2 tbsp olive oil (26g)
1 punnet (11.6 oz) cherry tomatoes, quartered (330g)
1 green pepper, diced (160g)
1 red pepper, diced (160g)
1 red onion, very finely chopped (150g)
2 garlic cloves, crushed (6g)
50g (1.8 oz) mixed black and green olives, stoned and chopped (50g with stones)
Big bunch of parsley, chopped (20g)
Salt and pepper (3g)

Serves 4

These eggplants make a fabulous veggie supper for four.

Chop up the eggplants into very small dice. Don't bother salting them. Heat up the olive oil in a big saucepan and fry the onion and eggplants over a high heat. If you have to add a splash of extra olive oil, do. If your saucepan isn't big enough, then fry them in two batches. Add the rest of the ingredients except the cilantro, which you can save as a garnish, and keep on a high heat until the mixture becomes quite dry. Serve with some chopped cilantro on top.

PER PORTION

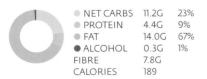

NET CARBS	11.2G	23%
PROTEIN	4.4G	9%
FAT	14.0G	67%
ALCOHOL	0.3G	1%
FIBRE	7.8G	
CALORIES	189	

Spiced eggplants

4 eggplants (1.2kg)
4 tbsp olive oil (52g)
1 onion, chopped (150g)
4 garlic cloves, sliced (12g)
1 chilli, deseeded and finely diced (20g)
Good knob of ginger, peeled and finely sliced (10g)
50ml (¼c) rice wine vinegar (50g)
50ml (¼c) rice wine (50g)
2 tbsp tamari (36g)
Freshly ground black pepper (1g)
Handful of cilantro, chopped (20g)

Serves 4

Roast eggplant, tomato and parsley 'smash'

3 large eggplants (1kg)

4 large, ripe tomatoes, quartered (800g)

1 onion, finely chopped (150g)

2 red chillies, deseeded and finely chopped (40g)

100g (3.5 oz) parsley, very finely chopped (100g)

3–6 (depending on your tastes!) garlic cloves, finely chopped (12g)

100ml (⅜c) olive oil (100g)

Juice and zest of 2 lemons (80g + 4g)

Serves 6–8

This is a great alternative to rice for dishes that are Middle Eastern in flavour.

Preheat the oven to 200°C (400°F).

Prick the eggplants with a fork, place on a baking tray and cook in the oven for 40 minutes, until the skin is blistered and the flesh inside is softened. Leave them aside to cool.

Meanwhile, pulse the tomatoes in a food processor until they're soft but not soupy. In a large bowl, mix the tomatoes with the chopped onion, chillies, parsley, garlic, oil and lemon juice.

When the eggplants have cooled, cut them in half lengthways and scoop out all the soft, smoky flesh within. Chop it roughly and add to the tomato mixture, mixing well to blend all the flavours. Let it stand for about an hour before serving at room temperature.

PER PORTION (⅛ OF THE RECIPE)

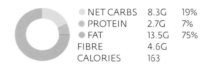

NET CARBS	8.3G	19%
PROTEIN	2.7G	7%
FAT	13.5G	75%
FIBRE	4.6G	
CALORIES	163	

This recipe makes far too much miso butter, but it's a revelation. Tasty, savoury, fabulous. So use what you need for this recipe and keep the rest for another day. It keeps really well in your freezer.

First make the butter by mixing it in a food processor with the miso. Wrap it in cling film and roll it up into a sausage shape. That way you can freeze it and cut slices from it to use at your leisure.

You can cook the asparagus in one of two ways. Rub the trimmed spears in a little olive oil and season with salt. Heat up your chargrill pan until it's really hot and cook them until they're nicely charred on all sides, then add a good chunk of miso butter and let it sizzle. Plop it onto a large platter and let everyone dig in. Alternatively, you can preheat the oven to 220°C (430°F), put the asparagus in a small roasting tray with a good slice of the miso butter and roast them in the oven for 6–8 minutes, until they are nicely starting to char.

Asparagus with miso butter

200g (⅞c) butter, softened (200g)
100g (3.5 oz) miso paste (100g)
2 bunches of asparagus, bases
   trimmed (470g)
1 tsp olive oil (4g)
Salt (2g)

Serves 4

PORTION OF ASPARAGUS WITH ⅓ OF THE MISO BUTTER (75G USED FOR 4 PEOPLE)

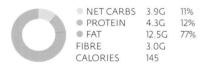

NET CARBS	3.9G	11%
PROTEIN	4.3G	12%
FAT	12.5G	77%
FIBRE	3.0G	
CALORIES	145	

Tomato salad

4 large, ripe beef tomatoes (1,120g)

Salt and pepper (3g)

1 red onion, finely diced (150g)

Small bunch of mint, finely chopped (12g)

1 garlic clove, crushed (3g)

100ml (⅜c) olive oil (100g)

Juice of 1 lemon or a splash of sherry vinegar (40g juice)

Serves 4

This is a great salad to serve with just about anything, but my preference is to accompany beef or grilled fish.

Slice the tomatoes into rounds, lay the slices out on a platter and sprinkle with salt. This will cause the tomatoes to release their own juices, which you then drain off and whisk together with the other ingredients. Season to taste, remembering that there will be residual salt on the tomatoes, and pour the dressing over the tomatoes before serving.

PER PORTION

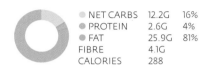

NET CARBS	12.2G	16%
PROTEIN	2.6G	4%
FAT	25.9G	81%
FIBRE	4.1G	
CALORIES	288	

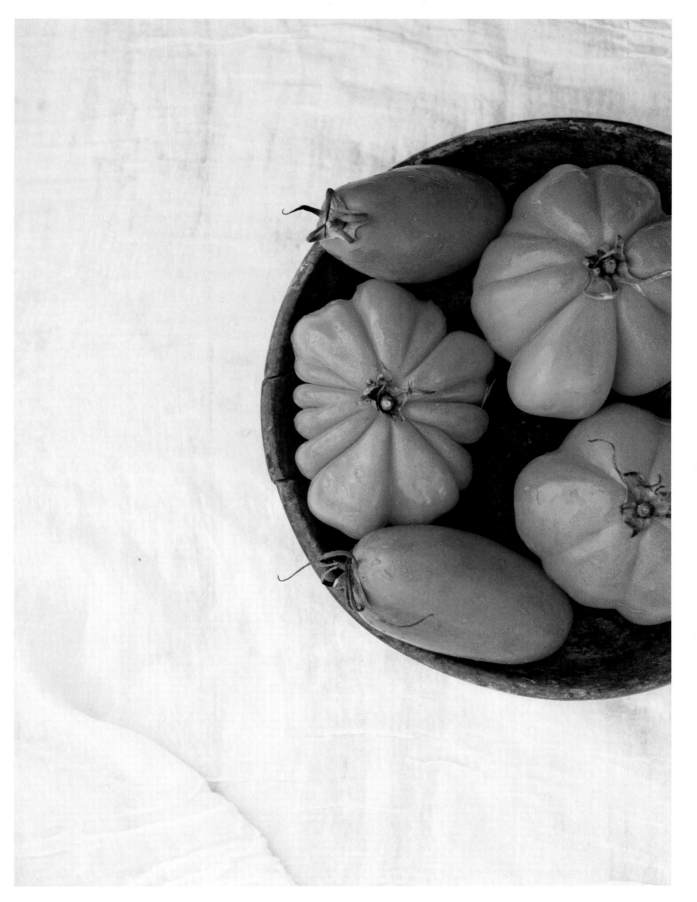

Artichoke dauphinoise

2 × 400g cans (28.2 oz) of whole
  artichoke hearts, drained (480g
  drained)
1 onion, finely diced (150g)
100g (1¾c) mayonnaise (100g)
70g (2.5 oz) grated Gruyère or
  Parmesan cheese (70g Gruyère)
1 tbsp wholegrain mustard (30g)
1 tbsp Worcestershire sauce (18g)
Salt and pepper (3g)

Feeds 4

I have always been eternally grateful for this crowd pleaser. People love this kind of party food, especially the golden brown melted cheese on top. Although it's basically vegetarian, don't forget that Worcestershire sauce contains anchovies. This is my alternative to pommes dauphinoise.

Preheat the oven to 180°C (350°F).

Drain the artichokes well or the dip will be very soggy. Chop the artichokes very finely and mix with the onion, mayonnaise, half of the grated cheese and the mustard, Worcestershire and salt and pepper in a large bowl. Taste and adjust the seasoning if necessary; you may want to add more mayonnaise.

Spoon into a gratin dish, smooth the top of the dip and scatter over the remaining grated cheese. Cook for about 30 minutes, until the topping is golden brown and the dip is piping hot.

PER PORTION

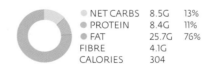

NET CARBS	8.5G	13%
PROTEIN	8.4G	11%
FAT	25.7G	76%
FIBRE	4.1G	
CALORIES	304	

This wild rice salad was one of those fantastic experiments that somehow came right the first time. With all that tahini, tamari and lemon, the dressing is certainly robust, but it's a good foil for any rich dish.

Cook the rice in boiling water for 35–40 minutes, until tender.

Meanwhile, whisk together the garlic, tahini, tamari and lemon juice in a bowl to make the dressing, which you can thin with a little hot water.

When the rice is cooked, drain it and leave to cool before tossing thoroughly in the dressing. Mix in the pistachios and chopped parsley and serve.

200g (7 oz) black rice (200g dry
   weight)
2 garlic cloves, crushed (6g)
2 tbsp tahini (36g)
2 tbsp tamari (36g)
Juice of 1 lemon (40g)
60g (2.1 oz) toasted shelled
   pistachios (60g)
Big bunch of parsley, chopped (20g)

Serves 4

PER PORTION

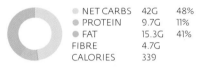

NET CARBS	42G	48%
PROTEIN	9.7G	11%
FAT	15.3G	41%
FIBRE	4.7G	
CALORIES	339	

'The emerging research that's just starting to come out . . . will demonstrate that ketone bodies are in essence a preferred fuel that the brain will use . . . in place of glucose.'
Dr Dominic D'Agostino

Baked sweet potatoes with smoked sweet paprika

3 sweet potatoes (714g)
50ml (¼c) olive oil (50g)
1 tbsp dried herbs (optional) (2g)
1 tsp smoked sweet paprika (2g)
Salt and pepper (3g)

Serves 4–6 as a nice accompaniment for dinner

Preheat the oven to 200°C (400°F).

Wash the spuds, leave the skin on and chop in half, then cut into quarters or eighths, depending on their size – you want chunky wedges. Drizzle with the olive oil, dried herbs, paprika and seasoning and bake for about 30 minutes, until tender and starting to brown. You may have to shake them about occasionally to stop them browning unevenly.

PER PORTION (¹/₆ OF THE RECIPE)

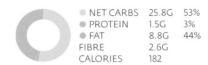

NET CARBS	25.8G	53%
PROTEIN	1.5G	3%
FAT	8.8G	44%
FIBRE	2.6G	
CALORIES	182	

Snazzy 'rice'

1 head of cauliflower (1kg)
Salt and pepper (3g)
1 bunch of scallions, finely chopped (60g)
Small bunch of cilantro, roughly torn or chopped (12g)

Serves 4

Blitz the cauliflower into 'crumbs' in a food processor. Bring 100ml (⅜c) water to the boil and add the cauliflower. Cook for a few minutes to let the water evaporate and the cauliflower steam-cook. Season well and add the scallions and cilantro. Serve with anything that you would normally serve with rice.

PER PORTION (¼ RECIPE)

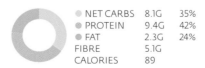

NET CARBS	8.1G	35%
PROTEIN	9.4G	42%
FAT	2.3G	24%
FIBRE	5.1G	
CALORIES	89	

Preheat the oven to 150°C (300°F).

Cook the walnuts in the oven for 5–10 minutes, until nicely toasted. Set aside.

Peel the apples and slice into little matchsticks and toss in the lemon juice to stop them discolouring. Peel the celeriac and also slice into very thin matchstick pieces and toss with the apple.

Mix the yoghurt with the parsley, olive oil, Dijon and horseradish. Remember that the lemon juice in the celeriac and apple mixture will sharpen up the flavours, but do season it and then mix with the apple and celeriac. Taste and adjust the seasoning. Keep this overnight if necessary, covered in the fridge. Sprinkle with the toasted walnuts just before serving.

Apple and celeriac salad

50g (1.8 oz) walnut halves (50g)
1 apple (100g)
Juice of 1 lemon (40g)
1 large celeriac (650g)
100ml (⅜c) Greek yoghurt (100g)
1 bunch of parsley, chopped (16g)
1 tbsp olive oil (13g)
1 tbsp Dijon mustard (24g)
Knob of fresh horseradish, finely grated (10g)
Salt and pepper (3g)

Serves 4 plus leftovers

PER PORTION (¼ OF THE RECIPE)

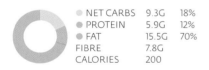

NET CARBS	9.3G	18%
PROTEIN	5.9G	12%
FAT	15.5G	70%
FIBRE	7.8G	
CALORIES	200	

Dressings and condiments

I'm always grateful when I open the fridge and find a jar of something on the shelf that I know will give everything it lands on a delicious kick up the rear, taste wise. Making a big batch of dressing takes barely any more time than making a small batch and they last really well in the fridge. Although there are some nice store-bought pestos available, I don't think anything can beat the delicious hit of herbs that you get from your own versions, especially things like salsa verde. Herbs are full of magnificent goodness, but eating a big handful of parsley is not high on my to do list. But blitzing it into something to be slathered on dinner . . . well, now you're talking.

Remember that egg yolks must be at room temperature or else they won't thicken. Add the oil very slowly at the start. Once it has started to thicken, you can speed up the oil flow. Make it with a whisk, as it's easier to keep an eye on it. If it curdles or splits, stop mixing. Start off with a fresh egg yolk and add the curdled mixture back to it very slowly.

Mix the egg yolks with the Dijon and add less than a teaspoon of olive oil. Keep whisking and add a few drops more. Add a few more – you should feel it start to change consistency. Literally add droplets until you can feel a definite change in texture. Once it has stared to thicken, you can start pouring the oil in a very light stream. Add about 200ml (⅞c) of the oil and then add the remaining ingredients except the cheese. It will get slightly watery again with the addition of liquid. Resume whisking in the remaining oil, again slowly at first, then pour in a steady stream. Decide on a consistency you like. Sometimes if it's too thick, I add a few tablespoons of water. Taste it. Add the Parmesan if you like. Leave the flavours to develop for an hour or so, then taste it again. Keep refrigerated for up to a week, provided your eggs were pretty fresh.

Caesar salad dressing

4 egg yolks, at room temperature (72g)
1 tbsp Dijon mustard (24g)
400ml (1⅝c) olive oil (400g)
Juice and zest of 2 lemons (80g juice + 4g zest)
6 garlic cloves, crushed (18g)
1 tbsp white wine vinegar (11g)
1 tbsp Worcestershire sauce (18g)
1 tsp fine sea salt (5g)
Tons of black pepper (3g)
100g (3.5 oz) finely grated Parmesan (optional) (100g)

Makes a big batch – should get enough to do 8 salads' worth

PER TABLESPOON (36G)

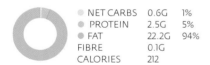

NET CARBS	0.6G	1%
PROTEIN	2.5G	5%
FAT	22.2G	94%
FIBRE	0.1G	
CALORIES	212	

Anchovy vinaigrette

2 egg yolks (36g)

2 garlic cloves, crushed (6g)

1 tbsp Dijon mustard (24g)

5 anchovy fillets, mashed with the back of a spoon (15g)

150ml (⅝c) olive oil (150g)

Juice of 2 lemons (80g)

Salt and pepper (3g)

Makes 6 servings of dressing

The lemon juice in this anchovy vinaigrette for torn bitter leaves like chicory or endive stops a robust dressing from being overwhelming. With a few shavings of Parmesan or Manchego cheese thrown in, it's a perfect salad, a homage to one of the (many) starters I had in a great New York restaurant called Charlie Bird. If you get to go there, get a glass of the Albariño, order plenty of sides and say hi from me.

I like to make this by hand rather than in a blender. In a medium bowl, whisk together the egg yolks, garlic and mustard before adding the mashed-up anchovies. Steadily but slowly pour in the olive oil, whisking all the time. Add about half the olive oil, then loosen it up with the lemon juice and go back to whisking in the olive oil again. Season well. Strong and robust.

PER 53G PORTION OF DRESSING ONLY:

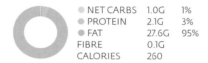

● NET CARBS	1.0G	1%
● PROTEIN	2.1G	3%
● FAT	27.6G	95%
FIBRE	0.1G	
CALORIES	260	

SALAD PORTION WITH 53G DRESSING, 15G PARMESAN, 100G CHICORY AND ENDIVE:

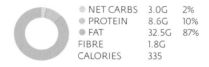

● NET CARBS	3.0G	2%
● PROTEIN	8.6G	10%
● FAT	32.5G	87%
FIBRE	1.8G	
CALORIES	335	

In the nutritional information below, each portion is one tablespoon, so bear this in mind if you use more per portion.

Put all the ingredients in a glass jar with a lid and shake, shake, shake. Use to dress a simple salad of green leaves. Stores perfectly well in your leftover jars and there's no need to wash up any utensils from making the dressing!

PER TABLESPOON (10G)

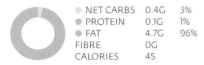

NET CARBS	0.4G	3%
PROTEIN	0.1G	1%
FAT	4.7G	96%
FIBRE	0G	
CALORIES	45	

Tarragon dressing

1 small red onion, very finely chopped (60g)
Handful of tarragon, very finely chopped (12g)
100ml (⅜c) olive oil (100g)
2 tbsp red wine vinegar (22.8g)
2 tsp Dijon mustard (16g)
Salt and pepper (3g)

Makes approx. 200g (7 oz)

This makes 24 × 25g (1½tbsp) servings. If you are using more than that, bear in mind you will need to double or treble the nutritional info below.

I find this easiest to do by blitzing everything in a food processor, but you could equally dice everything up finely and mix it all together. The dressing can be as thick or loose as you want it, but remember that by adding more water, you're asking for it to taste a little bland, so you may have to up the salt or tamari.

PER PORTION (¹/₂₄ OF THE RECIPE OR 25G)

NET CARBS	0.8G	6%
PROTEIN	1.0G	8%
FAT	5.0G	87%
FIBRE	0.6G	
CALORIES	52	

Tahini dressing

1 white onion, peeled (150g)
Few sticks of celery (120g)
2 garlic cloves (6g)
Handful of chopped parsley (16g)
Juice of 2 lemons (80g)
5 tbsp light tahini (90g)
5 tbsp cold-pressed olive oil (63g)
2 tbsp tamari (36g)
A few tbsp warm water to let the whole thing down (25g)
Salt and pepper (3g)

Makes approx. 600ml (2½c)

Simple dressing

1 heaped tbsp Dijon mustard (26g)
200ml (⅞c) olive oil (200g)
4 tbsp red wine vinegar (46g)
Salt and pepper (3g)
1 red onion, very finely diced (150g)

Makes approx. 20 × 1 tbsp portions

Whisk the mustard and add the olive oil in a steady, slow stream so that it thickens up. Add the vinegar, season and mix in the diced onions. Set aside till ready to use.

PER TABLESPOON (15G)

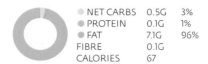

NET CARBS	0.5G	3%
PROTEIN	0.1G	1%
FAT	7.1G	96%
FIBRE	0.1G	
CALORIES	67	

Crushed tomato sauce

Approx. 500g (1.1lbs) ripe cherry or
   vine tomatoes (500g)
200g (7 oz) black olives, roughly
   chopped (200g)
3 garlic cloves, crushed (9g)
Big bunch of parsley, finely chopped
   (20g)
80ml (⅓c) olive oil (80g)
2 tbsp Dijon mustard (48g)
Few splashes of hot sauce (no sugar)
   (10g)
Salt and pepper (3g)

Serves 4

Preheat the oven to 200°C (400°F).

Slice the tomatoes in half and scatter them on a roasting pan, cut side up. Drizzle with a splash of olive oil. Roast the tomatoes for 15–20 minutes, until they are slightly charring. Transfer to a bowl. Add the rest of the ingredients and mix well, but try not to break up the tomatoes too much. Taste, season and serve with anything that goes well with tomatoes!

PER PORTION (¼ OF THE RECIPE)

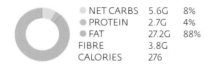

NET CARBS	5.6G	8%
PROTEIN	2.7G	4%
FAT	27.2G	88%
FIBRE	3.8G	
CALORIES	276	

The basic principle here is to chuck it all in and either use it up within a couple of days, or make a double quantity and freeze some in plastic containers. Works well with the zucchini 'spaghetti' on page 149. Add herbs, more or less garlic and anything else you can think of that you would like to sneak in. I sometimes add a few anchovies too.

Peel, wash and chop up the vegetables as roughly as you like. Heat the olive oil in a large saucepan and chuck everything in. Cook until soft, then purée in a food processor. Use the sauce straight away or else let it cool, then transfer into plastic containers and freeze. It's fine in the freezer for a month or two. Simply thaw out and heat in a small saucepan with a little water and check the seasoning. I usually add salt at this stage, plus a little pepper. I have left it out of the ingredients list as this can be a great sauce for young children, so I tend to go easy on the salt and add it later.

PER 100G PORTION (COOKED WEIGHT)

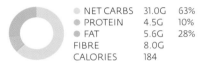

NET CARBS	31.0G	63%
PROTEIN	4.5G	10%
FAT	5.6G	28%
FIBRE	8.0G	
CALORIES	184	

Gotcha! RDA pasta sauce

8 ripe tomatoes (1,040g)
4 carrots (400g)
2 sweet potatoes (475g)
2 zucchinis (400g)
2 red onions (300g)
2 sticks of celery (120g)
Bunch of parsley (16g)
2 garlic cloves, crushed (6g)
2 tbsp olive oil (26g)

Makes enough to fill a 500g (17.6 oz) jar, plus a bit extra

Romesco sauce

2 red peppers (320g)

2 tomatoes (260g)

1 head of garlic (36g)

60ml (¼c) olive oil (60g)

Salt and pepper (3g)

50–80g (1.8–2.8 oz) flaked or ground
   almonds (65g)

3 tbsp sweet sherry vinegar (34g)

Good pinch of smoked sweet
   paprika (1g)

Serves 6 generously

Delicious with grilled fish, grilled vegetables or frittatas.

Preheat the oven to 220°C (430°F).

Cut the red peppers into big chunks and discard the seeds and stems. Slice the tomatoes in half and cut the garlic head in half horizontally. Place the peppers, tomatoes and garlic in a roasting pan, drizzle with half of the olive oil and season well with salt and pepper. Roast in the oven for 20 minuets, until the peppers are just starting to burn. Remove from the oven and cover with foil to let the steam continue to cook them for another 20 minutes.

In a blender, whizz the roasted tomatoes and peppers with the almonds. Squeeze out the garlic cloves and add them too. Add the vinegar, smoked paprika and the rest of the olive oil and whizz until it forms a thick purée. Taste and season. If it's too thick, add more vinegar or oil. This will last a few days in the fridge.

PER PORTION

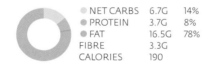

NET CARBS	6.7G	14%
PROTEIN	3.7G	8%
FAT	16.5G	78%
FIBRE	3.3G	
CALORIES	190	

Basil sauce

Lovely with lamb or grilled fish or chicken.

In a small bowl, mix the egg yolk with the garlic and mustard. It will form the base to which you slowly whisk in a few drops of olive oil. Continue adding the oil in a thin stream – you should feel it start to thicken. Add about half the olive oil, then season with the red wine· vinegar and anchovy essence. Start adding the rest of the oil, which will thicken it up a bit more.

Season really well and add the basil leaves and hot sauce. Taste and adjust the seasoning; you can tone it down by adding 25ml (1¾tbsp) sunflower oil or more olive oil. You can make this a few hours ahead of time and keep it in the fridge until ready to serve.

1 egg yolk, at room temperature (18g)
1 garlic clove, crushed (3g)
2 tsp Dijon mustard (16g)
75ml (⅓c) olive oil (75g)
1 tbsp red wine vinegar (11g)
Splash of anchovy essence or ½ tsp Worcestershire sauce (3g)
Salt and pepper (3g)
Few basil leaves, very finely sliced (3g)
½ tsp hot sauce (no sugar) (5g)

Serves 4

PER PORTION (¼ OF THE RECIPE)

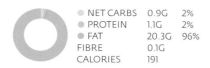

NET CARBS	0.9G	2%
PROTEIN	1.1G	2%
FAT	20.3G	96%
FIBRE	0.1G	
CALORIES	191	

Vi-coise dip

200g (7 oz) sunflower seeds, soaked in water for 30 minutes (200g before soaking)
125–150g (4.4–5.3 oz) green olives (140g)
100g (3.5 oz) sun-dried tomatoes (100g)
25g (0.9 oz) flat-leaf parsley, roughly chopped (25g)
2–4 garlic cloves, roughly chopped (12g)
Pepper (1g)
1 tbsp olive oil (13g)

Serves 4–6

This is delicious not only on its own as a dip, but also tossed through a big pile of the zucchini 'spaghetti' on page 149. Deliciously 'meaty', this recipe is a great addition to anything that needs a bit of a lift, such as grilled chicken or fish.

Put everything in a food processor and blend till smoothish. Let down with more olive oil or a tiny drop of water if required.

PER PORTION (¼ OF THE RECIPE)

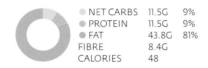

NET CARBS	11.5G	9%
PROTEIN	11.5G	9%
FAT	43.8G	81%
FIBRE	8.4G	
CALORIES	48	

Quick fish pâté

500g (1.1lbs) smoked fish, very finely diced (500g smoked salmon)
Approx. 250g (8.8 oz) crème fraîche (250g)
Small bunch of tarragon, finely chopped (12g)
Small bunch of dill, finely chopped (10g)
Juice and zest of 1 lemon (40g + 2g)
2 tbsp Dijon mustard (48g)
2 tbsp fresh horseradish, peeled and grated (50g)
Salt and pepper (3g)

Makes 10 portions

Mix all the ingredients together, adjust the seasoning and serve. This still tastes great after two days in the fridge, although you may need to give it a really good stir. The crème fraîche sauce on its own is a great condiment for roast beef or anything with beetroot.

PER PORTION (¹/₁₀ OF THE RECIPE OR 50G)

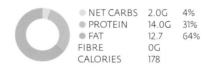

NET CARBS	2.0G	4%
PROTEIN	14.0G	31%
FAT	12.7	64%
FIBRE	0G	
CALORIES	178	

I am always making and experimenting with versions of salsa verde. This is another favourite.

Place all the ingredients in a food processor and blitz for about 1 minute, or until it's a smooth sauce. Store in jars with a thin layer of extra virgin olive oil on top to stop it oxidising. It should last a few days in the fridge, although I've often used this up to two weeks later and it's been fine.

PER 50G PORTION (⅛ OF THE RECIPE)

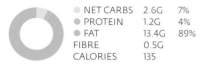

● NET CARBS	2.6G	7%
● PROTEIN	1.2G	4%
● FAT	13.4G	89%
FIBRE	0.5G	
CALORIES	135	

Handy green sauce

1 bunch of scallions (60g)
Big bunch of flat-leaf parsley (40g)
Big bunch of cilantro (40g)
2 green chillies (40g)
3 garlic cloves, peeled (12g)
100ml (⅜c) olive oil (100g)
2 tbsp Dijon mustard (48g)
2 tbsp capers (in vinegar, not salt) (17g)
1–2 tsp honey (11g)
1 tsp cumin seeds (2g)
1 tsp coriander seeds (2g)
Salt and pepper (3g)

Makes 8 portions

Grind the mustard seeds in a pestle and mortar. Place the mustard powder in a bowl and add in the ground mustard seeds. Whisk in the water, horseradish cream and vinegar. Season and taste. If it's too fiery, add some honey.

PER TEASPOON (8G)

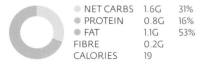

● NET CARBS	1.6G	31%
● PROTEIN	0.8G	16%
● FAT	1.1G	53%
FIBRE	0.2G	
CALORIES	19	

Homemade mustard

3 tbsp black or brown mustard seeds (19g)
3 tbsp dry mustard powder (54g)
40–50ml (2¾–3⅓tbsp) cold water, depending on the consistency you like (45g)
2 tbsp horseradish cream (48g)
1 tbsp white wine vinegar (11g)
Salt and pepper (3g)
1–2 tsp honey (optional) (11g)

Makes 1 small jar

Pesto

1 × 100g (3.5 oz) pack of basil (100g)

100g (3.5 oz) pistachio nuts, shelled
(100g)

50g (1.8 oz) pine nuts (50g)

50g (1.8 oz) grated Parmesan cheese
(50g)

6 garlic cloves, peeled (18g)

Salt and pepper (3g)

300ml (1¼c) olive oil (300g)

Makes approx. 600g

You can use any type of nut you like for making pesto. I like a combination of pine and pistachio nuts, but walnuts are also good, especially if you are serving it with chicken. This is a great one for kids to make.

Put all the ingredients except the olive oil into a food processor and blitz until the mixture is as smooth as you want it. I prefer to leave it on the chunky side, so I tend to process the pesto using the pulse button on my machine. Add as much olive oil as you like, depending on what you are using it for. If the pesto is for a pasta sauce, then you may want to use all the oil. Continue to process on the pulse mode.

PER TABLESPOON (26G)

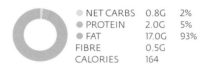

NET CARBS	0.8G	2%
PROTEIN	2.0G	5%
FAT	17.0G	93%
FIBRE	0.5G	
CALORIES	164	

Salsa verde

Large handful of flat-leaf parsley
(26g)

Smaller handful of mint leaves (16g)

100ml (⅜c) olive oil (100g)

4 tsp capers (12g)

2 good tsp Dijon mustard (18g)

Salt (2g)

Lots of black pepper (2g)

Makes 4 very generous portions

One of my favourite sauces to slather on anything.

Blitz everything in a food processor and serve. Season as necessary.

PER 44G SERVING (¼ OF THE RECIPE)

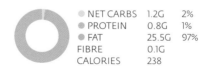

NET CARBS	1.2G	2%
PROTEIN	0.8G	1%
FAT	25.5G	97%
FIBRE	0.1G	
CALORIES	238	

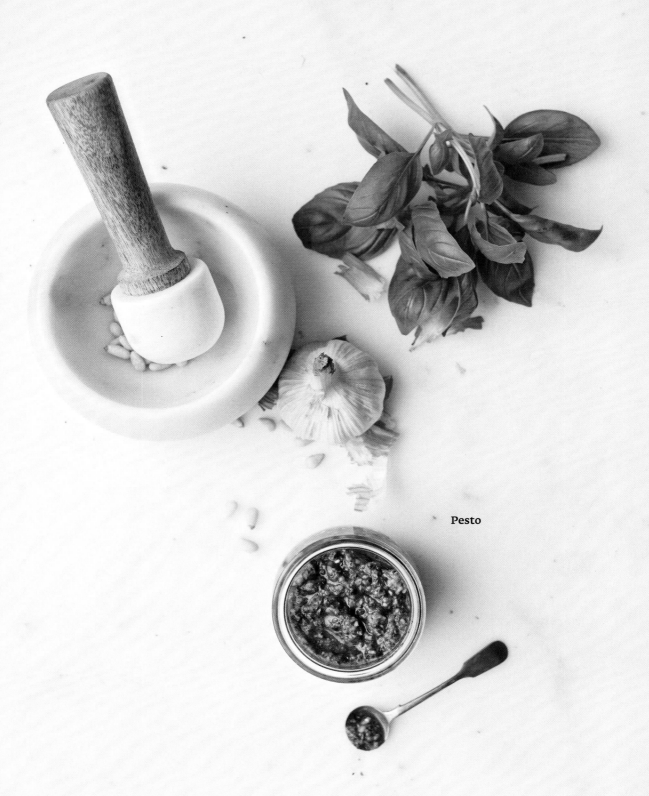

Pesto

Sun-dried tomato tapenade

100g (3.5 oz) sun-dried tomatoes, strained (100g)
2 garlic cloves, peeled (6g)
Juice of 1 lemon (40g)
100ml (⅜c) olive oil (100g)
1 good tbsp capers (10g)
1 good tbsp pitted green olives (10g)
1 good tsp Dijon mustard (10g)
1 tsp chopped rosemary (2g)

Makes enough for 6 generous portions

Uber tasty.

Pulse everything in a food processor until fairly smooth. Season and taste as necessary. This will keep for about a week in the fridge.

PER PORTION (¹/₆ OF THE RECIPE OR 46G)

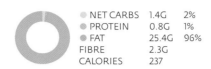

NET CARBS	1.4G	2%
PROTEIN	0.8G	1%
FAT	25.4G	96%
FIBRE	2.3G	
CALORIES	237	

Tapenade, of a sort

250g (8.8 oz) pitted black olives (250g)
100g (3.5 oz) sun-dried tomatoes (100g)
Large bunch of parsley (20g)
2 garlic cloves, crushed (6g)
Good few sprigs of rosemary (3g)
3 tbsp capers (26g)
2 tbsp olive oil (26g)
2 tsp Dijon mustard (16g)
Zest of ½ orange (2g)
Pepper (1g)

Makes 22 portions (to spread on a cracker, for instance)

Whizz or pulse everything in a food processor and adjust the seasoning, adding more pepper or garlic as required. This will keep for about a week in the fridge.

PER PORTION (¹/₂₂ OF THE RECIPE OR 20G)

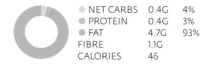

NET CARBS	0.4G	4%
PROTEIN	0.4G	3%
FAT	4.7G	93%
FIBRE	1.1G	
CALORIES	46	

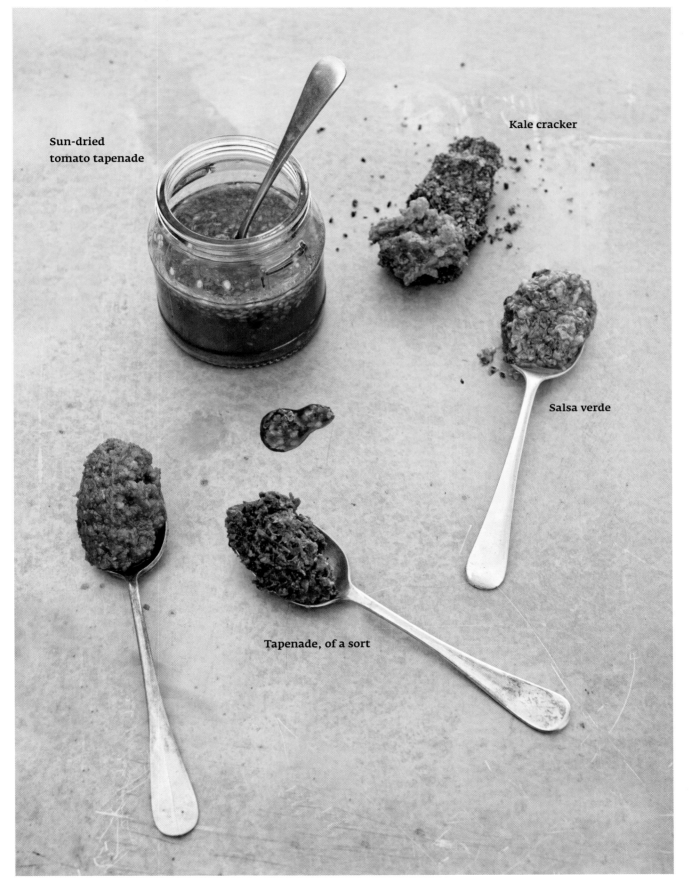

Sun-dried
tomato tapenade

Kale cracker

Salsa verde

Tapenade, of a sort

Tomato and scallion miso salsa

Gently mix the olive oil and miso together in a bowl until you get something dressing-like in consistency, then add the chopped tomatoes, red onion and scallions. Toss well to mix together and serve.

1 tbsp olive oil (13g)

1 tbsp miso (10g)

1 punnet (11.6 oz) cherry tomatoes, quartered (330g)

1 red onion, finely diced (150g)

1 bunch of scallions, chopped (60g)

Serves 4 as an accompaniment

PER PORTION

NET CARBS	6.4G	37%
PROTEIN	1.7G	10%
FAT	3.8G	53%
FIBRE	1.9G	
CALORIES	65	

Quick olive salsa

Mix all the ingredients together and chill until ready to serve. Give it a good mix and spoon onto each plate.

Small bunch of flat-leaf parsley, chopped (12g)

1 garlic clove, crushed (3g)

4 tbsp tapenade (100g)

2 tbsp chopped raisins (36g)

1–2 tsp sherry or balsamic vinegar (17g sherry vinegar)

Makes 8 portions

PER PORTION (⅛ OF THE RECIPE OR 21G)

NET CARBS	3.4G	33%
PROTEIN	0.4G	4%
FAT	2.8G	63%
FIBRE	0.7G	
CALORIES	40	

Celery and olive salsa

A nice, simple salsa that goes really well served with some pan-fried trout or salmon. Just heat up a knob of butter and a splash of olive oil in a frying pan. Fry the fish skin side down, then turn it over when the fish stops sticking to the pan (which will happen if you give it some time!) and season well. When it's golden brown on both sides, remove from the pan and serve with a big spoonful of this salsa.

I make this recipe using fairly average olives and it's fine, but if you have some gourmet ones you've just brought home from your own private olive grove in Tuscany, go for it and consider me for adoption. If your raisins have been sitting in your cupboard since 1982, put them in a bowl with some boiling water to plump them up, then drain and proceed as below.

Mix the raisins, capers, olive oil and vinegar together and leave to marinate for at least 10 minutes or up to an hour if you have time to spare. Mix with the remaining ingredients and season well. This will last for a few hours in the fridge.

40g (1.4 oz) raisins (40g)
3 tbsp capers (26g drained)
50ml (3⅓ tbsp) olive oil (50g)
2 tsp white wine vinegar (8g)
1 big head of celery, chopped (500g)
Approx. 200g (7 oz) green olives, stoned and chopped (200g with stones)
Handful of chopped parsley (20g)
1 tsp ground black pepper (2g)

Makes enough for 4 garnishes

PER PORTION

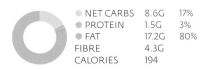

- NET CARBS 8.6G 17%
- PROTEIN 1.5G 3%
- FAT 17.2G 80%
- FIBRE 4.3G
- CALORIES 194

Sweet stuff
Domini's low-carb treats

We hear many nutritionists telling us that as far as the body is concerned, sugar is sugar is sugar whether it occurs naturally in fruit or in highly manufactured concentrations in certain substances like corn syrup, which we can't really consider a 'good' food. But they would be equally keen to point out that you can't compare pineapples to corn syrup, as you need to look at the entire package. Natural foods have plenty of goodness in them. Something like corn syrup or white sugar does not.

Be aware, though, that things like maple syrup, honey and coconut sugars, although less processed than something like high-fructose corn syrup, caster sugar or even fruit juices, is still sugar in terms of how your body deals with it, i.e. once it's in your system, it turns to glucose in the bloodstream.

But for many of us, life would be a little less sparkly without the occasional treat. Sometimes I am torn about providing 'healthy' treat recipes, as spoon for spoon – from a sugar point of view – you might be no better or worse off with a scoop of Häagen-Dazs.

I've provided plenty of truly bold recipes in my books and columns over the years, however, and I do think that when we eat at home, we feel better using natural and less processed ingredients. And Patricia has even included some sweet recipes that are entirely suitable for a keto diet, so I don't feel too guilty about popping in a few low-carbish ones for those of you who, as Patricia says, simply cannot imagine life without a foodie treat every now and then.

I know what you're thinking – 'but that's not baking as I know it' – and you'd be right. It *is* different and, I think, all the better for it, at least nutritionally speaking. Most traditional baked goods are not exactly abounding in nutrients and vitamins, which makes them no less delicious or desirable, of course, just not as kind to our bodies' systems. And with a better balance of ingredients comes the good news that you need to eat less of it to satisfy your cravings. Job done, I say.

Raw blondie balls

These sweet dessert balls use prunes and goji berries instead of sugar. Even better, they don't have to be cooked, hence the 'raw' of the title. Pretty good trick, I reckon!

The blondies are full of walnuts but also a few more ingredients that are becoming more mainstream, like lúcuma and maca powder for their sweetness and added nutrients. These powders work just as well in cooking terms, and many are really nutritious to boot. Maca, for example (or Peruvian ginseng, as it is better known), is full of fatty acids and amino acids. Traditionally it has been used medicinally, including for balancing hormones, so it's a good idea to use it sparingly.

In a food processor, blitz together the walnuts, hemp seeds and the two powders until it reaches a crumb-like consistency. Remove from the processor and set aside in a large bowl. Don't bother washing the food processor out – instead, blitz the soaked, drained prunes and let the processor break them down a bit before adding the cacao nibs, goji berries, cinnamon and vanilla extract. Then mix the dry, crumbly walnut mixture and the sweet prune paste together. At this stage you could always add in a few finely chopped dried apricots or even some lemon zest – this is relaxed baking. It's up to you.

Either way, when the mixture is ready, you have two choices. You can either form it into little balls or you can press the mixture into a lined baking pan and put it in the freezer before slicing it up later to form little bars.

185g (6.5 oz) walnuts (185g)
60g (2.1 oz) hemp seeds (60g)
40g (1.4 oz) maca powder (40g)
40g (1.4 oz) lúcuma powder (40g)
400g (14.1 oz) prunes, soaked in water for 10 minutes (400g unsoaked)
50g (1.8 oz) cacao nibs (50g)
20g (0.7 oz) goji berries (20g)
Good pinch of ground cinnamon (1g)
Splash of vanilla extract (2g)

Makes about 25 and they freeze well

PER BALL

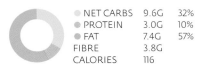

● NET CARBS	9.6G	32%
● PROTEIN	3.0G	10%
● FAT	7.4G	57%
FIBRE	3.8G	
CALORIES	116	

Baked pear crumbles

2 large pears, peeled (360g)
50g (1.8 oz) flaked almonds (50g)
50g (1.8 oz) dried apricots (50g)
50g (1.8 oz) stoned dates (50g)
Zest and juice of 1 lemon (2g + 40g)
1 tbsp maple syrup (20g)
Knob of butter (12g)

Serves 4

I had a hard time not eating the topping on its own. I kept rolling it into balls and having it with cups of tea. Again, this is the sort of trap we can fall into. Oooh, but it's healthy! Yes, compared to a white chocolate biscuit bar, but it's still got lots of sugar in it, so go easy!

Preheat the oven to 180°C (350°F). Line a baking tray with non-stick baking paper.

Start by cutting the peeled pears in half lengthways and scooping out the seeds to create a little crater that will take the topping. Next, blitz all the other ingredients together in a food processor on pulse – you want it to be chunky-ish, not a paste. When it's ready, just top each pear with about a quarter of the 'crumble' mixture.

Place the pears on the lined baking tray and loosely cover with foil. Bake for 20 minutes before removing the foil and cooking for a final 10 minutes or so, uncovered. Serve with cream, yoghurt or ice cream.

PER PORTION

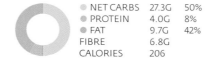

● NET CARBS	27.3G	50%
● PROTEIN	4.0G	8%
● FAT	9.7G	42%
FIBRE	6.8G	
CALORIES	206	

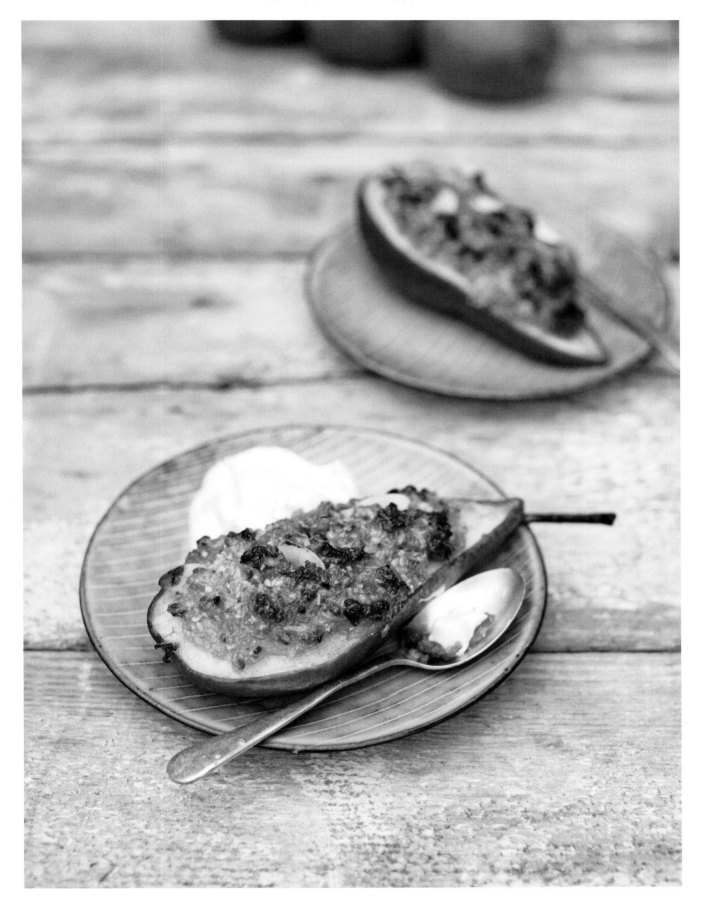

Rhubarb clafoutis

8 stalks of rhubarb, chopped (400g)

90g (3.2 oz) coconut or palm sugar or maple syrup (90g coconut sugar)

Few leaves of fresh rosemary, finely chopped (1g)

100g (3.5 oz) ground almonds (100g)

2 large eggs (130g)

2 egg yolks (40g)

250ml (1c) coconut milk (250g)

2 tbsp brown rice flour (24g)

½ tsp vanilla extract (3g)

Serves 6

I use coconut milk for the batter instead of ordinary milk and coconut sugar instead of refined white sugar, though you could also use palm sugar or maple syrup. Either way, the end result is very tasty indeed.

Preheat the oven to 180°C (350°F).

Toss the chopped rhubarb with the coconut sugar and rosemary and place in the bottom of a pie dish.

Next, make the batter by blitzing the remaining ingredients together in a blender. Pour over the rhubarb/sugar mixture and bake for 45 minutes. Serve with the banana 'ice cream' on page 206 or just cream.

PER PORTION

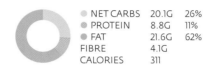

NET CARBS	20.1G	26%
PROTEIN	8.8G	11%
FAT	21.6G	62%
FIBRE	4.1G	
CALORIES	311	

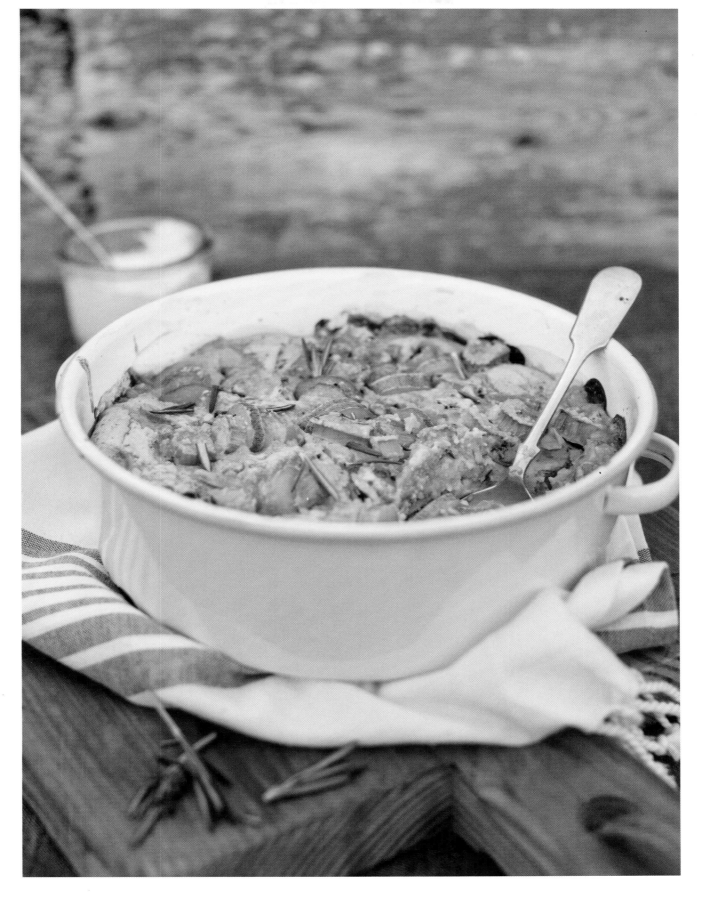

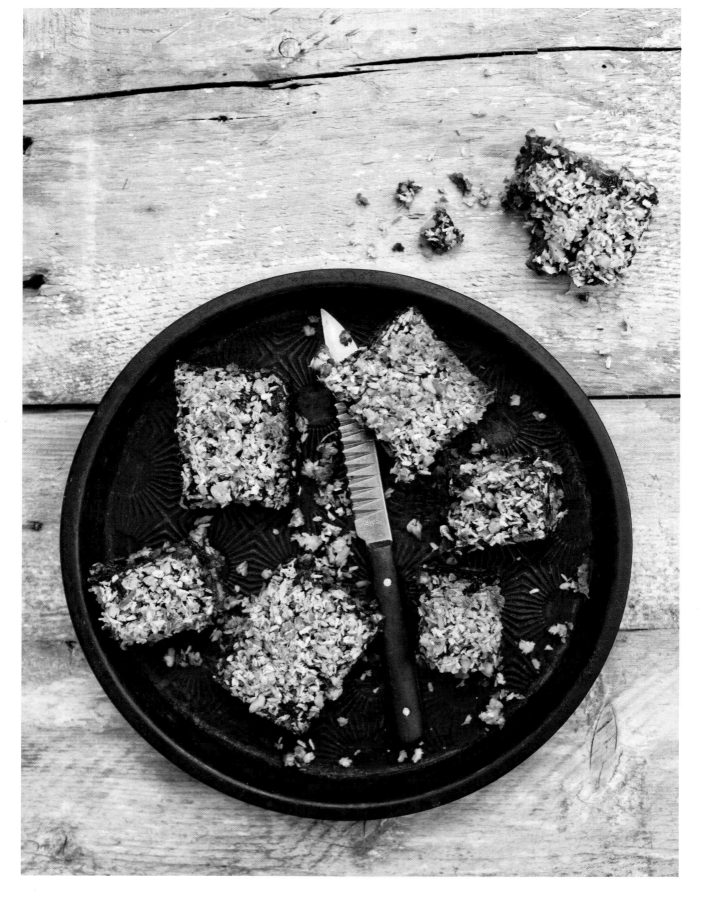

The first version of this recipe I attempted was too dry, so to make it hold together better I added more fat and reduced the quantity of nuts. The filling needed no tweaking, though; it's yummy. They emerge from the oven all warm and golden brown, so you'll be pleased you made the effort.

Preheat the oven to 170°C (340°F). Line a 20cm (8in) square baking pan with non-stick baking paper.

In a food processor, blitz together all the crust ingredients except the butter/oil and the chia seeds until they reach a loose, crumb-like consistency. Then take three-quarters of the mixture out and mix with the chia seeds and butter or oil; you will need the remaining quarter as a topping. Smooth the larger portion of the mixture into the lined pan.

To make the filling, simply blitz all the ingredients together in a food processor and spoon onto the crust mixture in the pan. Top with the remaining crust mixture and bake for 30 minutes, until golden. Serve the bars on their own or, if you must (and really, sometimes you must), with vanilla ice cream or cream.

PER PORTION (⅛ OF THE RECIPE)

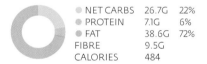

● NET CARBS	26.7G	22%
● PROTEIN	7.1G	6%
● FAT	38.6G	72%
FIBRE	9.5G	
CALORIES	484	

Walnut, fig and prune bars

Crust:
240g (8.5 oz) walnuts (240g)
150g (5.3 oz) desiccated coconut (150g)
60g (2.1 oz) applesauce (60g)
2 tbsp maple syrup (40g)
1 tsp vanilla extract (5g)
50ml (3⅓tbsp) melted butter or olive oil (50g butter)
2 tbsp chia seeds, soaked in 50ml water so that they swell (and yes, they do resemble frogspawn – of tiny frogs, though) (20g seeds)

Filling:
200g (7 oz) prunes (200g)
100g (3.5 oz) dried figs (100g)
2 apples, grated (200g)
Zest and juice of 1 lemon (2g + 40g)
Good pinch of ground cinnamon (1g)
Good pinch of ground ginger (1g)

Serves 6–8

Banana 'ice cream'

280g (9.9 oz) cashew nuts, soaked for 4 hours or overnight and then drained (280g)

100ml (⅜c) water (100g)

4 ripe, chopped, frozen bananas (400g without skins)

140ml (⅝c) maple syrup (140g)

1 good tbsp olive oil or liquid coconut oil (27g coconut oil)

Splash of vanilla extract (2g)

3 tbsp cacao nibs (available in most health stores) or a little bit of chopped-up dark chocolate (54g cacao nibs)

Serves 6

I was so impatient to get to the end result that I didn't soak the nuts for as long as I should have, and amazingly, the sky didn't fall in – the texture was just a bit grainier. I'd also run out of coconut oil so used olive oil instead, and it still worked. This recipe also allowed me to use up my store of over-ripe bananas that I'd consigned to the freezer months ago in a fit of 'waste-hate' enthusiasm. Dairy-free ice cream is mega pricey and so is this homemade version, but it's a little better in price if you don't factor in your own labour!

You'll need a good blender for this. Place the soaked, drained cashew nuts in the blender along with the water and blitz until smooth. Add the frozen banana bits, maple syrup, olive or coconut oil and vanilla extract and blitz again; it will thicken nicely, but taste it. Add the nibs and give one final blast to evenly distribute them. Decant the whole lot into a plastic container and freeze for a few hours or overnight.

PER PORTION

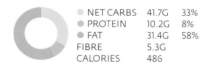

	NET CARBS	41.7G	33%
	PROTEIN	10.2G	8%
	FAT	31.4G	58%
	FIBRE	5.3G	
	CALORIES	486	

Patricia's keto treats

When we came together to write this book, we were adamant that nothing sweet would get in, especially not in the keto section of the book. Why encourage folks to eat sweet stuff (note: if you use certain sweeteners, there aren't many carbs!) when the whole point of the book was to encourage exactly the opposite?

Then it dawned on us that some people genuinely cannot hack any kind of diet unless there are treats somewhere along the way. Patricia often observes that treats can be the 'make or break' of somebody's compliance with a ketogenic diet. So we've caved and included some of the better-for-you sweet treats, some of which are borderline low-carb and some of which are very low-carb, suitable for ketogenic diets, to ensure you have the bit of sweet support you may need. Again, this section is not here to encourage you to eat treats, but to help you make this lifestyle more enjoyable and sustainable.

There is a lot of information regarding 'healthy' sweeteners out there, and it's important to pick the ones that aren't sending you on a blood sugar rollercoaster. Generally good choices are erythritol or on some rare occasions xylitol, which both come in powdered form and can add some bulk to baked goods. They're both so-called sugar alcohols and can cause digestive issues in sensitive people, especially when consumed in larger quantities. Patricia has observed that although sugar alcohols don't raise blood sugar levels, they can interfere with ketosis in some of her clients.

If you're looking for a liquid form of sweetener, Patricia's preferred options are stevia glycerite or yacón syrup. When you use stevia, you typically use very small amounts, i.e. 1 teaspoon of stevia glycerite is the equivalent of 1 cup of sugar. Yacón syrup has a very low glycaemic index of 0.5 and can therefore also be used in small amounts. You wouldn't go overboard with it anyway, as it's very pricey!

Truffles

75g (2.6 oz) cacao butter (75g)

80g (2.8 oz) hazelnut butter (80g)

15g (0.5 oz) ready-to-eat pitted prunes (15g)

2 tbsp maca root powder (15g)

1 tsp chaga powder (5g)

½ tsp ground cinnamon (1g)

1 pinch of rock salt or sea salt (1g)

Makes 20 small truffles

This recipe has been adapted from a wonderful truffle recipe of a colleague of mine, Doris Rabe. I threw in the prunes instead of some other sweeteners and found the combination of hazelnut, prunes and chaga really nice and different. The maca root adds some sweetness too, but if you suffer from a hormone-related cancer you might want to omit it and use lúcuma.

Melt the cacao butter in a pan. Mix the hazelnut butter with all the other ingredients, then blend well with the cacao butter. Place in the freezer for about 30 minutes, then roll into small balls between the palms of your hands. Store in the fridge.

PER PORTION (10G)

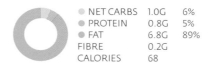

● NET CARBS	1.0G	6%
● PROTEIN	0.8G	5%
● FAT	6.8G	89%
FIBRE	0.2G	
CALORIES	68	

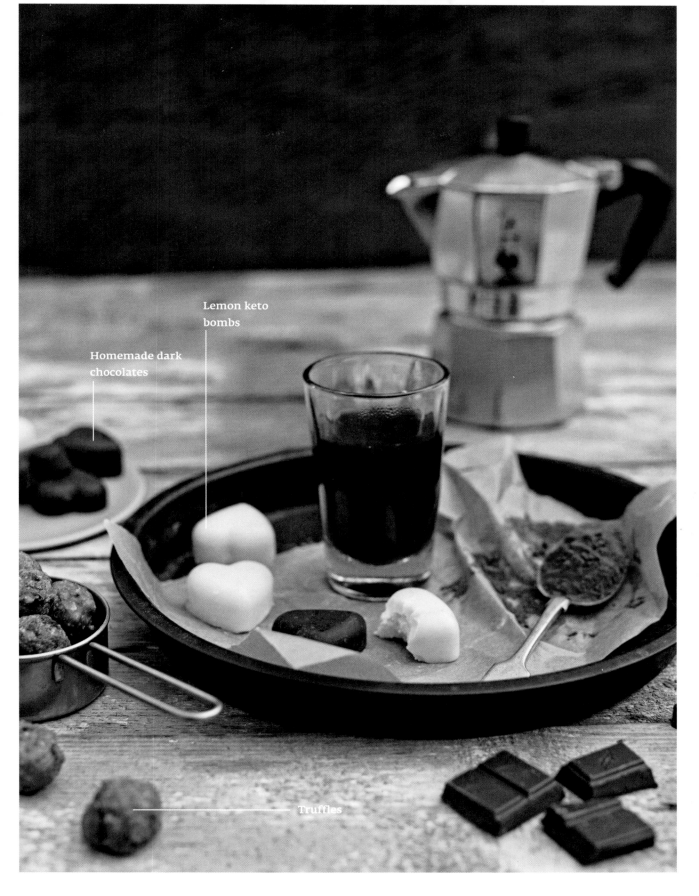

Homemade dark
chocolates

Lemon keto
bombs

Truffles

White chocolate

200g (7 oz) desiccated coconut,
 lightly toasted (200g)
60g (2.1 oz) cacao butter (60g)
30g (1.1 oz) erythritol (30g)

Makes 20 bites

This is incredibly easy if you have a good blender, otherwise it could be challenging to turn the desiccated coconut into a nice butter. If you lightly toast the desiccated coconut (or you can also buy toasted coconut flakes), it makes this process somewhat easier.

Make coconut butter by creaming the desiccated coconut in a strong blender – this can take up to 5 minutes. Alternatively, you can just use creamed coconut.

In the meantime, melt the cacao butter and mix it into the coconut butter. Sweeten as required with erythritol or stevia and put in a flat silicone baking dish. Let it set in the fridge, then break it up into pieces. Store in the fridge thereafter.

PER PORTION (13G)

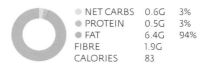

NET CARBS	0.6G	3%
PROTEIN	0.5G	3%
FAT	6.4G	94%
FIBRE	1.9G	
CALORIES	83	

Homemade dark chocolate

50g (1.8 oz) cacao butter (50g)
30g (1.1 oz) cacao powder (30g)
20g (0.7 oz) erythritol (20g)
½ tsp vanilla essence (optional) (3g)

Makes 6 portions

Have you heard about the amazing health benefits of cacao? It's not only nutritious, but also a powerful source of antioxidants. Raw, unprocessed cacao beans are among the highest-scoring foods ever tested in terms of ORAC, which stands for oxygen radical absorbance capacity, a measure of the antioxidant activity of foods. The bioactive compounds in cacao can also improve blood flow in the arteries and can lower blood pressure. These are just a few of the many beneficial properties of cacao!

Melt the cacao butter in a pan on a low heat, then add the cacao powder, erythritol and vanilla essence. Whisk well and pour into a silicone ice cube tray. Put in the freezer or fridge to set, then store in the fridge.

PER PORTION (17G)

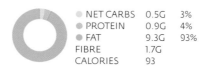

NET CARBS	0.5G	3%
PROTEIN	0.9G	4%
FAT	9.3G	93%
FIBRE	1.7G	
CALORIES	93	

A three-ingredient cheesecake by Japanese YouTube host Ochikeron went viral recently and I wondered if it was possible to 'ketofy' it. Here's my keto version – try it, it's super easy and light.

Preheat the oven to 170°C (340°F). Line a small round baking pan or springform pan with oiled non-stick baking paper.

Separate the egg yolks from the whites and put the whites in the fridge.

Melt the white chocolate in a pan on low heat, then mix with the cream cheese and beat in the egg yolks. Whisk until you have a smooth paste.

In a separate clean, dry bowl, beat the egg whites until stiff peaks form. Fold one-third of the egg whites into the white chocolate mixture with a spatula and mix gently, then add the next third, mix gently again and then fold in the rest. Gently pour the mixture into the lined baking pan. Tap the pan onto the countertop a few times to get rid of any air bubbles.

Put the cheesecake into a roasting pan and pour in enough water around the cheesecake until it reaches halfway up the sides of the pan. Bake in the oven for 15 minutes. After 15 minutes, reduce the heat to 160°C (320°F) and bake for another 15 minutes. After that, turn the heat off but let the cake sit in the oven for another 15 minutes, as it will continue to bake. Remove from the oven and let it cool on a wire rack.

White chocolate cheesecake

3 eggs, separated (150g)
120g (4.2 oz) white chocolate (page 210) (120g)
120g (4.2 oz) full-fat cream cheese (120g)

Serves 6

PER PORTION (65G)

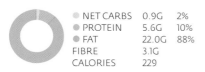

NET CARBS	0.9G	2%
PROTEIN	5.6G	10%
FAT	22.0G	88%
FIBRE	3.1G	
CALORIES	229	

Lemon keto bombs

125g (4.4 oz) desiccated coconut or toasted coconut flakes (125g)
120g (4.2 oz) butter or ghee, melted (120g)
55g (1.9 oz) coconut oil, melted (55g)
Zest of 1 lemon (2g)
1 tbsp lemon juice (15g)

Makes 12 bites

So-called fat bombs are a way of increasing your fat and calorie intake if you know you have consumed a fairly low-fat meal and need to boost your intake a bit. If I go to a restaurant, for instance, I sometimes take one or two of these with me because it can be difficult to get enough fat unless I have access to some good-quality olive oil that I can drizzle over a salad or vegetables. The only downside when you take them with you is that they can melt when they get warm. Feel free to adapt the proportions of the different fats to your liking.

Make coconut butter by blending the desiccated coconut or coconut flakes in a food processor until smooth. This might take up to 5 minutes, depending on your food processor. Try to buy toasted coconut flakes because they turn into coconut butter a lot more easily. Mix the melted butter or ghee with the melted coconut oil and the coconut butter, then add the lemon zest and juice. Pour into a silicone ice cube tray and freeze for 30 minutes. Keep in the fridge thereafter.

PER PORTION (27G)

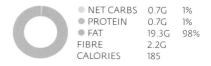

NET CARBS	0.7G	1%
PROTEIN	0.7G	1%
FAT	19.3G	98%
FIBRE	2.2G	
CALORIES	185	

If you like a bit of alcohol in your food, this is perfect. For those who can't stand it, use the same quantity of orange juice and grate the zest into the batter. It will increase the carbohydrate count slightly, but it's equally delicious.

Preheat the oven to 170°C (340°F). Grease a 23cm (9in) baking pan and line with non-stick baking paper.

Melt the chocolate and butter in a small pan over a low heat, then remove from the heat and allow to cool slightly.

Whisk the eggs, erythritol, ground almonds and cognac together in a separate bowl and mix well. When the chocolate mixture has cooled slightly, add it to the egg mixture. Pour into the prepared pan, cover with tin foil and bake for 25 minutes. Put in the fridge once it has cooled down and serve with crème fraîche or whipped cream.

Brandy chocolate torte

175g (6.2 oz) dark chocolate,
 e.g. Lindt 90% cocoa solids or
 homemade (page 210) (175g)
90g (2.1 oz) butter (90g)
3 eggs (150g)
130g (4.6 oz) erythritol (130g)
50g (1.8 oz) ground almonds (50g)
30g (1.1 oz) cognac, e.g. Hennessy
 (30g)

Serves 8

PER PORTION

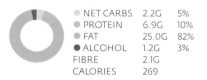

● NET CARBS	2.2G	5%
● PROTEIN	6.9G	10%
● FAT	25.0G	82%
● ALCOHOL	1.2G	3%
FIBRE	2.1G	
CALORIES	269	

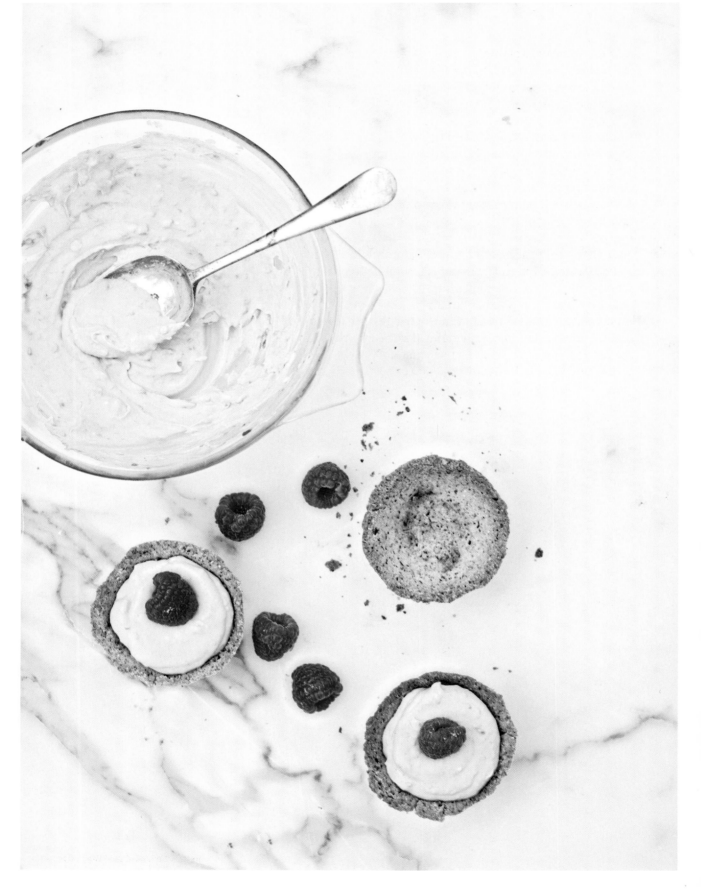

You can use any type of berry for this, it doesn't have to be raspberries. Does the crust recipe look familiar? It's similar to the one we used for the savoury crust for the asparagus quiche on page 278, except that we swap the cashew nuts for hazelnuts here. By the way, you can use this crust recipe to make yummy biscuits too.

Preheat the oven to 180°C (350°F).

To make the crust, mix the ground hazelnuts and coconut flour together. Add the soft butter and knead everything until you can form a firm dough. Press the dough into six holes of a muffin pan and bake for 15–20 minutes, until lightly brown. Allow to cool on a wire rack.

Meanwhile, mix the mascarpone, fresh raspberries and xylitol with a hand blender until you have a smooth, creamy mixture. Fill into the nut crust once it has cooled down. Refrigerate for about 30 minutes before serving.

Raspberry cupcakes

90g (3.2 oz) hazelnuts, ground to a fine flour (90g)
50g (1.8 oz) coconut flour (50g)
60g (2.1 oz) butter, softened (60g)
200g (7 oz) mascarpone cheese (200g)
100g (3.5 oz) fresh raspberries (100g)
1 tbsp xylitol (13g)

Makes 6 cupcakes

PER PORTION (86G)

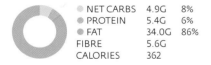

● NET CARBS	4.9G	8%
● PROTEIN	5.4G	6%
● FAT	34.0G	86%
FIBRE	5.6G	
CALORIES	362	

Peanutty chocolate torte

This tart is absolutely decadent and a great party piece. It is tried, tested and much loved by kids, too. It does contain a good amount of dairy and is full of calories, but trust me, it's totally worth it every now and then. If you're reluctant to use peanut butter, you can use almond butter or a mix of almond and cashew butter.

To make the base, melt the butter in a small pan over a medium heat, then stir in the erythritol and cacao powder and mix until it thickens. Remove from the heat and stir in the ground almonds, desiccated coconut, walnut flour and vanilla essence. After mixing everything really well, press the mixture flat into the base of a small round pan and refrigerate.

To make the filling, mix the cream cheese and peanut butter together. Add the whipped cream, erythritol and vanilla essence and whisk well until smooth. Take the base out of the fridge and spoon the filling on top.

To make the topping, melt the coconut oil and chocolate together in a small pan. Add the cacao powder and erythritol and stir until smooth. Add the stevia, then spread the topping over the filling and refrigerate for at least 30 minutes.

Base:

55g (1.9 oz) butter (55g)
80g (2.8 oz) erythritol (80g)
35g (1.2 oz) cacao powder (35g)
100g (3.5 oz) ground almonds (100g)
100g (3.5 oz) desiccated coconut (100g)
40g (1.4 oz) walnuts, ground to a coarse flour (40g)
1 tsp vanilla essence, no alcohol (5g)

Filling:

220g (2.8 oz) full-fat cream cheese (220g)
165g (5.8 oz) smooth peanut butter (165g)
105g (3.7 oz) cream, lightly whipped (105g)
60g (2.1 oz) erythritol (60g)
2 tsp vanilla essence, no alcohol (10g)

Topping:

75g (2.6 oz) coconut oil (75g)
55g (1.9 oz) dark chocolate, e.g. Lindt 90% cocoa solids (55g)
35g (1.2 oz) cacao powder (35g)
25g (0.9 oz) erythritol (25g)
20 drops of liquid stevia (1g)

Serves 12

PER PORTION (96G)

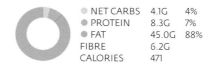

NET CARBS	4.1G	4%
PROTEIN	8.3G	7%
FAT	45.0G	88%
FIBRE	6.2G	
CALORIES	471	

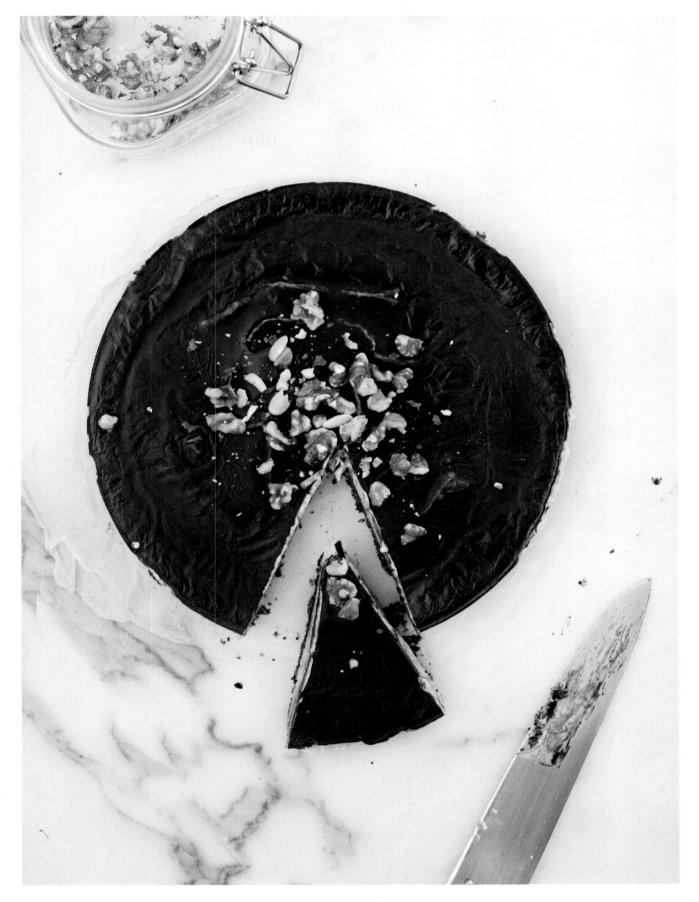

Sunny chocolate chip biscuits

55g (1.9 oz) butter, softened (55g)
1 duck egg (66g)
55g (1.9 oz) erythritol (55g)
2 tbsp yacón syrup (25g)
2 tsp vanilla essence, no alcohol (10g)
150g (5.3 oz) sunflower seeds, ground to a fine flour (150g)
2 tbsp coconut flour (20g)
½ tsp baking soda (2g)
½ tsp salt (3g)
60g (2.1 oz) dark chocolate, e.g. Lindt 90% cocoa solids, chopped (60g)

Makes 12 biscuits

These are quite addictive! Don't be turned off by the slightly greenish colour they turn into after baking – it's just the sunflower seeds. But if this is an issue for you, you can easily substitute the sunflower flour with ground almonds.

Preheat the oven to 180°C (350°F). Line a baking tray with non-stick baking paper.

Using a hand-held blender, process the butter and egg in a large bowl for a few seconds. Add the erythritol, yacón syrup and vanilla essence and whisk well.

In a separate bowl, mix together all the dry ingredients except the chocolate. Add the dry ingredients to the wet ingredients and incorporate to a firm dough, then gently fold in the chopped chocolate pieces. With your hands, form the dough into 12 flat biscuits, place them on the lined tray and bake for 12 minutes. Cool them on a wire rack and enjoy while they're still a bit warm.

PER PORTION

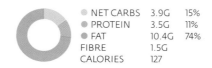

NET CARBS	3.9G	15%
PROTEIN	3.5G	11%
FAT	10.4G	74%
FIBRE	1.5G	
CALORIES	127	

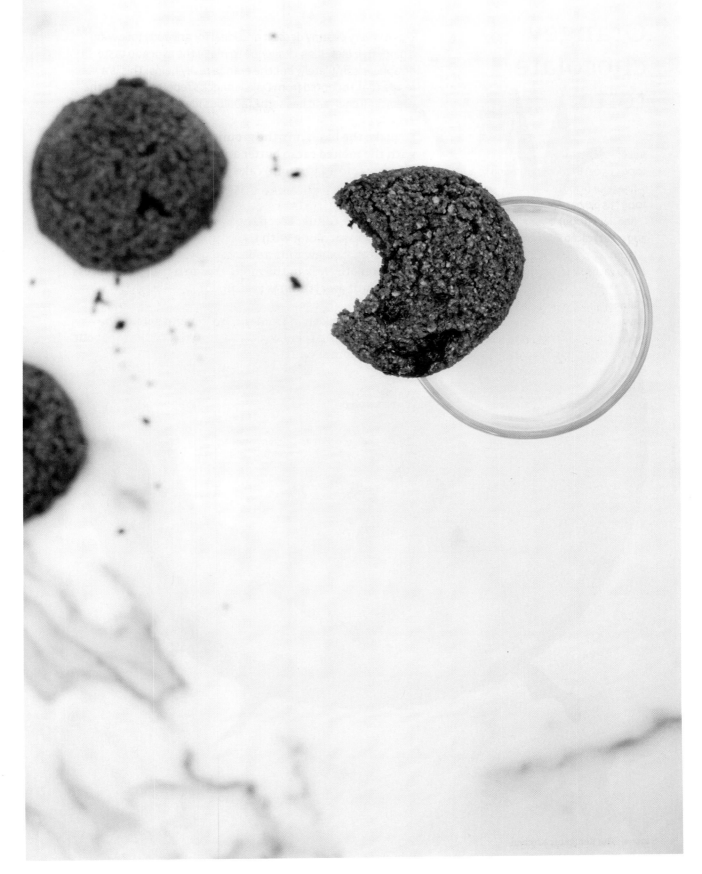

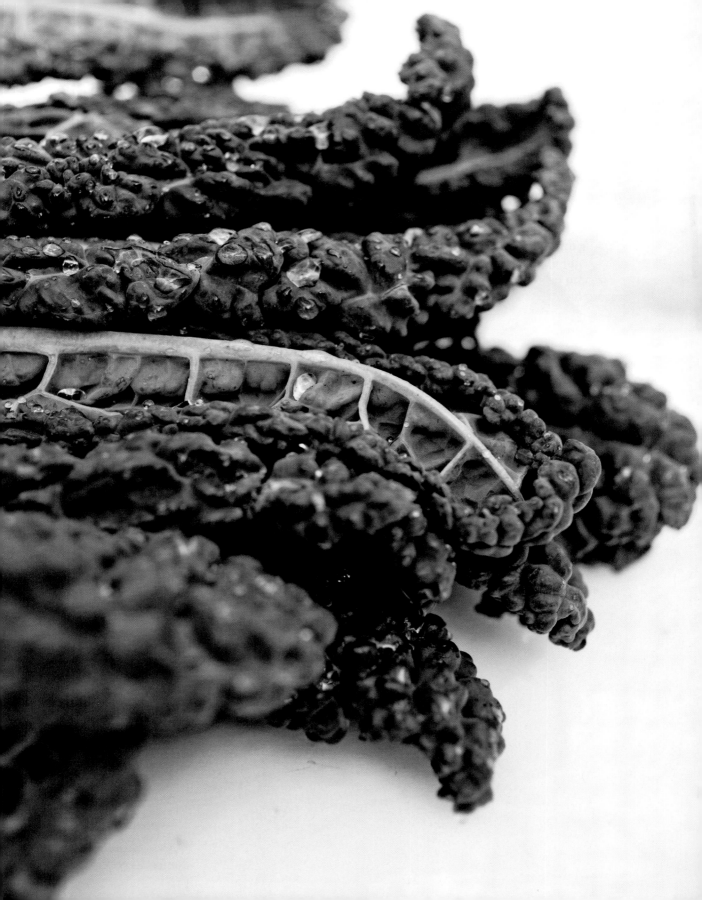

Part 3: The Ketogenic Way

Introduction to the ketogenic way

We've said it before, but we'll say it again: first and foremost, the benefits of a ketogenic diet have been shown when it is used *alongside conventional treatments*. There is no data to support that the diet by itself can treat, cure, maintain or manage cancer. Hopefully more data will become available soon, but as of yet, there is no evidence to support the comments made by those claiming that this diet in itself is a treatment for cancer.

The preclinical data is compelling, but this data is for animals and is case study based. While we are targeting many of the pathways that we know are vital to cancer survival, there are no randomised trials in humans showing these benefits. However, numerous clinical trials are currently underway (www.clinicaltrials.gov).

Overview

Ketogenic diets have been effective for seizure control in epileptic children for almost a century (Groesbeck, Bluml and Kossoff, 2006) and from the 1960s onwards they have been used for the treatment of obesity-related disorders in supervised clinics (Paoli et al, 2013). Researchers are investigating the ketogenic diet as a cancer therapy mainly due to the fact that cancer cells rely primarily on glucose to fuel their metabolism (Hamanaka and Chandel, 2012; Ho et al, 2011). This characteristic is the basis for tumour imaging using labelled glucose analogues (FDG-PET scans) and has become an important diagnostic tool for cancer detection and management (Hsu and Sabatini, 2008).

We also know that:
- A high glycaemic load is associated with increased cancer risk (Champ et al, 2012).
- Hyperglycaemia leads to poorer prognosis for cancer patients (Goodwin et al, 2012).
- There is a positive correlation between blood sugar levels and tumour growth in selected cancers (Hu et al, 2012).
- Downregulation, or the slowing down of several pathways, leads to better results in chemo- and radiotherapy (Klement and Champ, 2014). Downregulation is the process by which a cell decreases the quantity of a certain cellular component, for instance the number of receptors to a molecule, in response to an external variable (e.g. food).

- A ketogenic diet is likely safe, with minimal toxicity (Champ et al, 2014). It is more than likely that this will never be demonstrated in a large-scale trial because it is incredibly challenging to run a dietary study with hundreds of cancer patients.

The cornerstone of a ketogenic diet for cancer patients involves the **severe restriction of carbohydrates.** Generally, this means restricting carbohydrate intake to 3–4% of total calorie intake. However, for some patients this can increase to 10% as long as the effects on blood glucose are minimised. Carbohydrates are replaced with high amounts of fats (75–85% of total calorie intake) in the form of coconut oils, avocados and oily fish, for example, and adequate intake of vegetable and animal protein (12–20% of total calorie intake) (Davis, 2013). Excessive protein consumption can also result in elevated blood glucose levels through a process called gluconeogenesis (Westman et al, 2003). A ketogenic diet causes the body to enter a state called ketosis, where ketone bodies are produced by the liver as a by-product of fat breakdown when blood glucose is low (Maurer et al, 2011).

It has been theorised that because tumour cells do not seem to have the metabolic flexibility to use ketones for energy, the result of a ketogenic diet would be destabilisation of tumour tissue DNA, reduction of tumour size over time and therefore enhanced survival rates for cancer patients (Derr et al, 2009; Seyfried, 2012).

Ketogenic diet as part of cancer treatment: How does it work?

There are several potential mechanisms that explain why a ketogenic diet can be added as a type of dietary intervention in cancer treatment. The following points outline a few of them.

- A ketogenic diet may work simply through limiting available glucose to malignant cells. This is not a new concept. In the 1920s, German Nobel Prize winner Professor Dr Otto Warburg demonstrated that cancer cells generate their energy predominantly by a high rate of glycolysis (the breakdown of sugar), followed by lactic acid fermentation in the cytosol, even in the presence of plentiful oxygen (Warburg, Wind and Negelein, 1927). This process, called the Warburg effect or aerobic glycolysis, has been confirmed in many studies and has now been accepted as a robust hallmark of most tumours (Hanahan and Weinberg, 2011).

- Contrary to our normal cells, data shows that cancer cells are unable to effectively generate energy from ketone bodies and rely heavily on glucose (Westman et al, 2003). This increased appetite for glucose could result from the fact that most malignant cells have deficient or defective mitochondria (Klement and Kaemmerer, 2011), the powerhouses of the cell that create energy. Research carried out by US biologist Dr Thomas Seyfried and his team indicates that genomic instability and essentially all hallmarks of cancer, including the Warburg effect, can be linked back to impaired mitochondrial function and therefore energy metabolism (Seyfried and Shelton, 2010). Malignant cells are able to reprogramme their glucose metabolism, and thus their energy production, by limiting their energy metabolism largely to glycolysis in the cytoplasm. However, this process is very inefficient for generating energy: mitochondria can create around 20 times more ATP (the energy currency of the cell) than the process of glycolysis. To compensate for this lower efficiency, cancer cells have developed the ability to upregulate glucose transporters, notably GLUT1, which significantly increases glucose transport into the cell (Hsu and Sabatini, 2008). Rapidly growing tumour cells typically have glycolytic rates up to 200 times higher than those of their normal tissues of origin (Paoli et al, 2013).

- Due to their faulty mitochondria, cancer cells also depend on glucose to fix free radical damage. Much like our normal cells, cancer cells are under constant attack of free radicals. Since their mitochondria do not function properly, they rely on even more uptake of glucose to counter free radical damage. Limiting this glucose will inhibit their capacity to repair damaged cells (Aykin-Burns et al, 2009). This may also be one of the reasons why restricting glucose through a ketogenic diet may enhance the effects of radio- and chemotherapy (Allen et al, 2013; Abdelwahab et al, 2012).

- Like any cell, malignant cells require signalling hormones that tell them to grow and survive. They have receptors such as the insulin-like growth factor receptor (IGF-1R). Insulin-like growth factor (IGF) can bind to this, as can insulin, which is secreted in our bloodstream in response to carbohydrate consumption. Insulin then activates several pathways that may increase cancer growth and survival (Klement and Kaemmerer, 2011). A recent study in advanced cancer patients tested the hypothesis that a carbohydrate-restricted diet will slow cancer growth in patients by reducing the secretion and circulating levels of insulin (Fine et al, 2012). Minimising the pathways that lead to cancer growth or indeed activating those that limit it, like the AMP-K pathway, is another potential mechanism by which a ketogenic diet can be effective.

- It's also worth mentioning that inflammation is a key player in the development and proliferation of cancer cells (Coussens and Werb, 2002). The ketogenic diet reduces inflammation, as outlined on page 252, and ketone bodies prevent free radical production (unstable molecules that can cause havoc) on a cellular level (Youm et al, 2015).

Practical aspects of the ketogenic diet

It seems to be a reasonable possibility that a ketogenic diet could help to reduce the progression of some types of cancer, although at present the evidence is preliminary. Most of the trials have been animal studies and case reports, though a few larger randomised, controlled trials are currently underway.

The ketogenic diet also has its drawbacks. It is a therapy that requires total compliance and careful monitoring by a trained nutrition professional who is familiar with the required metabolic testing, contraindicated health conditions and medication. A ketogenic diet for cancer patients cannot be thought of as reduction of macronutrients (carbohydrates, fats or protein). Micronutrients (vitamins, minerals) and anti-cancer nutraceuticals (e.g. curcumin, omega-3 fatty acids, green tea polyphenols) are equally important and their content must be addressed when discussing and evaluating a ketogenic diet (Klement, 2013).

As with any dietary intervention during cancer treatment, a multidisciplinary approach is vital, i.e. looking for synergistic interactions between different therapies that may increase the efficacy of treatment (Poff et al, 2013). A low-carbohydrate diet is one of many nutritional and lifestyle interventions that can be used in the management of cancer, and certainly a very promising one.

What is the ketogenic diet?

People are often intrigued by the term *ketogenic diet* and wonder what it is exactly, as it does sound very technical and scientific. This curiosity is natural given that *ketone* and *ketogenic diet* have become something of a buzzword in the nutritional and medical world recently. But what exactly is a ketone body, and what happens in the body when we enter the state of so-called nutritional ketosis?

Our cells need a constant flow of oxygen and an energy source to survive. To put it simply, they run either on sugar (glucose) or fat. Sugar in the blood will provide a small amount of energy, as will proteins and fats. But when sugar isn't around, the body turns to ketone production to feed the brain, organs and cells. Most of us produce ketone bodies on a regular basis, in fact, including early in the morning after a night's sleep.

If we weren't able to turn fatty acids into ketone bodies in times of starvation, carbohydrate restriction or fasting, the human race most likely wouldn't exist any more. We sometimes have to smirk when the media talk about 'a brand new, revolutionary' diet when talking about the high-fat, low-carb approach. In fact, it has been around for 2 million years! Probably the biggest advantage of burning fat instead of sugar is that the body has access to up to 100,000 calories or more, depending on body weight and composition, instead of only about 2,000 calories of stored glucose. This is a serious advantage over other species when it comes to survival.

Keto and clinical trials: The evidence

We know quite a lot about cancer cell metabolism (i.e. how they generate energy) and also the mechanisms of the ketogenic diet. Pre-clinical data in favour of the diet is compelling (the 'pre-clinical' stage of research takes place before clinical trials in humans can start, and aims to collect data in support of the feasibility and safety of a treatment).

What we're lacking at the moment are randomised controlled trials on humans that confirm the safety and effectiveness of this approach. The good news is that numerous clinical trials are currently underway and these will hopefully help incorporate the ketogenic diet into existing treatment protocols.

Because of this current (and frustrating) lack of the kind of rock-solid evidence that the medical community requires to implement any new approaches, for a long time I was reluctant to guide clients through the ketogenic diet. I take my job very seriously and want my recommendations to be as evidence-based and safe as possible. The penny dropped, however, when a client who I had initially refused to set up on the ketogenic diet stated, 'Patricia, I honestly don't have the luxury of time to wait for clinical trials. If you don't help me, I'm going to start the ketogenic diet anyway, all by myself. Chances are that I might seriously mess myself up, though.'

That was about three years ago, and she was right – she would have had to wait a long time to confirm her decision to go keto, along with many other people for whom this diet has turned out to be a lifesaver.

The cornerstone of a ketogenic diet is the severe restriction of carbohydrates. This causes the body to enter a state called nutritional ketosis, in which the liver produces ketone bodies when blood glucose is low. Those on the diet replace carbohydrates with fat in the form of foods such as coconut oils, avocados and oily fish. It isn't enough to keep an eye just on carbohydrates, though. Protein intake needs to be moderate too, and this includes both vegetable and animal protein. This is important to remember because excessive protein consumption can also result in elevated blood glucose levels (through a process called gluconeogenesis).

The main goal of the ketogenic lifestyle, then, is to teach the body to run on fat instead of glucose. This takes time. Through fasting and reducing carbohydrates, sugar levels drop and the amount of ketones feeding the brain and body rises. Not only is this a clinically proven method of weight loss, but it also holds a great deal of promise for patients suffering from cancer, diabetes, epilepsy and neurological and cardiovascular disease.

Pitfalls of the ketogenic diet

I always talk about potential pitfalls with clients before we start implementing the diet. It's not because I like scaring people – I do it because many potential complications can be prevented with some knowledge of the kind of metabolic changes that can be expected. There are a number of factors to consider before implementing the ketogenic diet. Here's a list of the most helpful and common ones.

1. Fat phobia

To enter ketosis in a successful and sustainable way, I've observed that many people have to overcome a lifelong fat phobia. I was exactly the same. It was so ingrained in me to eat the bulk of my food in the form of carbohydrates that I had a mental block when it came to increasing my fat calories. There was this little voice in my head that kept nagging that 'fat makes you fat', 'fat is unhealthy' and that I should have a 'balanced, healthy diet'. It took lots of reading, education and mindset-changing to get my head around the fact that fat is doing me good, helping me manage my cancer and improving my general well-being. For many people, the time between the initial stages of the ketogenic diet and the first blood tests or scans can be one of great uncertainty and doubt. But once you see tangible results like improved scans, better markers and benefits like more energy, clearer skin or optimised weight management, you won't need any more convincing that you're on the right path.

2. High protein consumption

A common misconception is that simply lowering carbohydrate intake is enough to go into sustained ketosis. While this is a big and important step on the ketogenic diet, it's often not enough. Protein intake has to be adjusted too. Some people, especially those transitioning from a vegan diet, need to get used to eating more protein, but the majority have to reduce it.

Many people are surprised when they start weighing their food according to my meal plans and realise how little protein they actually need to eat on a ketogenic diet. This is because your need for protein decreases with a high fat intake.

There are several reasons why we need to keep an eye on protein, and we go into more detail on this in the FAQ section on page 244.

3. Carbs creeping in

In the initial stages of going on a ketogenic diet people are really focused, but then sometimes they relax a bit over time. Depending on what your goals are, that's totally okay, but if you're in nutritional ketosis for medical reasons, it's a good idea to keep an eye on carbs.

The thing is that carbohydrates can quickly add up, especially if you're keen to get your veggies, herbs and spices in. They're also in products you'd never think would contain carbs. Good examples are any processed foods (we'll talk about them later), shop-bought salad dressings, milk substitutes (many coconut and almond milks have added sugar), tomato sauce, some meats like duck confit, starchy vegetables and even herbal tea, to name just a few. Eating out can also be a challenge because many restaurants like to use sauces, dressings and dips that have added honey or other sources of sugar. It tastes nice, but sadly it's not keto-friendly.

Having solid, reliable information is the key to carbohydrate restriction, especially in the initial stages when metabolic changes happen. Running your daily food intake through a calculator from time to time can be helpful.

4. Giving up too early

The quicker you go into nutritional ketosis, the more side effects you might suffer from initially. The metabolic changes can be dramatic because every single cell in the body needs to make the switch from glucose to fat metabolism.

The dietary changes have a big impact on insulin, for instance. Insulin is a hormone with many functions in the body (it makes fat cells store fat, for example), but the other thing that insulin does is tell the kidneys to hold on to sodium. If your insulin levels are low, your body starts to shed extra sodium and water along with it, which is why people often get rid of bloating and shed weight within a few days of going on a low-carb ketogenic diet.

But this can also be a problem. Sodium is a very important electrolyte, and when the kidneys get rid of too much, it can potentially have consequences, with common symptoms including light-headedness, fatigue, constipation and headaches. This is why it's so important that you add sufficient sodium to your diet and keep well hydrated, especially in the first few days of starting to reduce carbohydrates. This will help to make sure you don't suffer from any of the symptoms of the dreaded 'keto flu': shivers, foggy brain, headaches or nausea are some of the possible symptoms. Actually, it's probably more appropriate to call them 'carbohydrate withdrawal symptoms' because of the effects on hormonal and electrolyte balance.

Other things that help overcome these initial obstacles are strong bone broth with good-quality salt (flaky sea salt or Himalayan pink salt), lots of rest, no intense exercise and plenty of mineral-rich water, such as San Pellegrino. Take things slowly and don't give up when you're feeling a bit off in the initial stages, provided, of course, that you've done blood tests to exclude any underlying health issues prior to starting a ketogenic diet.

5. Boredom

Many people feel overwhelmed in the initial stages of implementing a low-carb and ketogenic diet, and because they have very little experience with certain new foods, they keep eating the same 'safe' low-carb stuff: bacon and eggs for breakfast and nuts for snacks.

Of course, this means that you are still eating low-carb, but as a nutritionist guiding some very ill patients through the diet, my first priority is always to improve their health, and this is possible only with a nutritious, varied and individualised approach. Eating the same things over and over again isn't just boring, it may also set you up for developing nutrient deficiencies or food intolerances. This happens quite often, especially if you're a little stressed, your gut function isn't optimal or you're on medication.

Food intolerances can have an impact not only on your gut health by causing bloating, cramps, diarrhoea, constipation or other symptoms, but also on your immune system. My best advice is to keep experimenting with new foods, even if they seem utterly strange to you, like, say, chicken liver, which is much easier to find and prepare than you'd think. There's a nice recipe out there for every single food – we hope you'll find loads that take your fancy in this book.

6. Focusing on quantity rather than quality

Some ketogenic dieters only think of macronutrients and whether they are in ketosis by measuring their ketone bodies, but they forget about the bigger picture. Yes, there are (processed) foods that are low-carb friendly, keep you within the carbohydrate limits that you choose and which may make life a lot easier. But they may also be of poor quality and full of artificial flavours, colouring, polydextrose, sucralose and other artificial sweeteners that can mess with your mental and physical health. My rule of thumb is: if you wouldn't be able to bake or cook a meal based on the ingredients list (because you don't recognise half of them or wouldn't know where to buy them), stay away from it.

How to eat is as important as *what* to eat, but I know that the big focus of most 'ketoers' is on what to eat and how to keep the carbs down.

First of all, it's really important to eat in a relaxed way rather than on the go, but a lot of people don't do that. They're very busy, they're at work and they eat on the go or in front of their computer. I also recommend pausing for a few minutes before starting a meal. Prayers or any ritual before a meal don't just have a spiritual reason; they also have a very important physiological function. They prepare your digestive tract for what is to come – when you start to think about food, hormones kick in that tell your pancreas and other digestive organs to start producing enzymes, bile and hormones that you need for good digestion and absorption.

Also, the more slowly you take it and the better you chew, the better you support your digestive system and reduce the risk of developing food intolerances. Food intolerances are nothing but the inability to digest food properly, which can also be a result of eating in a stressed state without chewing properly. This can actually be a common cause of food sensitivities. Eating slowly is a challenge for many people, especially for those who grew up in big families.

Another important point to be aware of is that you should try to drink *in between* rather than *during* meals. The gastric juices that we produce while we're eating can get diluted by drinks. As a result, absorbing and digesting nutrients can be more difficult.

7. Not having a plan or obsessing too much

Lack of planning and obsessing too much can both be stumbling blocks. If you don't plan, you're much more likely to fail and give up on your lifestyle changes, whereas obsessing too much can stress you out.

Baseline blood tests are the first step towards a ketogenic diet. Monitoring blood markers is equally beneficial for making sure you're on track and that your body agrees with the ketogenic diet. For example, at the very beginning of implementing the ketogenic diet, lipid markers (e.g. cholesterol) can go off the charts, and if they don't settle after a few weeks, more tests need to be done to find out why this is happening.

Lack of planning can also be problem when you realise you haven't got all of the ingredients you need for a low-carb recipe. Although we do our best do use ordinary ingredients in our recipes, you might not find some of them in your corner shop. Some of the staples on a low-carb or ketogenic diet (like coconut oil, olives, oily fish or ghee) might only be found in health food shops or online. More and more supermarkets are starting to stock them, but this really depends on where you live. If you plan a bit ahead and know that you need certain things to follow the meal plans in our book, then you won't get stressed because you'll already have them in your cupboard. Planning also makes it easier to cook in bulk and therefore save time and money.

On the other hand, I often work with clients who start obsessing too much and plan every single bite they eat. Obviously, it's a slightly different story for somebody following a ketogenic diet for medical reasons, for instance in the case of epilepsy, where the diet has to be well calculated and any mistake has a serious consequence. But sometimes people tell me they're so stressed out about dietary changes that they wake up in the middle of the night and can't go back to sleep. They worry about what their next meal would look like, how they could further increase ketones or what to eat on a holiday. In this case, it's time to take a (big) step back, relax, try some recipes without weighing and counting and maybe give it another go after a few weeks with a different mindset. Stressing about food can cancel out all the positive effects of good nutrition – I'll discuss this again a bit further on.

8. Not tuning in

People who obsess over dietary changes can get caught up in measuring blood glucose and ketones, weighing their food all the time and creating exact meal plans and they can get really scared of eating out, where things are out of their control. In my experience, they are also likely candidates to ignore their body's warning signs.

I used to be an 'expert' in this. Even though there were foods I couldn't stand because they tended to bloat me, I still ate them because I'd read somewhere that they're really good. Or I'd do another high-intensity training just because it was on my training plan, even though I felt absolutely exhausted and just wanted to take it easy.

Please don't forget that you know your body best and that no meal plan can beat your own innate knowledge and intuition. Take warning signs seriously and don't override them because you have it in your head that you need to stick to a particular regime.

Low-carb and ketogenic diets aren't for everyone. If you feel worse than before – even after getting over the initial symptoms I talked about earlier – then it's probably time to stop and reconsider.

9. Social pressure

This is a big one and shouldn't be underestimated! I've lost count of the number of times I've been at a party and have to listen to someone saying, 'Oh come on, surely one piece of cake won't hurt, don't be so extreme!' Seriously, the last thing I want to do is go into a scientific monologue about metabolism at a party. Even three years into following a ketogenic diet, I still get comments from family and friends even though they all know how miraculous the diet has been for my health.

But ketogenic diets are still poorly understood, even by the medical profession. People don't understand that you can't follow the famous 80/20 rule, where some treats are allowed in moderate amounts. Quite simply, you're either in ketosis or you're not. It's pretty black or white, actually.

And trust me, once you've been keto adapted for a while and you eat a piece of cake, you will feel pretty shoddy and not remotely in a party mood afterwards anyway.

10. Being too stressed

It's essential to have a good balance between exercise and rest, but also mental stimulation and meditation. I'm sure you know about the detrimental health effects of stress. But sometimes we get overly paranoid because it's not so much the fact that we're being stressed that's a problem – it's how we *respond* to stress or stressful situations. The goal isn't to be completely relaxed and unstressed all the time. Human evolution is very much based on stress – if we don't experience some stressful situations, we basically don't progress. The point is that we need really good breaks on a regular basis. Stress can become a problem if it's chronic, i.e. ongoing and prolonged.

If we experience short periods of stress, if we know how to handle it and if we can relax again in between, then our adrenal glands that produce the stress hormones can replenish. Chronic stress is associated with persistently high levels of cortisol, one of the stress hormones. Cortisol and glucose levels usually go hand in hand, so even just for this reason it's crucial to have those downtimes. Being chronically stressed will make it challenging to control your blood sugar levels and therefore achieve ketosis. And that's also the reason why you shouldn't start the ketogenic diet when you're going through a very hectic phase of your life and you know you probably won't have enough time to take it easy. This could be a major change in your life like moving house, changing job or anything that can trigger a stress response. You know you probably won't be able to cope if you also make big dietary and lifestyle changes.

One point I'd like to get across – and I already talked about this earlier on – is that if you're getting stressed out by a diet plan and/or lifestyle changes, you will definitely cancel out the effects of good nutrition. For instance, I had a client recently who called me and said, 'Patricia, I can't even sleep. I wake up in the middle of the night worrying about what I will have for breakfast or what I will cook for lunch. I'm so stressed out and just can't cope with all these changes.' That's when it's time to take a step back, relax and not think about food too much. Get support, re-evaluate and then maybe start again when you feel more ready. I know we're all really keen to make the ketogenic diet work for us and go into nutritional ketosis as quickly as possible, but please be aware that it could take time. You need to be patient and go at the pace of your body.

History of the ketogenic diet with a focus on cancer

Though it didn't earn the name *ketogenic* until the last century, this diet has been around for a surprisingly long time.

For centuries, fasting, the precursor to the ketogenic diet, has been used to treat a variety of human diseases. Probably the first written account of successfully using a high-fat, high-meat, low-carb approach was delivered by Dr John Rollo, a surgeon in the British Royal Artillery, who in 1797 used it with two diabetic and obese army officers. This 'meat diet' became very popular, because at the time there was no option other than fasting to treat this deadly disease (insulin wasn't discovered until 1910).

Similarly to Rollo, the overweight undertaker and coffin maker William Banting described his remarkable weight loss success using a low-carb, high-fat way of eating in his 'Letter on Corpulence' in 1863. This diet had been recommended by the British physician William Harvey and subsequently became one of the most popular weight-loss diets, also called banting. In recent years, banting has seen a renaissance, especially in South Africa, under the guidance of Professor Tim Noakes.

In 1921, Dr Rollin Woodyatt reported that three water-soluble compounds, known collectively as ketone bodies, became prevalent in the blood, urine and breath of otherwise healthy people when they were fasting or consuming a low-carb, high-fat diet. It became apparent that these ketone bodies were being used as an alternative fuel source when glucose wasn't available. Based on these findings, Dr Russell Wilder at the Mayo Clinic came up with the term *ketogenic diet* for the first time to describe a way of eating that produces high amounts of ketone bodies in the blood. His colleague Mynie Peterman further developed this concept and defined the classic ketogenic diet used to treat patients with epileptic seizures. He also documented improvements in behaviour and cognitive effects in his patients following a ketogenic diet. The use of this dietary approach was outlined in detail in every comprehensive textbook on epilepsy in children that was published between 1941 and 1980, but with the discovery of anticonvulsant drugs in 1938, a new era of medical therapy for epilepsy began and the ketogenic diet fell by the wayside.

Over the past 15 years, scientific interest in the use of the ketogenic diet has taken off again, and not only in the area of epilepsy. In the area of cancer research in particular, a debate has started as to what the origins of the disease really are.

After a cancer diagnosis, many people ask themselves what the cause of their

Keto foods

Yes Foods

All meat and fish (ideally grass-fed meat and wild fish)
including but not limited to:
Beef
Chicken
Duck
Eggs
Game
Goat
Lamb
Lobster
Mussels
Scallops
Shrimp
Small oily fish*
Turkey
Veal
White fish
Small fish are preferred, e.g. anchovies, freshwater trout, mackerel, sardines, wild salmon

Vegetables
Alfalfa sprouts
Artichokes
Asparagus
Bamboo shoots
Beet greens
Bok choy
Broccoli
Brussels sprouts
Cabbage
Cauliflower
Celery (root)
Chives
Collard greens
Cucumbers
Dandelion
Eggplant
Fennel
Green beans
Kale
Kohlrabi
Leeks
Lettuces and green leafy veg
Mushrooms
Olives
Radishes
Sauerkraut
Scallions
Snow peas
Spinach
Scallions
Swiss chard
Turnips
Water chestnuts
Zucchini

Nuts, seeds & butters
Cacao (100%)
Coconut
Flax, hemp and chia seeds

Fats and oils
Animal fats (ghee, (goat) butter, lard, duck and goose fat)
Avocado oil
Cacao butter
Coconut oil/milk/cream (unsweetened)
Macadamia oil
Olive oil

Beverages
Almond milk (unsweetened)
Filtered or bottled water
Herbal teas (unsweetened)

Fruit
Avocados
Lemon
Lime

Condiments
Fermented foods
Mayonnaise (ideally homemade with olive oil, not sunflower oil)
Mustard
Pesto (see page 192)
Spices and herbs

Limit Foods

Meat and fish

Pork: good-quality sausages once a week, bacon and chorizo as a condiment or snack but not in large amounts

Vegetables

Bean sprouts
Beetroot
Bell peppers
Carrots
Garlic
Onions
Parsnips
Pumpkin
Shallots
Squash
Tomatoes

Nuts, seeds & butters

Almonds
Brazil nuts
Cashews
Hazelnuts
Macadamia nuts
Peanuts
Pecans
Pumpkin and sunflower seeds
Sesame seeds
Tahini
Walnuts

Oils

Fish oil as a supplement
Flax oil (store in the fridge)
Sesame oil (store in the fridge)

Grains and legumes

Edamame
Nattō
Tempeh

Beverages

Coffee if tolerated
Protein powder drinks (low-carb)
Dry wine (1 small glass twice a week max)
Soy milk (when no alternative)

Fruit

Small amounts of fresh berries, cherries, ½ kiwi, ½ small apple or a small amount of papaya

Dairy

Organic cheese, ideally unpasteurised
Goat and sheep cheese
Cream cheese
Cream
Mascarpone
Kefir (homemade)

Sauces and dressings

Coconut aminos
Sea vegetables
Tamari

Treats

Coconut yoghurt (unsweetened)
85–99% dark chocolate

Condiments

Extra-dark chocolate
Zero-carb sweeteners (stevia, erythritol)

No Foods

Meat and fish

Meat and fish in a batter
Processed meat or fish with preservatives and additives

Vegetables

Corn
Peas
White and sweet potatoes

Beverages

Alcohol
Coconut juice or water
Coffee drinks or shakes
Fruit juices
Milks except those in the above column

Oils

Margarine
Vegetable oils (see page 245)

Grains and legumes

Barley
Black beans
Buckwheat
Chickpeas
Kamut
Lentils
Pinto beans
Quinoa
Red beans
Rice
Soy/tofu
Spelt

Unrefined carbohydrates

Processed bread
Bagels

Breadsticks
Brownies
Cake
Candy
Cereal/granola
Chips
Cookies
Couscous
Crackers
Croissants
Cupcakes
Muffins
Oats/porridge
Pasta
Pastries
Pita
Popcorn
Processed pizza
Rolls
Tortillas
Tortilla chips
Wheat product

Fruit

All except for those in the above column

Dairy

Milk
Processed or low-fat dairy products

Sauces and dressings

Bottled salad dressing
Ready-made sauces
Relishes

Anything diet or sugar-free

Or artificially sweetened food or beverage items of any kind

Before you start

Here are some tips on getting the most out of this section of the book.

Who might benefit from a ketogenic diet and who should stay away from it?

I don't recommend going straight from a standard Western diet to a strict ketogenic diet without any transition phase. In my experience, the best approach is to start with a low-carb diet and then reduce your carbohydrate intake over at least two weeks from 50 grams of net carbohydrates a day and then maintain the 12 grams for as long as necessary. This book will show you how this is doable. It is paramount to do a complete blood chemistry panel (see below) before attempting to go into nutritional ketosis. And be sure to check the text box on page 239 to ensure you don't suffer from one of the conditions described (contraindications).

While supervised carbohydrate restriction during pregnancy is safe, I don't recommend attempting ketosis when you're expecting. There is only limited research available, but one (admittedly poorly designed) study shows that there might be a risk of birth defects. Until more conclusive evidence emerges, I advise waiting until the baby is on solid food and not exclusively breastfed any more. I started the ketogenic diet when my son was 10 months old (and breastfeeding) and he clearly thrived on it.

Cancer patients who are at risk of developing cachexia (excessive weight and muscle loss) should not attempt these meal plans without strict medical supervision. They might also have to adapt their protein intake to maintain weight and make other important adjustments to the meal plans. Finally, don't forget that **the ketogenic way does not suit everybody**. Some people absolutely thrive on it while others struggle with (fat) digestion, hormone imbalances or other issues. That's why it's so important that you tune in to your body, listen to the signs and also do functional testing with an appropriately trained professional.

Educate yourself as best you can on health and nutrition

There are some great books by some brilliant scientists, and I particularly rely on the work of Dr Thomas Seyfried (*Cancer as a Metabolic Disease: On the Origin, Management, and Prevention of Cancer*) and Dr Dominic D'Agostino. Ellen Davis's e-book *Fight Cancer with a Ketogenic Diet* is full of information based on their research. Another e-book with some great information, written by Miriam Kalamian, is available on www.dietarytherapies.com. Miriam has a wealth of experience when it comes to the implementation of a ketogenic diet, and we are in touch on a regular basis to update each other on the latest research and developments in the ketogenic cancer world. I also recommend Jeff Volek and Stephen Phinney's *The Art and Science of Low Carbohydrate Living* and Jimmy Moore and Eric Westman's *Keto Clarity*.

Whether or not you suffer from any health conditions, I always recommend having a complete blood chemistry panel done before starting the diet. This is to ensure there are no underlying issues (e.g. impaired liver function, kidney or blood cell issues, low levels of vitamin D, lipid imbalances or thyroid issues) that might pose a problem while you are on the ketogenic diet. You will find a full list of the blood panel I usually do on page 432. Please find an experienced nutrition professional who can monitor your progress instead of embarking on the journey on your own. Trained professionals will also be able to tell you if a ketogenic diet is suitable in your case and how much monitoring you require.

Contraindications

Nobody denies that cancer metabolism is currently a hot area of research. The goal is to find ways to target the common metabolic abnormalities of cancer cells. A number of drugs and therapies are currently on the market that target the same or similar pathways as the ketogenic diet, but they all come at a price: side effects. If the ketogenic diet can be a powerful tool, doesn't it come with side effects too?

The answer is yes. There are potential dangers to the ketogenic diet, especially if the diet isn't implemented correctly and important blood markers are not being monitored. It's also important to note that there are contraindications and situations where somebody shouldn't go keto (Kossoff et al, 2009).

Absolute contraindications

This is when the ketogenic diet is an absolute no-no. Yes, this is quite a long list, but there's no need to be worried. To be honest, I haven't come across any of these conditions in my clinical practice and I don't know anybody among my friends and family who suffers from any of them either.

Often these conditions are diagnosed early in life, with the exception of porphyria, which can also develop at a later stage in life, so the likelihood of having one of these conditions and not being aware of it is really small.

- Carnitine deficiency (primary)
- Carnitine palmitoyltransferase (CPT) I or II deficiency
- Carnitine translocase deficiency
- β-oxidation defects
- Medium-chain acyl dehydrogenase deficiency (MCAD)
- Long-chain acyl dehydrogenase deficiency (LCAD)
- Short-chain acyl dehydrogenase deficiency (SCAD)
- Long-chain 3-hydroxyacyl-CoA deficiency
- Medium-chain 3-hydroxyacyl-CoA deficiency
- Pyruvate carboxylase deficiency
- Porphyria

Health conditions that need special attention

But what about other health conditions that could make it difficult, impossible or just harmful to go into nutritional ketosis? There are a number of conditions that can put a spanner in the works, so it is very important that you're getting extra support if you suffer from any of these.

- **Abnormalities in blood chemistry:** My first step with any client is to do a full blood count and other relevant baseline blood tests to exclude any underlying conditions (see page 432 for common blood tests). Impaired liver function, for instance, can be a problem when implementing a ketogenic diet because the liver will be in charge of producing ketone bodies and also larger amounts of bile than usual (due to the high fat intake on the ketogenic diet).
- **History of pancreatitis:** Case studies show that elevated levels of triglycerides in the blood can lead to acute pancreatitis. Prolonged hypotension and acidosis can eventually lead to cardiac arrest.
- **Active gall bladder disease:** The gall bladder is responsible for storing and concentrating bile produced by the liver. There are various types of gall bladder disease and you need professional advice before starting the ketogenic diet.

- **History of kidney failure:** Although there are studies suggesting that low-carb approaches can be very beneficial in renal failure, caution is advised when there are or have been issues with the kidneys.
- **Poor nutritional status:** If you already suffer from poor nutritional status, you definitely need individual guidance and special care. Poor nutritional status can be assessed via blood work, as suggested earlier, but also via physical signs. There is also a functional test called NutrEval that is outstanding when it comes to determining and analysing nutrient deficiencies.
- **Gastric bypass surgery:** This is obviously a unique situation where the patient needs an individualised nutrition protocol.
- **Abdominal tumours and/or impaired gut function:** The high fat consumption can pose a problem for patients with abdominal tumours or impaired gut function. Gut healing or an adapted form of ketogenic diets can be an option. I'm currently looking into a GAPS keto approach for people with seriously compromised gut function.
- **Decreased gastrointestinal motility:** This can be caused by conventional cancer treatments and also certain medication. Because one of the first side effects of the ketogenic diet can be constipation, you need to be cautious if you suffer from this condition.
- **Liver tumours:** I often get asked if people with liver tumours (primary or secondary, i.e. metastatic) can do the ketogenic diet. This very much depends on liver function, which can be tested. I look after a number of clients who have large tumours in their liver but who successfully manage to be in ketosis. As always, it depends on the individual.

As you can see, the ketogenic diet is not for everybody and can in certain circumstances lead to serious complications. That's why it is so important to do baseline blood tests and have professional support from somebody who fully understands the ins and outs of the ketogenic diet and how to manage it successfully for optimal health.

The meal plans that follow are based on an individual with daily calorie requirements of 1,800–2,000 calories with an ideal body weight of approximately 75kg (165 pounds). It is important that you **work out your daily requirements** and make adjustments based on your weight and activity levels to ensure adequate nutrient intake. It's easy to add extra fat and calories in the form of fat bombs, olives, some nuts or seeds or a little bit more protein with your meals.

Prepare well before starting the plans
Here are a few tips to make the diet more practical and easier to integrate into family life.
- On a weekend day, spend some time making snacks, breads, pestos, spreads and anything else that you can **prepare in advance**. You can freeze almost anything in portions and then just take it out the night before if you know you won't have time the following day.
- **Involve your kids**. Mine love to crack eggs, stir vegetables, do small chopping jobs (with blunt knives) and I always find something to keep them busy while I do some bulk cooking. When you go shopping, make sure you have plenty of time and give your kids some small tasks. They learn about all the different fruit and vegetables, they can practise counting and when they beg to get flavoured yoghurts, processed ready meals or fish fingers, I explain why we're not buying them.
- If you don't have enough time to do the

shopping, **shop online**. There are more and more organic suppliers that deliver straight to your door too.

- If you follow the plan for the 28 days outlined here, use leftovers to create new meals and cook in bulk. With a little practice, this way of eating can be integrated into **family life**. You will see that breakfast and lunch are usually designed for one or two people and that dinners are for the whole family or more. You don't need to cook several meals – anybody who is not following the ketogenic diet can simply add some carbohydrates as side dishes (e.g. starchy vegetables, sweetcorn, quinoa, millet, wholegrain pasta, rice, potatoes) and reduce the size of the main (ketogenic) dish. I do my best to incorporate leftovers into lunches so that there is usually only one meal a day that needs to be cooked from scratch.

- The main idea of these meal plans is to show you that there are **many possibilities** to integrate it into your daily and family life. It *is* restrictive to reduce carbohydrate intake to 12g a day, so it's even more important to have as much variety as possible and include nutrient-dense foods. There might be a few meals that you don't like, but this is why I provide you with lots of nutritional information so that you can customise the plans if you do well on the diet and want to adopt it in the long term.

- Please take it easy at the beginning and **don't get overwhelmed**. For many people, eating in a ketogenic way is a huge change in eating habits and takes some adjustment, not just for your body, but also in terms of psychological barriers that might be in the way.

How to get started

It may have been around for decades, but the concept of the ketogenic diet is becoming more mainstream only now, as exciting evidence of its success and effectiveness continues to mount.

Because it is metabolic therapy rather than merely a diet, keto is a lifestyle, really, so choosing to commit to it, if only for a short time, can be a little daunting at first, especially if, like me, you were conditioned to regard fat as the ultimate dietary sin. But the rewards are great and long lasting, so please don't let worry stand in the way. Arm yourself with knowledge and prepare well, and success will be yours. Below are some pointers to help you get started and progress with confidence.

Clean up your diet

If you are a complete newbie to this way of eating, then rather than overwhelm yourself with carb counting and introducing new foods at every single meal, start by **cleaning up your diet**, as outlined below. By reducing carbohydrates gradually, your system has a chance to adapt, and you get plenty of opportunity to get your head around new foods, cooking methods and shopping lists. However, some people prefer making radical changes and starting the diet straight away, provided they don't have any underlying health issues (e.g. malnutrition, thyroid or cardiovascular problems). I have had good experience with the following steps before starting proper carbohydrate restriction (daily carbohydrate intake of 50g or lower). You choose the pace.

1. Eliminate **sugar** in all forms and shapes. This includes fruit juices, sports drinks, honey, agave and all the other sweeteners. Educate yourself on the subject.

2. Replace the sugar calories with **healthy fats** like avocados, coconut oil, olive oil, grass-fed butter, ghee and MCT oil.

3. Eliminate **gluten** in any shape or form. This includes wheat, spelt, kamut, rye, barley and oats. Remove grains in general as well as grain-derived and vegetable oils (corn, soy and rapeseed/canola).

4. Be careful not to overheat unstable polyunsaturated oils (walnut, flax, peanut oil) and always store them in the fridge.

5. Eliminate all **synthetic additives, colourings and flavourings** – basically, any names on an ingredient list that you don't recognise. This includes aspartame, MSG, dyes and artificial flavourings.

6. Eat **wild-caught seafood** and **pastured, grass-fed meat** within the limits recommended by the World Cancer Research Fund (see the myths on red meat in the FAQs on page 246 for more details). My favourite red meat is lamb, and in Ireland we are very lucky that it is grass fed, readily available and inexpensive. To balance this, also eat (oily) fish, free-range or organic eggs as well as some chicken, duck and shellfish.

7. Eliminate **legumes** such as beans and lentils. Small amounts of sprouted lentils or beans are fine. Use peanut butter as a condiment in sauces if you tolerate it well and are not following a paleo diet, but otherwise replace it with sesame paste (tahini), for instance.

8. **Limit processed dairy from commercially raised animals as best you can.** Choose full-fat products from goats, sheep or grass-fed cows instead.

9. Switch to **organic fruits and vegetables** as much as your budget allows. This is more important for some plants than others. We'll talk about the so-called dirty dozen and clean fifteen on page 411, where you will also find a list from the Environmental Working Group.

10. **Cook your food gently, if at all.** Always have a good amount of raw food in your daily diet if well tolerated. Opt for steaming, slow cooking or baking at 180°C or lower. Incorporate water into your cooking whenever possible and use low temperatures. **Burnt, blackened or charred foods** need to be thrown out.

11. Limit **fruit consumption** to one or two small servings (i.e. one handful) per day. Go for low-fructose fruits like berries and lemons over watermelon and apples.

12. **Add spices and other flavourings.** Start experimenting with herbs and spices such as turmeric, oregano, parsley, cilantro, thyme or rosemary. Bear in mind that these contain carbohydrates too.

13. **Enjoy your food**, preferably in great company.

Weigh your food

I strongly recommend buying a weighing scale for weighing your food, at least for the initial month. It will help ensure accuracy, which is important when you are trying to get into ketosis.

Counting calories

Calculate your daily calorie requirements based on your basal metabolic rate (BMR). I'm not a fan of counting calories at all, but some people get a lot of comfort out of knowing where they're at. You can use an online calorie calculator, such as this one: www.freedieting.com/tools/calorie_calculator.htm.

Fasting

In order to achieve a faster 'metabolic switch-over', some people prefer to do a two- or three-day fast (ideally under medical supervision). Intermittent fasting, where the window of time during which food is consumed is gradually restricted to 4–8 hours, can be another effective tool in reaching and maintaining nutritional ketosis. A realistic schedule would be to have dinner at 6pm, for instance, and then not eat anything until 10am the following day. Intermittent fasting is generally easier and more efficient for men, whereas it can pose problems for some women, especially if thyroid issues are present.

Daily carbohydrate intake

A diet is considered to be 'very low-carb' with a daily carbohydrate intake of **below 50g**. However, based on experience, ideally an intake **closer to 30g per day is better to reach ketosis**. The level of carbohydrate at which somebody goes into nutritional ketosis is very individual and also depends on how quickly your metabolism adapts. For some people it can take weeks to enter a state of nutritional ketosis, where others achieve it within days. To become an **efficient fat burner** easily takes weeks, if not months.

Based on Dr Thomas Seyfried's research, cancer patients should aim to lower their daily carbohydrate intake to 12g. This is very challenging, but it's exactly what this section of the book does: moving towards a 12g ketogenic diet that is well formulated and enjoyable.

Protein intake

Recommended protein intake on a ketogenic diet is between 0.8g and 1.2g per kilogram of ideal body weight, though some experts are of the opinion that it can be even lower. For example, a patient who weighs 75kg and is neither under- nor overweight should consume between 60g and 90g of protein on a daily basis. Cancer patients who suffer from low white blood count or weight loss, or who go through treatment or exercise quite a bit, should make sure their protein intake is at the higher end of the above calculation.

Fat intake

Fat intake makes up the balance of your daily calorie requirements. Don't be shocked when you see the figure. It took me a while not to feel guilty because the mantra that most of us were brought up with is that fat is bad and makes you fat and sick, so this is a huge thing for most people (including me). Educating yourself about it is the best way to get your head around it. You'll see that you may need to make adjustments to the meal plans based on your weight, calorie intake and activity level to ensure adequate nutrient intake.

A great resource is available for free at www.keto-calculator.ankerl.com. It guides you through the process of determining your macronutrient levels. Use it to help get on track initially if you feel you need it.

Monitor your progress

The best way to monitor progress and make sure you are in ketosis is to use a home monitor that allows you to measure your blood glucose and ketone levels. They are the same ones used by diabetics and are available online. Dr Dominic D'Agostino recommends Precision Xtra by Abbott Laboratories (in the UK and Ireland, it's called FreeStyle Optium Neo).

Myth-busting FAQs

So many questions come up during the first consultation with my patients about this dietary approach that I now spend time doing a lot of 'myth busting' during our first session. People often question how ketogenic diets can be healthy, especially in the context of cancer. So here are some of the most frequently asked questions.

Q. How can a diet that cuts out an entire food group (carbohydrates) and their corresponding nutrients be healthy and beneficial for me? We're always told to eat a balanced diet, so doesn't an elimination diet cause nutrient deficiencies?

We're very keen to emphasise that whichever way you choose to eat – be it low-fat, vegetarian, Mediterranean or anything else – you need to choose the best-quality, most nutrient-dense foods to optimise your health. This is no different with a diet that is high in fat and low in carbohydrates. Unless you're on a very strict ketogenic diet for medical reasons where you're ideally also supervised by a medical professional, you will still have some carbohydrate-containing foods in your diet, for instance in the form of vegetables or some fruit, nuts and seeds.

Many people don't know that many plant-based foods such as legumes and grains may contain so-called anti-nutrients (e.g. lectins or phytates), meaning they reduce the body's ability to absorb essential nutrients. That's why ancient tribes whose diet relied on grains and legumes found methods to reduce these anti-nutrients, for instance by soaking, sprouting or fermenting foods. But in our industrialised society, this is not being done any longer and those anti-nutrients can be a problem for people who are ill or malnourished.

Don't forget that only fat and protein are essential nutrients, meaning that they can't be produced by the body and *must* be part of our diet. Carbohydrates, on the other hand, are not essential and can be made by our liver, for instance, out of other components. For the geeks amongst you, this process is called gluconeogenesis.

Q. Doesn't eating so much fat (also in the form of saturated and animal fat) raise my cholesterol?

The simplified answer is that the body regulates how much cholesterol it requires in the blood for optimum function at any given time. Dietary cholesterol has very little effect on blood cholesterol and is made from the products of glucose rather than fat metabolism. Rising insulin levels lead to increased cholesterol production (via HMG-CoA) (Ness and Chambers, 2000).

Cholesterol is found in all animal foods because it is what makes the cell membranes stable. It is such an important substance that life simply wouldn't exist without it. It's no surprise that there are warning signs emerging that low cholesterol is actually more of a risk factor than high cholesterol for conditions like mental health disease as well as for cancer (Ancelin et al, 2010; Mabuchi et al, 2002; Martinez-Carpio et al, 2009).

Cholesterol is used to make sex and stress hormones. You need more cholesterol when you're working hard, ill, injured or pregnant, but you can get by with a lot less when you're relaxed and well. There are two ways it can get into your blood: most of it is made by your liver (but virtually every cell in the body can produce cholesterol), and a maximum of 20% comes from your food. Even if you eat absolutely no cholesterol, which is likely if you follow a vegan diet, you'd still have the exact right amount your body needs at any time because your liver compensates by working harder and producing more. If you eat a lot of cholesterol, your digestive system will stop absorbing it, your liver produces less and starts excreting more via bile into your bowels.

As always, there are a few exceptions to this rule. One is the genetic condition called familiar hypercholesterolemia. Another is if someone suffers from low cholesterol, which is often associated with a hypocaloric state (i.e. somebody who doesn't eat enough calories). If your cholesterol is low because you suffer from liver disease, hyperthyroidism or cancer, it can be improved by eating more cholesterol.

Bottom line: Blood cholesterol levels can fluctuate regularly, but if they are chronically elevated, then this is a cause for concern and needs medical attention. In the long term, it is advisable to have your cholesterol and its components (e.g. HDL, LDL) in a healthy range (although there is ongoing debate on what this range is). High cholesterol is absolutely a risk factor for heart disease, but other factors like nutrient deficiencies, stress, inflamed arteries, obesity, autoimmune conditions, increased homocysteine, insulin resistance or elevated blood sugar also need to be taken into consideration.

Q: Wouldn't it be better to eat fats from plants, for instance vegetable oils that contain polyunsaturated fats?

For a long time, vegetable oils were deemed healthy (maybe because they have the word 'vegetable' in them?) and saturated fats were blamed for everything from clogging arteries and causing cancer to making you generally unwell. The tables are turning, though, as more and more compelling research acknowledges that saturated fat is no longer a 'nutrient of concern'.

While saturated fat was being demonised, the seed oil marketeers stepped in to convince the public and the medical establishment that seed oils, e.g. polyunsaturated 'vegetable' oils, were healthy. This opinion has been – and still is – deeply rooted in society and the myth persists to this day.

All three types of fat – saturated, monounsaturated and polyunsaturated – have different functions in the body and can be good for health. The vast majority of vegetable oil sold today is made from seeds like canola, sunflower, safflower, soya beans and corn. The oil from the seeds is extracted using high heat, solvents and chemicals. As it is predominantly polyunsaturated, it is very susceptible to damage (oxidation) by heat and light and is likely to turn into trans fats, which are not good for the body. Olive oil and coconut oil don't fall into this category, by the way.

If you're using cold-pressed versions of seed oils, this is less of an issue. However, the other problem is that they still contain a large amount of omega-6 fatty acids. An overabundance of omega-6 fatty acids, unless adequately balanced with omega-3s, can lead to inflammation and can contribute to heart disease (BMJ, 2013). Good sources of omega-3 fatty acids are oily fish (like sardines, anchovies, salmon, mackerel, pilchards or herring), hemp seeds and oil, flaxseeds and oil and chia seeds.

For these two main reasons – oxidisation by the extracting process and high omega-6 content – vegetable oils are not the best choice. Saturated fat, on the other hand, is much more stable when exposed to heat and light and thus is less prone to oxidation and rancidity. It's therefore more suitable for cooking and consumption than polyunsaturated oils.

Bottom line: Stick to coconut oil, olive oil, butter, ghee, avocado oil, macadamia oil or other animal fats (lard, tallow, bacon or beef dripping) for cooking and baking. These are oils that have a high smoke point (160°C and above) and a low percentage of polyunsaturated fats (15% or below).

If you are going to use seed or nut oils, try to buy cold-pressed ones and avoid heating them. In our recipes, for instance, we drizzle small amounts of sesame oil over Asian meals after cooking them.

Q: What about red meat? I've heard it's cancer-causing.

Red meat is another one of those highly controversial foods in the nutrition world, especially when it comes to the link to cancer. Although the human race has possibly been eating red meat throughout our entire history, in recent times it has received a lot of bad press.

Some of this kerfuffle might be completely justified, but mainly because the way we keep and feed animals has changed tremendously when we compare it with what our ancestors did. The meat of an animal that is free to roam and chew on grass and other plants is obviously very different to the one that is kept in a factory, grain fed and pumped full of antibiotics and steroids to accelerate growth. A lot of meat is then processed after the animal is slaughtered, and the products are smoked, cured and treated with various chemicals. It's easy to see that not all meat is created equal and that it does not have the same effects on the same body, but unfortunately not many studies have taken this into account yet.

There's no doubt that red meat, especially if it comes from organically raised and naturally fed animals, is one of the most nutritious foods. It is full of B vitamins, vitamin E and A, CLA (conjugated linoleic acid) and omega-3 fatty acids, zinc, iron and selenium, but also creatine and carnosine, which a lot of vegetarians can be deficient in unless they supplement.

Many observational studies claim that consuming red meat is linked to an increased risk of cancer, particularly of the colon. As mentioned earlier, the problem with these studies, apart from them being 'only' observational, is that they don't distinguish between processed and unprocessed meat. A recently published meta-analysis (Alexander et al, 2014), however, established that there is very little, if any, reliable evidence to suggest that eating fresh (as opposed to processed!) red meat contributes to colorectal cancer.

This is positive news for red meat eaters, but it doesn't mean they're completely off the hook. First of all, in terms of quantities, it's prudent to follow the guidelines of the World Cancer Research Fund, which recommends a weekly intake of no more than 500g (1.1lbs) of cooked meat, which is the equivalent to about 700g (1.5lbs) raw weight. You will see in the meal plans that our red meat intake is significantly lower than this because on a ketogenic diet, protein is restricted and therefore the overconsumption of red meat (and animal products in general) is almost impossible.

It's also very important to prepare meat with some caution. Avoid cooking it until it is well done and avoid eating charred, blackened parts. Trim them away (that applies to any food, by the way, not just red meat). Prepare the meat rare or medium or make stews and slow-cooked meals instead. Grilling, unfortunately, is not one of the healthiest ways to prepare your meat. Cooking at high temperatures results in the creation of toxic chemicals such as heterocyclic amines (HCAs), which are linked to cancer. Not charring meat can help to some extent, as the blackened section is the worst in terms of HCAs. It will not completely eliminate your risk, however. For instance, when fat drips onto the heat source causing excess smoke, the smoke surrounds your food.

Along with adding that 'flame-grilled' flavour to your meat, smoke can transfer cancer-causing polycyclic aromatic hydrocarbons (PAHs). Both HCAs and PAHs are mutagenic, which means they have the potential to initiate changes in DNA that may increase cancer risk and have been found to cause cancer in animals.

If you do enjoy a BBQ from time to time, you can marinate your meat in garlic, red wine, lemon juice or olive oil to reduce HCAs (Melo et al, 2008). Herbs and spices can also have a protective effect (Schor, 2010). Make sure you flip your meat frequently to prevent it from getting burned when cooking at high heat.

Finally, fry meat in stable fats like butter, coconut oil or lard. As discussed earlier, avoid polyunsaturated fats like sunflower oil, corn oil, rapeseed oil or margarines like the plague when cooking at high temperatures. These unstable polyunsaturated fats can't withstand heat and lots of potentially toxic substances are being formed.

Q. I was told to eat little and often. How come you recommend eating only three meals a day or even less?

Anybody who is not fat adapted (i.e. used to burning fat as a main source of fuel) probably needs to eat a lot more often because they rely on sugar for generating energy. In this case, eating little and often may help stabilise blood sugar levels or other metabolic functions, as it's often claimed.

I used to be somebody who 'grazed' all day long, every two to three hours, or I would get grumpy, irritable and feel weak. But as soon as I started to adapt to ketosis, I realised that this might not have been the most suitable way for me to eat and that my body actually thrived on long breaks in between meals.

It looks like science is changing in this area of nutrition, too, and that the 'eat little and often' paradigm has started to shift. 'There are many myths and presumptions concerning diet and health, including that it is important to eat three or more meals per day on a regular basis' (Mattson et al, 2014).

You will see that as you start incorporating more fat in your diet, you might be able to wean yourself off snacks after a little while.

Q. I've heard that ketosis is a potentially life-threatening state. How come you claim that ketosis has health benefits if it's so dangerous?

When people hear the word *ketosis*, many of them immediately jump to the conclusion that you're talking about ketoacidosis, which is a completely different thing. There is still a lot of ignorance surrounding this subject, and medical textbooks for students talk about this only very briefly and, unfortunately, often with lots of factual errors. Ketoacidosis is an unstable and dangerous condition that can be potentially fatal. Ketones can rise to 8 or 12 or even up to 20 mmol/l, while blood sugars are high at the same time. In nutritional ketosis, however, ketones go up and blood sugars come down, which is the whole point of following the ketogenic diet. It's about regulating blood sugars.

In type 1 diabetes and in late-stage type 2 diabetes, as well as for alcoholics, ketoacidosis can clearly be a problem as the pancreas starts to pack it in. That's why it's very important to bear in mind that if someone has type 1 diabetes, they need to monitor their bloods very carefully until they are in established nutritional ketosis. But for those patients whose pancreas is healthy, even just a tiny amount of insulin prevents ketoacidosis.

Nutritional ketosis is not dangerous. If it was, the human race would most certainly not exist any more. We wouldn't last long without food if it weren't for the fact that we can use fat for generating energy. Claims that ketosis is an 'unnatural or unsafe metabolic state' that 'should be avoided' should look into the research that has been done into the metabolic state of breastfed babies (Cunnane and Crawford, 2003).

One reason that suggests a ketogenic metabolism is natural and desirable is that babies go into ketosis very shortly after birth and remain so while they are exclusively breastfed. Breast milk is high in fat (55% of total calories come from fat), although it contains a reasonable amount of carbohydrates (about 39%) in the form of lactose. Ketone bodies are therefore used in humans as a fuel when the brain is growing particularly fast. Babies seem to be particularly efficient at using fatty acids and turning them into ketones.

Q. But many guidelines for cancer patients recommend avoiding fat and also animal protein.

Trust us, it took us a while to get our heads around the scientific fact that fat is the safest macronutrient that a cancer patient can eat. For both of us, the low-fat paradigm was so deeply ingrained that we initially had a mental block trying to increase fat intake. And we know we're not the only ones!

Digging into the work carried out by reputable scientists who don't have any vested interests certainly helped, and for me the penny definitely dropped when listening to Craig Thompson, CEO of Memorial Sloan Cancer Center in New York. In his YouTube video 'How Do People Get Cancer', he clearly states, 'It matters where your calories come from. If you overfeed somebody with fat, you don't increase their cancer risk at all. If you overfeed somebody with carbohydrates, you dramatically increase their cancer risk. And protein is halfway in between.'

Surprising, isn't it? But wait, what about the protein issue? He's implying it's still a risk factor. Well, here goes some more myth-busting. Protein intake is a tricky one. On the one hand, many bodily functions and the immune system in particular rely on amino acids, the building blocks of proteins. On the other hand, research shows that high levels of insulin-like growth factor 1 (IGF-1) can increase cancer risk. Lower protein consumption decreases IGF-1.

What we also know is that many tumours use glutamine, a type of amino acid, as a fuel alongside glucose. Casein is another amino acid that has potential cancer-promoting properties, which is why some people prefer to avoid or limit dairy. The evidence for cutting out dairy completely is not solid enough, however, and I recommend having small amounts of good-quality dairy unless you have an intolerance. If you want to be safe, focus on organic, grass-fed dairy products with little protein. Products that fall into this category include cream, cream cheese, crème fraîche and full-fat natural Greek yoghurt. Another good option is to opt for goat and sheep products.

Last but not least, excess consumption of protein can lead to gluconeogenesis, the production of glucose from amino acids and other substrates, which pushes up glucose levels.

To sum up, a sensible approach is to consume moderate amounts of protein without compromising immune and other functions in the body.

Q. Is soy safe for breast cancer patients?

One question that comes up over and over again, especially because it's a food low in carbohydrates, is whether soy is safe for breast cancer patients. There is certainly a lot of confusing information about the topic. Some sources claim that soy has adverse effects on cancer patients, whereas others tout its benefits.

Soy foods contain isoflavones, a phytoestrogen, which have both anti-oestrogenic and oestrogen-like properties. What causes the most confusion and controversy is that many studies have shown that isoflavones may protect against breast cancer development in the initial stages. However, in a few laboratory studies, certain isoflavone components of soy have been able to enhance the growth of breast cancer cells in select doses. In rats, soy isoflavones have been able to both promote and inhibit mammary tumour growth.

Confusing, right? So what do the results of these studies mean in practice?

Looking at the current evidence, there are three solid epidemiologic studies that report no adverse effects of soy foods on the prognosis of breast cancer. The most recent dates from 2011 (called Women's Healthy Eating and Living, or WHEL), and it was used to examine the effect of soy intake on breast cancer prognosis in 3,088 breast cancer survivors (Caan et al, 2011).

The women in this study were early-stage breast cancer patients who were followed for an average of 7.3 years. First, soy isoflavone intakes were measured after the diagnosis with a food frequency questionnaire and the association between soy intake and breast cancer recurrence and/or death was then tracked. Results showed that as soy isoflavone intake increased, the risk of death decreased. Women at the highest levels of soy isoflavone intake (> 16.3mg isoflavones per day) had a 54% reduction in the risk of death.

The other two studies report no adverse effects of soy foods on the prognosis of breast cancer. In 2009, some clarity began to emerge for breast cancer patients. One study in Asian women (the Shanghai Breast Cancer Survival Study) and the other in US women (the Life after Cancer Epidemiology Study, or LACE) both suggest that soy-containing foods do not negatively affect breast cancer prognosis. It's important to note that such foods do not counteract the effect of the breast cancer drug tamoxifen and may in fact provide potential benefits in decreasing the risk of recurrence or death from breast cancer.

Based on the results of these three studies, you should be reassured of the safety of soy consumption if you're facing a breast cancer diagnosis and that there is benefit in one serving per day for you. But I can't emphasise enough that the quality of soy foods needs to be high and that organic and non-GMO are preferable. Also, please bear in mind that although soy has a range of good health benefits, particularly for bones and cardiovascular health, in sensitive people it can cause digestive, skin and other issues. In such cases, as with any other food, it's important to avoid soy.

Q. I've heard that it's really important to have a good acid–alkaline balance in my body. Some experts also claim that cancer can't grow in an acidic environment. If I severely restrict carbohydrates, I have to limit my fruit and vegetable intake, which helps alkalising my body. Can this not cause problems?

Foods leave an acid or alkaline ash behind. What type of ash this is depends on acid-forming components (e.g. phosphate and sulphur) or alkalis (e.g. calcium, magnesium and potassium). Very generally speaking, animal products and grains are acid forming, whereas fruit and vegetables are alkali forming. Pure fats, sugars and starches are neutral because they contain neither protein, sulphur nor minerals.

Foods we eat have the power to change the pH of our urine and it's very easy to measure this. This might be one of the reasons why so-called alkalising diets have become so popular: because people can see what impact their food choices have on their urine pH.

It is a myth, however, that we can change the pH of our blood by changing the foods we eat or that acidic blood causes disease while alkaline blood keeps us healthy. The body tightly regulates the pH or our blood and extracellular fluid (7.35–7.45) regardless of what we eat or what our urine pH is.

There are a few exceptions. Sodium bicarbonate (also called baking soda), for instance, can temporarily increase blood pH. It is being used by many cancer patients to 'alkalise the body'. However, it needs to be used with caution because excessive and prolonged use can be unsafe. Many people who try sodium bicarbonate based on anecdotal evidence complain about bloating and other digestive discomfort. This could be due to changes in stomach acidity, which can interfere with digestion of protein in particular. Pre-clinical studies are underway to develop methods that monitor changes in acid content of tumours following treatment with sodium bicarbonate.

And, as we already saw, a state of acidosis (acid overload in the body) can happen when ketone bodies rise too quickly and too high, but it can also be caused by chronic renal insufficiency, for instance.

The kidneys are the ultimate regulator of blood pH in a sustainable cycle. For example, when we digest food, the acids that are produced are quickly buffered (neutralised) by bicarbonate ions in the blood. This reaction leads to the production of carbon dioxide (exhaled through the lungs) and salts, which are excreted by the kidneys. During the process of getting rid of these salts, the kidneys produce 'new' bicarbonate ions that then replace the bicarbonate that was initially used to buffer the acid.

Claims have been made with regards to bone health and alkaline diets. The theory of proponents is that blood pH is kept in a tight range by pulling minerals from bones to neutralise any excess acid from the diet. However, this 'acid ash hypothesis of osteoporosis' has been debunked by both clinical trials and observational studies (Bonjour, 2013). As we've explained, the kidneys are perfectly capable of dealing with the 'acid ash' from food without any involvement from the bones.

We've seen that our food choices can't substantially change the pH of the blood and extracellular fluid. The claim that alkaline diets can cure cancer is nothing more than that: a claim without any scientific basis. Cancer cells have also been shown to be perfectly capable of originating in a slightly alkaline environment of 7.4, which is the pH of normal body tissue (Martinez-Zaguilan et al, 1996).

You often also hear that cancer cells grow and metastasise better in an acidic environment, which is true. But we know that cancer cells use fermentation to generate energy and that this process creates a by-product called lactic acid, which, of course, is acidic. Hence, the causality is reversed: it's not an acidic environment that causes cancer, it's the cancer that causes the acidic environment.

To sum up, I quote Dominic D'Agostino, PhD, Assistant Professor at the University of South Florida, who stated in Ellen Davis's e-book *Fight Cancer with a Ketogenic Diet*, 'An alkaline diet can't hurt, but it won't do much to restore defective cancer cell metabolism or even change the tumour microenvironment.'

Adding alkaline foods to the diet usually means adding more fruit and vegetables, which increases carbohydrate content in the diet. Our advice is to include green leafy and other vegetables as much as you can within your carbohydrate allowance when following a ketogenic diet. If following a low-carb diet, you can certainly incorporate more vegetables and lower-carb fruits (like strawberries and blueberries, but not overeating bananas, for example), but remain conscious of quantities.

Q. Similar to the question above, I also want to make sure I have enough antioxidants in my diet, which also come from fruit and vegetables. Where do antioxidants come from on a ketogenic diet?

Many people are concerned that by cutting back on plant foods, they also reduce their body's ability to deal with oxidative stress. In our cells, oxidative stress can create molecules called reactive oxygen species (ROS), also called free radicals. These can damage internal cellular structures but also our genetic material. We're constantly under attack from free radicals produced by our environment, but they're also the by-product of normal cellular respiration.

That's where antioxidants come on the scene. They are chemicals – contained in antioxidant-rich foods, for instance – that are capable of repairing or preventing oxidative damage in the body. But if inflammation is present, large amounts of ROS are produced that will eventually overwhelm the cell's antioxidant defences and cause damage.

Food choices are closely linked to these processes. A diet high in foods that constantly increase glucose and insulin (i.e. carbohydrates and excessive amounts of protein) in the bloodstream leads to increased ROS and inflammation caused by AGEs (advanced glycation end products). Typically, a healthy individual has less than a teaspoon of sugar dissolved in the bloodstream at any given time, so you can imagine what happens in the body when a sugary soft drink containing 10 teaspoons of sugar is consumed.

On a well-designed ketogenic diet, where glucose and insulin levels are at a low, steady level, the risk of inflammation is reduced. Also, the presence of fat-derived ketone bodies in the mitochondria prevents reactive oxygen species (ROS) production (Youm et al, 2015) and makes energy production more effective.

As you can see, a ketogenic diet reduces oxidative stress, and as always, the compounded effect of your overall diet is what really counts. But of course it's a good idea to incorporate antioxidant-rich foods into the ketogenic diet, such as green leafy and rainbow-coloured vegetables, sulphur-rich foods and nuts, but also nutrient-dense animal foods like grass-fed lamb or chicken liver. Plants don't necessarily have higher amounts of vitamins and minerals. In fact, Mathieu Lalonde, PhD, an organic chemist from Harvard University, has made a ranking of various foods according to their vitamin, mineral and other essential nutrient density and has clearly shown that organ meats/oils, herbs and spices, cacao, fish and other animal products like eggs and meat outrank fruit and vegetables. Of course, we have to put this into perspective because plants contain nutrients (called phytonutrients) that aren't necessarily essential but have been proven to be extremely beneficial for health. But still, it's a good demonstration that good-quality animal foods can and should have their place in a well-formulated low-carb and ketogenic diet, even if it's 'only' in the form of eggs and oily fish, maybe with the addition of some organ meat.

There is no doubt that certain dietary regimes are the consequence of the environment we live in and that this also has an impact on our gene expression, as we discussed earlier. Again, your body usually gives you clear signs if you tune in. For the majority of us, it's beneficial to have a healthy mix of plant- and animal-based foods and to focus on quality.

Introduction to the meal plans

The reason we present such detailed meal plans with nutritional info and instructions doesn't mean that we like obsessing over numbers or bossing you around (well, okay, we *can* be bossy sometimes). This approach draws on Patricia's extensive experience working with clients, which has shown that most people need very clear guidance, at least in the initial stages of implementing a ketogenic diet, and lots of recipes to try.

Of course, these meal plans need to be tailored to an individual's unique needs – height, ideal weight, activity levels, stage of recovery – and also take account of the level of support from family and friends. That's why the meal plans here will apply to some but not all people and may need a few tweaks for some of you.

Meal plans need to be realistic too, so another important factor we've considered is how to use leftovers from dinner to make simple lunches so that you can avoid cooking three meals a day from scratch. You'll see that we tell you in advance if certain ingredients or meals are being used again for another day or need to be frozen. We try to keep things as simple as possible, and we're particularly fond of recipes with the instructions 'put in a blender and whizz'! We know you're busy, be it with work, feeding a family, treatment, hobbies or, like us, juggling all of the above as best you can.

We do warn you, though, that until you get the hang of this new way of eating, you will definitely be spending more time in the kitchen. The recipes might be very different to what you're used to and you will cook almost everything from scratch. And to really optimise nutrient intake and ensure the best-quality produce, we don't advocate using ready-made meals, even though some of them might be keto friendly. The meal plans and calculated recipes will take a ton of work off your plate, but you still need to do the shopping and cooking yourself (or some willing minion, if you're lucky to have one about the place!).

It's important to understand that a ketogenic diet isn't just another dietary approach like going on a gluten-free diet or becoming a vegetarian. It is metabolic therapy, and like any other therapeutic approach, it can come with its own challenges and side effects. Many of those occur when blood glucose levels remain high, whether as a result of consuming too many carbs, protein or excessive calories. There is quite a bit of controversy going on about calories, though. Some weight loss experts claim that they're crucial, while others argue they are totally irrelevant. In my experience, we have to aim for something in between: not obsessing about calories, but certainly not totally ignoring them, especially if weight management is a challenge (whether it's to lose or gain weight). This is the case with many cancer patients.

According to Dr Thomas Seyfried (Meidenbauer, Nathan and Seyfried, 2014), excessive calorie consumption on a ketogenic diet for prolonged periods of time can lead to insulin insensitivity, elevated blood glucose and dyslipidemia (e.g. high LDL and low HDL cholesterol). In my experience, the important thing is to shift the focus from quantity to the *quality* of calories that come from unprocessed, whole, nutrient-dense foods. It is very rare that somebody who follows a well-designed and monitored ketogenic diet consumes too many calories.

For all the above reasons, we give the following exact nutritional information for every single meal:

- Net carbs (= total carbs – fibre)
- Protein
- Fat
- Fibre (for anybody who wants to count total carbs, you just add fibre back to net carbs)
- Calories

Giving this detailed information will allow you to design your own meal plans with all your favourite recipes.

To make it easier to go into ketosis, we recommend that you get prepared by spending a morning or two in the kitchen. This is how we usually do it:

- Check the meal plans and make, say, some kale crackers (page 268), zucchini crackers (page 294 and also a bread or two. Cut them into the portion size we suggest in the recipes and freeze them in batches.
- Pestos, pâtés or guacamoles are also easy to freeze and can be a quick snack or lunch if you're stuck.
- In the initial stages, having some treats to hand can be really helpful. You might get strong carbohydrate and sugar cravings at the beginning when your body adapts, but if you have something to hand that is keto friendly, you will sail through these phases. Try the lemon keto bombs, white chocolate cheesecake or any of the treats on pages 208–220.

And now, you should be ready to get started.

References

Abdelwahab, M.G. et al (2012) 'The ketogenic diet is an effective adjuvant to radiation therapy for the treatment of malignant glioma', *PLoS One*, 7(5), p. e36197.

Alexander, D.D. et al (2014) 'Red meat and colorectal cancer: A quantitative update on the state of the epidemiologic science', *Journal of the American College of Nutrition*, 5, pp. 1–23.

Allen, B.G. et al (2013) 'Ketogenic diets enhance oxidative stress and radio-chemo-therapy responses in lung cancer xenografts', *Clinical Cancer Research*, 19(14), pp. 3,905–3,913.

Ancelin, M.L. et al (2010) 'Gender and genotype modulation of the association between lipid levels and depressive symptomatology in community-dwelling elderly (the ESPRIT study)', *Biological Psychiatry*, 68(2), pp. 125–132.

Aykin-Burns, N. et al (2009) 'Increased levels of superoxide and H2O2 mediate the differential susceptibility of cancer cells versus normal cells to glucose deprivation', *Biochemical Journal*, 418, pp. 29–37.

BMJ (2013) 'Study raises questions about dietary fats and heart disease guidance', press release, 4 February, available online at: www.bmj.com/press-releases/2013/02/04/study-raises-questions-about-dietary-fats-and-heart-disease-guidance.

Bonjour, J.P. (2013) 'Nutritional disturbance in acid-base balance and osteoporosis: A hypothesis that disregards the essential homeostatic role of the kidney', *British Journal of Nutrition*, 110(7), pp. 1,168–1,177.

Caan, B.J. et al (2011) 'Soy food consumption and breast cancer prognosis', *Cancer Epidemiology, Biomarkers & Prevention*, 20(5), pp. 854–858.

Champ, C.E. et al (2012) 'Weight gain, metabolic syndrome, and breast cancer recurrence: Are dietary recommendations supported by the data?', *International Journal of Breast Cancer*, 2012.

Champ, C.E. et al (2014) 'Targeting metabolism with a ketogenic diet during the treatment of glioblastoma multiforme', *Journal of Neuro-Oncology*, 117(1), pp. 125–131.

Coussens, L.M. and Werb, Z. (2002) 'Inflammation and cancer', *Nature*, Dec 19–26, 420(6,917), pp. 860–867.

Cunnane, S.C. and Crawford, M.A. (2003) 'Survival of the fattest: Fat babies were the key to evolution of the large human brain', *Comparative Biochemistry and Physiology*, Part A, 136, pp. 17–26.

Davis, E. (2013) 'Fight cancer with a ketogenic diet', available online at www.ketogenic-diet-resource.com.

Derr, R.L. et al (2009) 'Association between hyperglycemia and survival in patients with newly diagnosed glioblastoma', *Journal of Clinical Oncology*, 27, pp. 1,082–1,086.

Fine, E.J. et al (2012) 'Targeting insulin inhibition as a metabolic therapy in advanced cancer: A pilot safety and feasibility dietary trial in 10 patients', Nutrition, 28(10), pp. 1,028–1,035.

Goodwin, P.J. et al (2012) 'Insulin- and obesity-related variables in early-stage breast cancer: Correlations and time course of prognostic associations', Journal of Clinical Oncology, 30(2), pp. 164–171.

Groesbeck, D.K., Bluml, R.M. and Kossoff, E.H. (2006) 'Long-term use of the ketogenic diet in the treatment of epilepsy', Developmental Medicine and Child Neurology, 48, pp. 978–981.

Hamanaka, R.B. and Chandel, N.S. (2012) 'Targeting glucose metabolism for cancer therapy', Journal of Experimental Medicine, 209(2), pp. 211–215.

Hanahan, D. and Weinberg, P.A. (2011) 'Hallmarks of cancer: The next generation', Cell, 144(5), pp. 646–674.

Ho, V.W. et al (2011) 'A low carbohydrate, high protein diet slows tumor growth and prevents cancer initiation', Cancer Research, 71(13), pp. 4,484–4,493.

Hsu, P.P. and Sabatini, D.M. (2008) 'Cancer cell metabolism: Warburg and beyond', Cell, 134(5), pp. 703–707.

Hu, J. et al (2012), 'Glycemic index, glycemic load and cancer risk', Annals of Oncology, 24(1), pp. 245–251.

Kalamian, M. (2014), 'Get started with the ketogenic diet for cancer', available online on www.dietarytherapies.com.

Klement, R.J. (2013) 'Calorie or carbohydrate restriction? The ketogenic diet as another option for supportive cancer treatment', Oncologist, 18(9), pp. 1,056.

Klement, R.J. and Champ, C.E. (2014) 'Calories, carbohydrates, and cancer therapy with radiation: Exploiting the five R's through dietary manipulation', Cancer Metastasis Review, 33(1), pp. 217–229.

Klement, R.J. and Kaemmerer, U. (2011) 'Is there a role for carbohydrate restriction in the treatment and prevention of cancer?', Nutrition & Metabolism, 8(75), pp. 1–16.

Kossoff, E.H. et al (2009) 'Optimal clinical management of children receiving the ketogenic diet: Recommendations of the International Ketogenic Diet Study Group', Epilepsia, 50(2), pp. 304–317.

Mabuchi, H. et al (2002) 'Large-scale cohort study of the relationship between serum cholesterol concentration and coronary events with low-dose simvastatin therapy in Japanese patients with hypercholesterolemia', Circulation Journal, 66(12), pp. 1,087–1,095.

Martinez-Carpio, P.A. et al (2009) 'Relation between cholesterol levels and neuropsychiatric disorders', Revue Neurologique, 48(5), pp. 261–264.

Martinez-Zaguilan, R. et al (1996) 'Acidic pH enhances the invasive behavior of human melanoma cells', Clinical & Experimental Metastasis, 14(2), pp. 176–186.

Mattson, M.P. et al (2014) 'Meal frequency and timing in health and disease', Proceedings of the National Academy of Sciences of the United States of America, 111(47), pp. 16,647–16,653.

Maurer, G.B. et al (2011) 'Differential utilization of ketone bodies by neurons and glioma cell lines: A rationale for ketogenic diet as experimental glioma therapy', BMC Cancer, 11(315), pp. 1–17.

Meidenbauer, J.J., Nathan, T. and Seyfried, T.N. (2014) 'Influence of a ketogenic diet, fish-oil, and calorie restriction on plasma metabolites and lipids in C57BL/6J mice', Nutrition & Metabolism, 11, p. 23.

Melo, A. et al (2008) 'Effect of beer/red wine marinades on the formation of heterocyclic aromatic amines in pan-fried beef', Journal of Agricultural and Food Chemistry, 56(22), pp. 10,625–10,632.

Ness, G.C. and Chambers, C.M. (2000) 'Feedback and hormonal regulation of hepatic 3-hydroxy-3-methylglutaryl coenzyme A reductase: The concept of cholesterol buffering capacity', Proceedings of the Society for Experimental Biology and Medicine, 224(1), pp. 8–19.

Paoli, A., Rubini, A., Volek, J.S. and Grimaldi, K.A. (2013) 'Beyond weight loss: A review of therapeutic uses of very-low-carbohydrate (ketogenic) diets', European Journal of Clinical Nutrition, 67, pp. 789–796.

Poff, A.M., Ari, C., Seyfried, T.N. and D'Agostino, D.P. (2013) 'The ketogenic diet and hyperbaric oxygen therapy prolong survival in mice with systemic metastatic cancer', PLoS One, 8(6), pp. 1–9.

Schor, J. (2010) 'Marinades reduce heterocyclic amines from primitive food preparation techniques', Natural Medicine Journal, 2(7).

Seyfried, T. and Shelton, L. (2010) 'Cancer as a metabolic disease', Nutrition & Metabolism, 7(7), pp. 1–22.

Seyfried, T.N. (2012) Cancer as a Metabolic Disease: On the Origin, Management, and Prevention of Cancer. New Jersey: John Wiley & Sons.

Seyfried, T.N. (2015) 'Cancer as a mitochondrial metabolic disease', Frontiers in Cell Development and Biology, 3(43).

Warburg, O., Wind, F. and Negelein, E. (1927) 'The metabolism of tumours in the body', Journal of General Physiology, 8, pp. 519–530.

Westman, E.C., Mavropoulos, J., Yancy, W.S. and Volek, J.S. (2003) 'A review of low-carbohydrate ketogenic diets', Current Atherosclerosis Reports, 5, pp. 476–483.

Youm, Y.H. et al (2015) 'The ketone metabolite-hydroxybutyrate blocks NLRP3 inflammasome-mediated inflammatory disease', Nature Medicine, 21(3), pp. 263–269.

Patricia Daly
My story

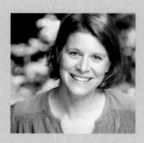

It was an ordinary morning in the office of the Bank of Ireland on a warm summer's day in July 2008. *Almost* ordinary, I'd say, because I had this odd flickering in the corner of my right eye that seemed to be determined to stay there, day and night, even when I closed my eyes. Initially I didn't give it much thought, but because I'd had some temporary loss of vision for a good while the previous evening, I finally decided to pick up the phone and call an optician.

When I described my symptoms to the assistant who answered, I was told to make my way to their practice immediately. I got a bit concerned because in Ireland, it can sometimes take forever to get a doctor's, consultant's or any appointment.

I left work and cycled over to the optician. Then everything happened very quickly. As soon as the optician looked at the back of my dilated eye, I knew something wasn't right. Apparently, I had a detached retina that needed to be operated on immediately, which is why I was referred to one of the top ophthalmic surgeons in the country. A few hours later, I sat on a chair enduring more gruesome eye tests. Finally, I was told that yes, I did indeed have a detached retina, but that wasn't all. It was detached because a large tumour was growing underneath it – a melanoma.

To be honest, at the time I was not very well versed in medical language and I didn't realise straight away that I was dealing with a cancer diagnosis. I guess it was a mix of denial and ignorance.

Because my type of tumour was still very rare in Ireland at the time, I had to get treatment abroad. We travelled to Liverpool in the UK three weeks later, where I went through eye surgery twice within four days and had radiotherapy.

One of the key moments during this time – and probably one of the key moments in my life – was when I asked my consultant if there was anything I could do to recover from surgery and treatment, to feel better and to protect myself from a possible relapse. He looked at me with a mix of slight bemusement, pity and impatience. 'No, there's nothing you can do apart from taking it easy for a little while and then get back to your old life.'

Now, this answer totally piqued my curiosity. Did I really want to go back to the same lifestyle that had got me where I was now, with cancer at the age of 28? Don't get me wrong – I was never filled with guilt and I never beat myself up that I had brought cancer upon myself or anything like that – but deep down I knew that it was time for a change.

This is when my journey started, a journey of learning more about myself and of researching everything that had to do with cancer, nutrition, the mind–body link and other lifestyle aspects. So in a way, I thank my consultant for his answer because ultimately it pushed me into taking action myself.

Just four weeks after finishing my treatments, I started to study nutritional therapy. Initially this was with a view to supporting myself, but very quickly I realised that my life really had been turned upside down. I tried to go back to work in the bank about two weeks after returning from the UK, with disastrous results. Working on a computer screen for longer than 15 minutes proved to be impossible and resulted in vomiting and headaches.

I had to seriously think about a new job that would take the pressure off my eyes and an office job didn't seem to be the right choice any more. That's when I started to study even harder – by recording all the study material so that I wouldn't put any strain on my eye – because I felt that becoming a nutritional therapist wasn't just a way to help myself, it was also an amazing opportunity to build a new career that I was genuinely passionate about.

About eight months after my treatments, I got pregnant and a beautiful baby girl was born in November 2009. My life was great: a new baby, a loving partner, we had just moved house and I had a new career perspective. But then my old symptoms returned; my baby was just two months old when I went for check-ups. I voiced my concerns over the flickering in my eye, the floaters and the fatigue, but the scans were clear and I thought it was probably just the tiredness that motherhood brings.

I left the hospital with a bad feeling that something was terribly wrong. At that stage, I was so in tune with my body that I knew I could trust myself more than a scan. And four months later, my worst nightmare came true: another set of scans confirmed that the tumour had doubled in size and was growing aggressively. I was shocked and a lot more shaken than when I had initially been diagnosed.

More surgery and strong external radiotherapy had to be performed immediately. I was told that because the tumour had moved so close to the optic nerve, I would lose the sight in my right eye within 12 to 18 months of finishing treatments.

I went through radiotherapy while feeding my six-month-old baby and everything felt like defeat. Although I had worked hard, educated myself and had made a lot of lifestyle changes, I found myself in the same place as I had been 18 months before, but this time with a baby in tow.

I felt that I had done everything I could, including dietary adjustments. My diet was full of healthy whole grains, lots of fruit and vegetables, juices and smoothies; I ate oily fish and hardly any meat; and I had replaced all sugars in my treats with dried fruit. In April 2012, when my second baby was eight months old, I was struggling with a lot of side effects from the radiotherapy and surgery. I had developed radiotherapy-related retinopathy and there was lots of swelling in the eye. On top of everything else, I had to learn to adjust to major sight loss. My consultant told me that I was at risk of developing more serious conditions and eventually losing my eye itself, not just the sight. The one option I had was to try Avastin injections to stop excessive blood vessel growth, and if that didn't work, we'd have to consider removing the eyeball.

But I wasn't prepared to give up just yet. I asked for a grace period of a few weeks and went back to researching more frantically than ever. And this is when I came across the emerging concept of cancer as a metabolic disease. I read studies conducted by a German researcher, Dr Johannes Coy, showing that most cancer cells rely heavily on glucose for generating energy and promoting growth. The suggested therapy to cut off this constant supply of sugar to the tumour was a radical dietary change: adopting a so-called ketogenic diet.

It sounded very counterintuitive to me initially: I had to start cutting down on carbohydrates. I'm not just talking about white pasta, bread, rice, cakes and biscuits. This also included whole and gluten-free grains like my beloved millet, quinoa or buckwheat. To compensate, I had to increase my fat intake drastically to 75–80% of total daily calorie intake. I started to eat avocados, olives, oily fish, duck and other fatty meats, and treats made with coconut oil and cacao butter. Getting my head around it wasn't easy in the initial stages, even though I was almost a fully qualified nutritional therapist at that stage.

I had nothing to lose. According to studies, it was safe to follow a diet that had been used for epileptic patients for a long time, and if it didn't have any effects, at least I could reassure myself that I had tried everything to save my eye.

Admittedly, at the beginning it felt really odd to eat that much fat after being 'low-fat' for all my life, especially saturated animal fat; thank goodness this myth has been largely debunked, along with many others. For me, turning the food pyramid upside down (with the very top chopped off, of course) was radical, but the results were astonishing. At my next check-up a few weeks later, my consultant said that the inside of my eye looked like 'the calm after a big storm'. My eyesight had also started to come back. He said that if this development continued, I might move myself out of the danger zone and could possibly save my eye.

Ever since then, my eye has been stable. Five years after treatment, I still have my eyesight and I've regained my health in general. My energy is great and my digestion and hormones have finally settled, which makes my skin glow. And my tumour hasn't grown back.

In the past two years, I've guided many cancer patients through the implementation of a ketogenic diet. The nutrition world is changing fast, governments are finally starting to change their food pyramids and oncologists are now getting interested in how nutrition can support their work.

Although research into nutrition is and will remain challenging, I'm hopeful that we will get more and more clear on how to use food as an invaluable tool in the support of cancer patients and people affected by chronic illness in general.

I'm a big fan of using evidence-based information and I research everything before making recommendations. But there is one big lesson that I've learned on my journey: despite all the modern technology and science, we mustn't forget our own inner wisdom and intuition. I will never forget the day when all my scans were clear but my inner voice told me that my tumour was growing again. A client of mine who had a similar experience couldn't have said it better: 'My oncologist is a body of knowledge, but I have knowledge of my body.'

It is now my greatest passion – and privilege – to support and guide clients on how to safely combine science with their own intuition and experience so they can become as healthy as possible, whether or not they are living with cancer. And it is my hope that this book will inspire many of you to become as healthy as you can be, too.

– Patricia Daly 2016

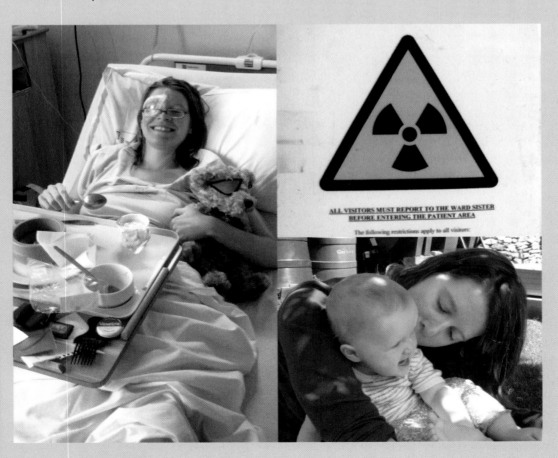

Meal Plan for Week 1 Day 1

RECIPE	QUANTITY		CALORIES	CARBS	PROTEIN	FAT
BREAKFAST						
Berry smoothie	433g		526	13.0g	21.0g	42.0g
		Meal total:	526	13.0g	21.0g	42.0g
LUNCH						
Turkey lettuce wrap	341g		595	8.0g	21.0g	51.0g
Avocado with lime	57g		150	0.9g	0.9g	15.3g
		Meal total:	745	8.9g	21.9g	66.3g
DINNER						
Zucchini and sweet potato frittata	326g		367	18.7g	16.5g	24.0g
Vegan superfood salad	168g		288	5.6g	7.1g	25.0g
		Meal total:	655	24.3g	23.6g	49.0g
PLAN TOTAL:			1,926	46.2g	66.5g	157.3g

Macronutrient Analysis

	CARBOHYDRATE	PROTEIN	FAT	ALCOHOL
INTAKE	46.2g	66.5g	157.3g	0g
	9% carbs	**15% protein**	**76% fat**	

Although they're not a whole food, high-quality protein powders can be a useful and quite often necessary addition to a ketogenic regime. It's not only a handy way to add protein to smoothies, like in this recipe, that is easy to calculate, but it's also incredibly practical for patients who need to (temporarily) increase their intake to support healing.

There are tons of different products on the market, but do make sure you only buy the best quality. In our book, we mostly use Nuzest because it is a very pure form of protein and available in many countries, but I do like to use different kinds of protein powders and rotate them during the week. I also use pure hemp or pea protein, which is a bit higher in carbs, though. Always check the label for sugar and 'nasty' ingredients and fillers.

A note on whey protein: I recommend that cancer patients steer away from whey protein unless it's incredibly pure (whey concentrate rather than isolate), hormone-free and preferably without the addition of IgG immunoglobulins, which I never supplement. Glutamine content tends to be higher, too, which is also a concern.

Put all the ingredients into a blender and whizz to combine.

Berry smoothie

2 handfuls of blueberries (48g)
10 raspberries (40g)
2 medium strawberries, hulled (52g)
125ml (½c) full-fat coconut milk (125g)
125ml (½c) water (125g)
1 scant scoop of protein powder (vanilla or natural) (20g)
9g (0.3 oz) coconut oil (9g)
1 tsp hazelnut butter (14g)

Serves 1

PER PORTION

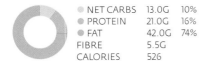

NET CARBS	13.0G	10%
PROTEIN	21.0G	16%
FAT	42.0G	74%
FIBRE	5.5G	
CALORIES	526	

Turkey lettuce wrap

Use your imagination and taste buds to create your favourite lettuce wrap. You can use any kind of leftovers, pâtés, guacamole or tapenade to add more flavour.

8 thin slices of roast turkey (80g)

8 large lettuce leaves (192g)

8 handfuls of spinach (80g)

110g (3.9 oz) sliced cucumber (110g)

8 strips of red pepper (64g)

8 tbsp red hemp pesto (see below) (156g)

Serves 2

Put a slice of turkey on each of the lettuce leaves. Add the spinach, cucumber, pepper and pesto and wrap it up.

PER PORTION

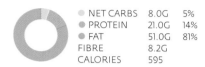

● NET CARBS	8.0G	5%
● PROTEIN	21.0G	14%
● FAT	51.0G	81%
FIBRE	8.2G	
CALORIES	595	

Red hemp pesto

This pesto is a firm favourite in our house and goes with almost anything. It's particularly handy for those who are looking for a dairy-free version of pesto. It freezes really well, so I always make a double batch. We will be using this pesto in other recipes throughout this book, so keep it in handy portions in the freezer.

120g (4.2 oz) sun-dried tomatoes, soaked (120g)

20g (0.7 oz) basil (20g)

120ml (½c) extra virgin olive oil (120g)

2 heaped tbsp shelled hemp seeds (30g)

1 tbsp balsamic vinegar (10g)

½ tsp cayenne pepper (1g)

½ tsp rock salt (3g)

Serves 6

Put all the ingredients into a blender and whizz to combine. Spoon into a clean glass jar, top with a thin film of olive oil and store in the fridge for up to five days.

PER PORTION

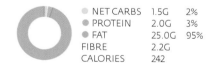

● NET CARBS	1.5G	2%
● PROTEIN	2.0G	3%
● FAT	25.0G	95%
FIBRE	2.2G	
CALORIES	242	

Arrange the avocado slices on a plate. Sprinkle with the olive oil, squeeze the lime over it and season to taste.

PER PORTION

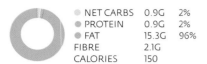

NET CARBS	0.9G	2%
PROTEIN	0.9G	2%
FAT	15.3G	96%
FIBRE	2.1G	
CALORIES	150	

Avocado with lime

90g (3.2 oz) avocado, thinly sliced (90g)
1 tbsp extra virgin olive oil (13g)
2 tsp lime juice (10g)
Salt and pepper (3g)

Serves 2

We're often asked about sweet potatoes and how they fit into a ketogenic meal plan. As you can see, they quickly add carbs to a meal but can be used in small amounts in the initial stages. They can also be useful for chemotherapy patients who suffer from nausea and have a craving for white potatoes. There's also a recipe for sweet potato chips on page 428.

Melt the butter in a large frying pan and caramelise the onion on a low heat for about 30 minutes.

Meanwhile, lightly steam the zucchinis and sweet potato for about 10 minutes.

Whisk the eggs in a bowl and add the olives, crushed garlic, rosemary, salt and pepper. When the vegetables are soft, add the egg mix, sweet potatoes and zucchinis to the pan and cook everything on a low to medium heat for about 15 minutes. You can finish off the frittata in the oven if you prefer a golden brown crust.

Zucchini and sweet potato frittata

60g (4tbsp) butter (60g)
1 large red onion, chopped (240g)
2 zucchinis, sliced (300g)
1 medium sweet potato, sliced (238g)
8 eggs (400g)
50g (1.8 oz) Kalamata olives (50g)
3 garlic cloves, crushed (9g)
1 tsp dried rosemary (1g)
Salt and pepper (3g)

Serves 4

PER PORTION

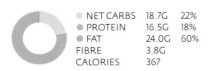

NET CARBS	18.7G	22%
PROTEIN	16.5G	18%
FAT	24.0G	60%
FIBRE	3.8G	
CALORIES	367	

Vegan superfood salad

14 cherry tomatoes, halved (168g)
80g (2.8 oz) scallions, chopped (80g)
40g (1.4 oz) mint, chopped (40g)
40g (1.4 oz) parsley, chopped (40g)
60g (2.1 oz) arugula (60g)
4 broccoli florets, steamed or
    blanched (132g)
2 handfuls of whole blanched
    almonds (40g)
4 tbsp sunflower seeds (40g)
Juice of 1 lemon (40g)
4 tbsp avocado oil (56g)

Serves 4

Vegans eat absolutely no animal or animal-derived products – no meat, fish, dairy, honey or eggs. It's possible to follow a vegan ketogenic diet, but it's not something I recommend. Unless it's for very strong ethical reasons and there is absolutely no way I can get somebody to eat animal products, I suggest at least having eggs and some oily fish, but ideally also meat in the form of organ meat.

My main problem with veganism – and I speak from experience! – is that it can lead to nutrient deficiencies, especially vitamin B12, iron, omega-3 fatty acids and vitamin D to some extent too. A vegan diet needs to be carefully designed, supplemented with nutrients and monitored. There can be health benefits of a vegan diet if it's well planned, but we don't know whether they are due to the elimination of 'harmful ingredients'. A lot of people who turn to veganism from a very processed diet also tend to start to eat a lot cleaner, and they don't have as much refined sugar or trans fats. While this is definitely positive, the question remains whether people who benefit from vegan diets feel better because they eliminate processed foods or because they avoid animal products. In my clinical experience, the consumption of animal fat and protein clearly accelerates recovery after treatment in most cancer patients – if they tolerate those foods well, of course.

You will need a lot of these same ingredients for lunch on Day 2, so you can save time in the morning by preparing everything now.

Mix the tomatoes and scallions together, then add the mint and parsley. Toss with the arugula and place in a bowl. Add the cooked broccoli to the salad, then mix with the almonds and seeds. Squeeze the lemon juice over it and drizzle everything with the oil.

PER PORTION

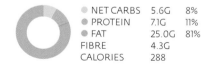

● NET CARBS	5.6G	8%
● PROTEIN	7.1G	11%
● FAT	25.0G	81%
FIBRE	4.3G	
CALORIES	288	

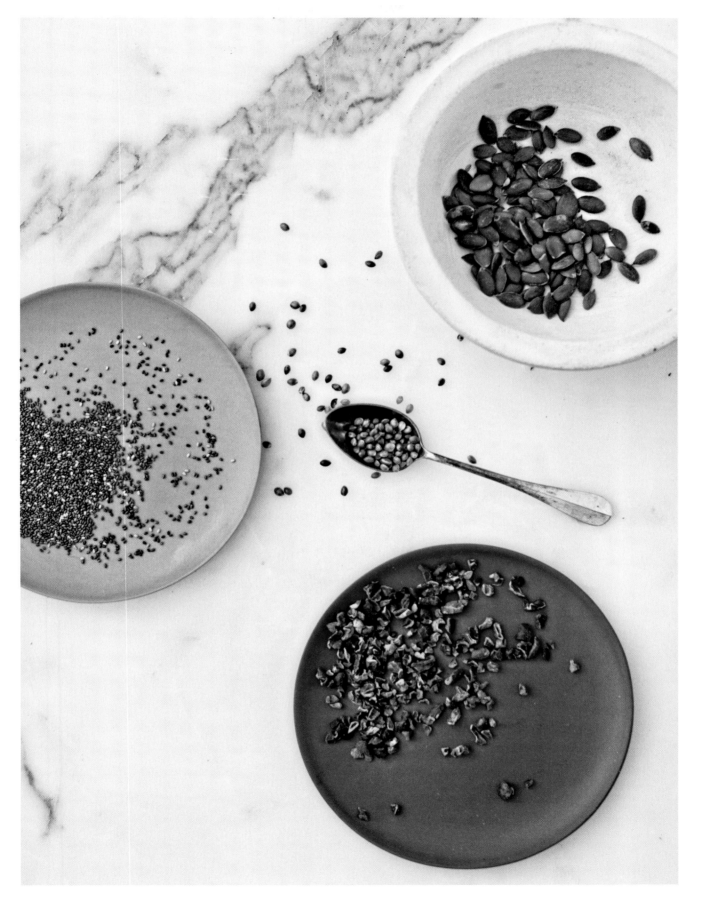

Meal Plan for Week 1 Day 2

RECIPE	QUANTITY		CALORIES	CARBS	PROTEIN	FAT
BREAKFAST						
Spinach, shiitake and tomato on 'toast'	245g		599	15.6g	15.1g	51.0g
		Meal total:	599	15.6g	15.1g	51.0g
LUNCH						
Superfood salad with mackerel	338g		637	13.9g	23.0g	53.0g
		Meal total:	637	13.9g	23.0g	53.0g
DINNER						
Beef stir-fry	241g		379	5.0g	24.0g	29.0g
Detox soup	370g		223	5.8g	6.1g	18.2g
		Meal total:	602	10.8g	30.1g	47.2g
PLAN TOTAL:			1,838	40.3g	68.2g	151.2g

Macronutrient Analysis

	CARBOHYDRATE	PROTEIN	FAT	ALCOHOL
INTAKE	40.3g	68.2g	151.2g	0.5g
	9% carbs	**15% protein**	**76% fat**	

Shiitake mushrooms have wonderful immune-enhancing properties and are therefore sometimes called an 'anti-cancer' food. They can be used in small amounts on a ketogenic diet, like in this yummy breakfast recipe.

Heat the olive oil in a frying pan on a medium heat. Fry the mushrooms, tomatoes, spinach and garlic until the mushrooms are well cooked. Season with turmeric, salt and pepper. Top the kale crackers with the mushroom mix and sprinkle with hemp seeds.

PER PORTION

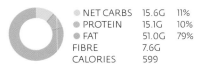

NET CARBS	15.6G	11%
PROTEIN	15.1G	10%
FAT	51.0G	79%
FIBRE	7.6G	
CALORIES	599	

Spinach, shiitake and tomato on 'toast'

2 tbsp olive oil (26g)

120g (4.2 oz) shiitake mushrooms, sliced (120g)

8 cherry tomatoes, halved (96g)

30g (1.1 oz) spinach (30g)

2 garlic cloves, crushed (6g)

1 tsp ground turmeric (2g)

Salt and pepper (3g)

6 kale crackers (see page 268) (192g)

2 tbsp shelled hemp seeds (18g)

Serves 2

'If our early ancestors hadn't developed a way to use ketones for energy, our species would have ended up on Darwin's shortlist eons ago!'
Dr Eric Westman

Kale crackers

135g (4.8 oz) curly kale (135g)
135g (4.8 oz) Brazil nuts (135g)
135g (4.8 oz) sunflower seeds (135g)
2 eggs (100g)
½ onion (75g)
2 good tbsp coconut oil (54g)
2 tsp five-spice powder (34g)
1–2 tsp salt (5–10g)

Makes 20 crackers

These crackers are fabulous with pestos, pâtés, guacamole and all kinds of spreads. We know for a fact that most people wouldn't go far without bread and crackers, which is why you'll find several recipes for them throughout the book. These crackers can be frozen, but they also keep for at least five days in an airtight container.

Preheat the oven to 150°C (300°F). Line a baking tray with non-stick baking paper.

Put all the ingredients into a strong blender and process to a smooth paste. Spread the paste onto the lined tray as thinly as possible. Bake for 55–70 minutes, depending on how crunchy you like the crackers. Allow to cool down, then break them into pieces by hand.

PER CRACKER (32G)

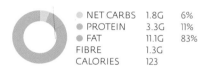

NET CARBS	1.8G	6%
PROTEIN	3.3G	11%
FAT	11.1G	83%
FIBRE	1.3G	
CALORIES	123	

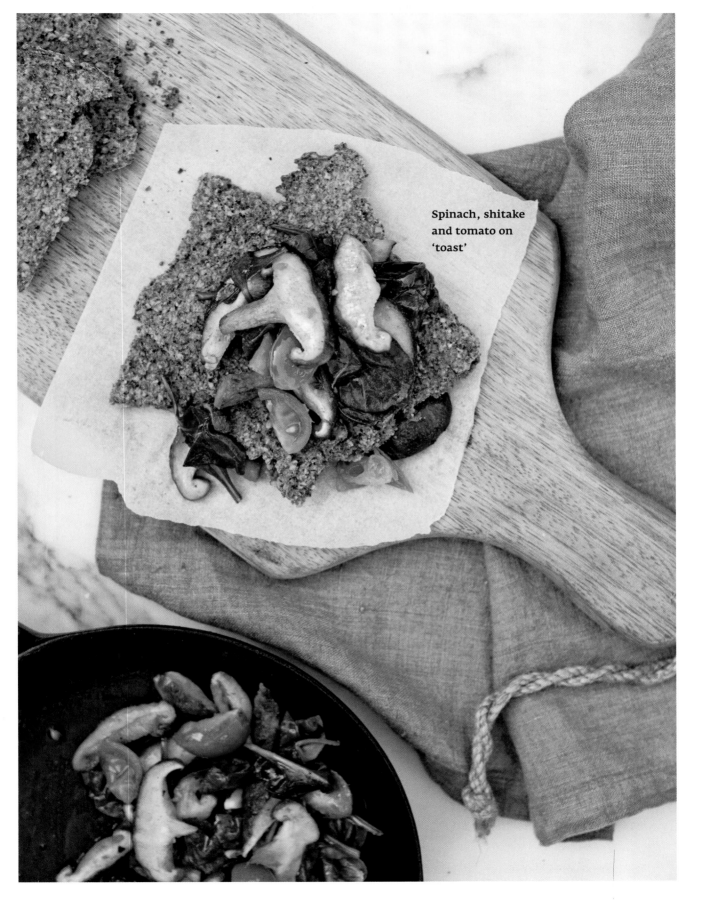

Spinach, shitake and tomato on 'toast'

Superfood salad with mackerel

3 cherry tomatoes, halved (48g)

20g (0.7 oz) scallions, chopped (20g)

10g (0.4 oz) mint, chopped (10g)

10g (0.4 oz) parsley, chopped (10g)

20g (0.7 oz) arugula (20g)

1 large broccoli floret, steamed or
  blanched (44g)

100g (3.5 oz) smoked mackerel
  (100g)

50g (1.8 oz) leftover cooked sweet
  potato (50g)

1 tbsp lemon juice (15g)

1½ tbsp avocado oil (21g)

Serves 1

This is a prime example of how you can use leftovers to make a quick, tasty and nutritious lunch. Once you get a good idea of what vegetables you can use, you'll be able to design your own favourite leftover salads.

Mix the tomatoes and scallions together, then add the mint and parsley. Toss with the arugula, then add the cooked broccoli to the salad, then top with the mackerel and sweet potato pieces. Squeeze the lemon juice over the salad and drizzle everything with oil.

PER PORTION

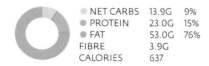

NET CARBS	13.9G	9%
PROTEIN	23.0G	15%
FAT	53.0G	76%
FIBRE	3.9G	
CALORIES	637	

Beef stir-fry

The beef can easily be replaced with lamb here, which is easier to digest for many people because of its different protein structure. Many people who are dairy-sensitive also have trouble with beef, which is important to bear in mind.

Mix together the garlic, ginger, sherry, soy sauce and sesame oil and marinate the steak in it for at least 20 minutes.

Heat the coconut oil in a frying pan until hot. Add the meat with the marinade and stir-fry for 3–4 minutes, until the meat is lightly browned. Transfer to a plate but leave the juices in the pan.

Stir-fry the snow peas and carrot strips for 4 minutes, then add the meat back in and mix everything well. Serve in the lettuce leaves.

2 garlic cloves, crushed (6g)

2cm (¾in) piece of ginger, peeled and grated (5g)

1 tbsp dry sherry (12g)

1 tbsp soy sauce or tamari (18g)

2 tsp sesame oil (8g)

400g (14.1 oz) sirloin steak, sliced thinly across the grain (400g)

2 good tbsp coconut oil (54g)

2 handfuls of snow peas, halved lengthways (160g)

1 large carrot, peeled and cut into matchsticks or strips (200g)

4 large salad leaves, such as butterhead (100g)

Serves 4

PER PORTION

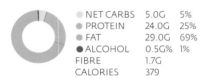

NET CARBS	5.0G	5%
PROTEIN	24.0G	25%
FAT	29.0G	69%
ALCOHOL	0.5G%	1%
FIBRE	1.7G	
CALORIES	379	

Detox soup

80g (2.8 oz) coconut oil (80g)

1 large leek, with leaves, chopped (250g)

1 small bunch of scallions, bulbs and tops chopped (30g)

190g (6.7 oz) broccoli, chopped (190g)

3 stalks of celery, chopped (180g)

60g (2.1 oz) spinach (60g)

3 garlic cloves, chopped (9g)

1 litre (4¼c) vegetable stock or bone broth (1kg)

1 × 50g can (1.8 oz) anchovies in oil, drained (50g)

Serves 6

We're not huge fans of the word *detox*. It's totally overused and sometimes used in the wrong context. But this recipe has so many liver-supporting foods like leeks, broccoli, garlic and omega-3s from the anchovies that we couldn't think of any other name! This soup will be also used for lunch on Day 5, so I recommend freezing the leftovers until then.

Heat 1 tablespoon of coconut oil on a medium heat and gently fry the leek and scallions until soft. Add all the other vegetables and the stock. Bring to the boil, then immediately reduce the heat and simmer for 15–20 minutes. Add the remaining 2 tablespoons of coconut oil and the anchovies. Blend the soup well in a food processor and serve.

PER PORTION

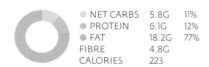

NET CARBS	5.8G	11%
PROTEIN	6.1G	12%
FAT	18.2G	77%
FIBRE	4.8G	
CALORIES	223	

Meal Plan for Week 1 Day 3

RECIPE	QUANTITY		CALORIES	CARBS	PROTEIN	FAT
BREAKFAST						
Nut porridge	254g		556	14.8g	21.0g	45.0g
		Meal total:	556	14.8g	21.0g	45.0g
LUNCH						
Prawn-filled avocado	265g		483	4.4g	18.3g	42.0g
Super quick zucchini salad (page 164)	236g		167	4.7g	4.0g	13.6g
		Meal total:	650	9.1g	22.3g	55.6g
DINNER						
Asparagus quiche	214g		602	8.6g	22.0g	51.0g
Arugula salad	72g		135	3.1g	1.0g	12.9g
		Meal total:	737	11.7g	23.0g	63.9g
PLAN TOTAL:			1,943	35.6g	66.3g	164.5g

Macronutrient Analysis

	CARBOHYDRATE	PROTEIN	FAT	ALCOHOL
INTAKE	35.6g	66.3g	164.5g	
	9% carbs	**14% protein**	**77% fat**	

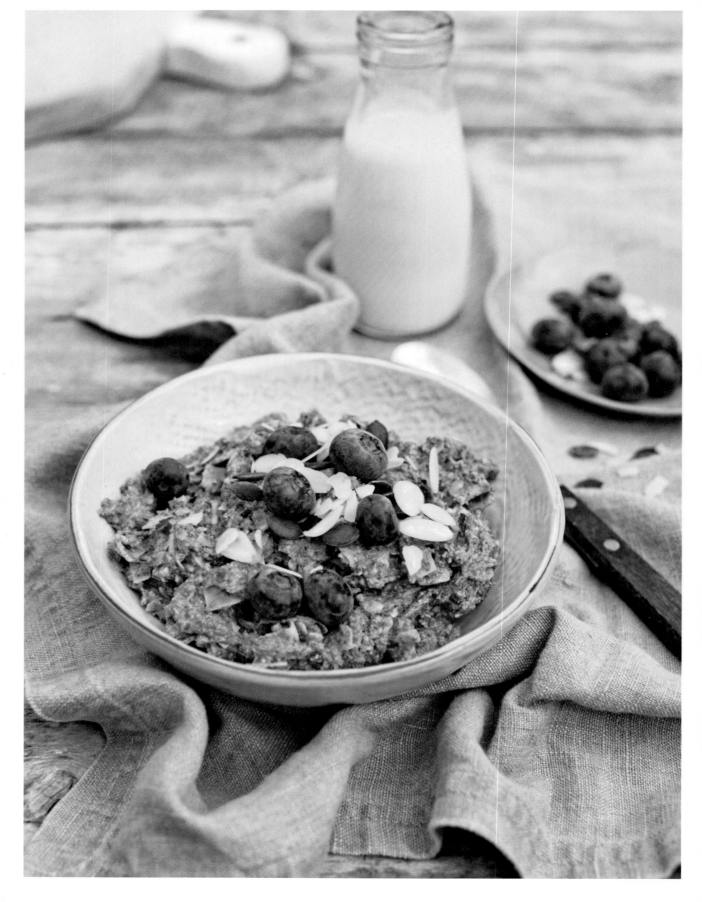

Nut porridge

Here in Ireland, oats – and porridge in particular – are an important part of our diet. Most people are completely lost when they hear they can't have porridge for breakfast any more. That's why we've come up with some different versions of porridge that are much lower in carbs and therefore more keto-friendly. Feel free to mix and match, try different types of nuts, and most importantly, experiment with the amount of liquids in it. As with 'regular' porridge, everybody prefers different textures.

Put all the ingredients except the blueberries in your food processor and blend. Add less water if you prefer a coarser texture. Pour into a bowl and garnish with the berries.

40g (1.4 oz) cashew nuts (40g)
30g (1.1 oz) ground almonds (30g)
25g (0.9 oz) desiccated coconut (25g)
125ml (½c) full-fat coconut milk (125g)
100ml (⅜c) hot water (100g)
½ scoop protein powder (20g)
2 tbsp pumpkin seeds (24g)
1 tbsp whole linseeds (flaxseeds) (14g)
2 tsp ground cinnamon (5g)
100g blueberries (100g)

Serves 2

PER PORTION

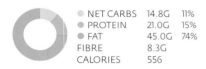

NET CARBS	14.8G	11%
PROTEIN	21.0G	15%
FAT	45.0G	74%
FIBRE	8.3G	
CALORIES	556	

Prawn-filled avocado

Prawns and avocado are a match made in heaven. Prawns are super high in protein, though, and should be eaten in small-ish amounts. They're pricey enough anyway, so maybe that's not a bad thing.

120g (4.2 oz) prawns, boiled (120g)

1 chilli, deseeded and finely chopped (12g)

4 garlic cloves, crushed (12g)

2 tbsp lime juice (30g)

2 tbsp sesame oil (24g)

2 tsp fish sauce (12g)

2 tsp soy sauce or tamari (12g)

2 small avocados, peeled and stone removed (300g)

2 tbsp cilantro leaves (8g)

Serves 2

Put all the ingredients except the avocado and cilantro into a food processor and blend. Fill the mixture into the holes of the halved avocado and top with cilantro leaves. Serve with Domini's super quick zucchini salad on page 164.

PER PORTION

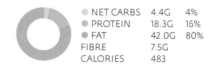

NET CARBS	4.4G	4%
PROTEIN	18.3G	16%
FAT	42.0G	80%
FIBRE	7.5G	
CALORIES	483	

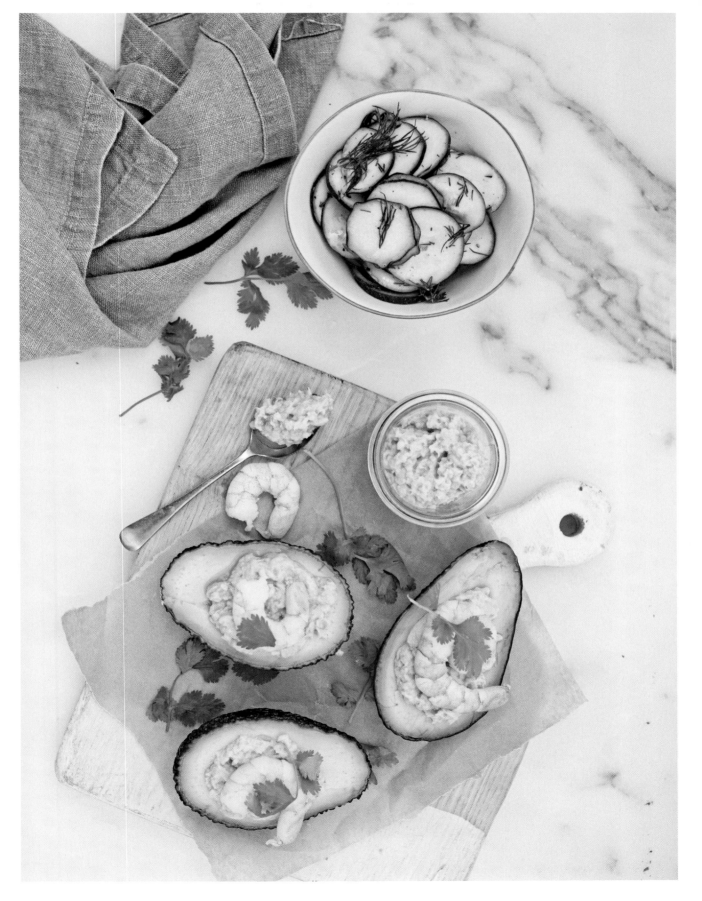

Asparagus quiche

1 tbsp olive oil (13g)

150g (5.3 oz) leeks, thinly sliced (150g)

1 × coconut quiche base (see page 279) (235g)

150g (5.3 oz) asparagus, chopped (150g)

3 heaped tbsp red hemp pesto (page 262) (100g)

6 eggs (300g)

1 tsp ground turmeric (2g)

Salt and pepper (3g)

120g (4.2 oz) cheese, e.g. Gruyère or Manchego, grated (120g)

Serves 5 (or 4 plus leftovers)

Asparagus is a typical keto food and is not only very tasty, but also good for liver support.

Preheat the oven to 180°C (350°F).

Heat the olive oil in a frying pan and gently sauté the leeks. Once the quiche base is in the oven for its 10 minutes (see the recipe on page 279) add the asparagus and pesto to the leeks and fry for another 3–5 minutes.

Whisk the eggs in a bowl and season well with turmeric, salt and pepper. Spread the asparagus mix onto the quiche base and top with the beaten eggs. Sprinkle the grated cheese over it and bake for 45 minutes.

While you're baking the quiche, cook the eggplant slices on page 284 for about 20 minutes so that your lunch on Day 4 will be ready in no time.

PER PORTION

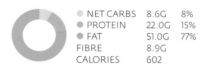

NET CARBS	8.6G	8%
PROTEIN	22.0G	15%
FAT	51.0G	77%
FIBRE	8.9G	
CALORIES	602	

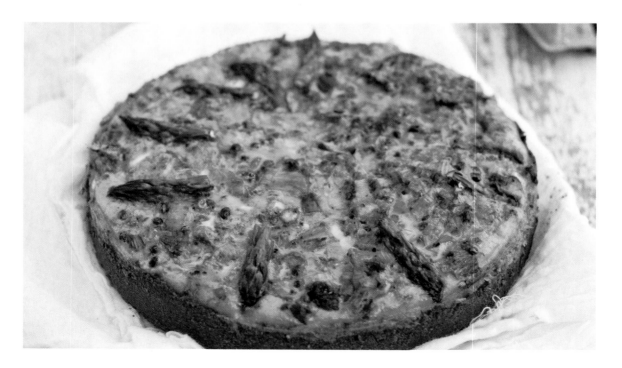

This coconut quiche base is super versatile. It was inspired by a good colleague of mine, Lily Nichols, a registered dietician and nutritionist who specialises in gestational diabetes (www.realfoodforGD.com). Make sure you make a big batch of it, as you can use it for lots of other things. My kids eat it as breadsticks, or you can add some sweetener and it can be the base for a sweet dish, like the raspberry cupcakes on page 215. Or you can just top it with your favourite spread.

Preheat the oven to 180°C (350°F).

Add the ground cashew nuts, coconut flour, garlic and salt to a bowl and mix well. With your hands, mix in the butter and press the batter into a small round baking pan lined with non-stick baking paper. Bake for 10 minutes.

Coconut quiche base

80g (2.8 oz) cashew nuts, ground to a fine flour (80g)
75g (2.6 oz) coconut flour (75g)
1 garlic clove, crushed (3g)
½ tsp salt (3g)
75g (2.6 oz) butter, at room temperature (75g)

Serves 5

PER PORTION

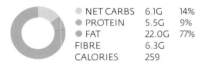

●	NET CARBS	6.1G	14%
●	PROTEIN	5.5G	9%
●	FAT	22.0G	77%
	FIBRE	6.3G	
	CALORIES	259	

'Humans went into ketosis every winter for thousands of generations. Being in a low level of ketosis is the more natural state for our metabolism. We do have metabolic flexibility and can operate on amino acids, glucose, or fat.'
Dr Terry Wahls

Arugula salad

5 portions vinaigrette recipe below
   (120g)
100g (3.5 oz) arugula (100g)
140g (5 oz) chopped carrots (140g)

Serves 5

Carrots aren't a common sight on a low-carb menu because like all other starchy vegetables, they're higher in carbs than their non-starchy counterparts. They are full of nutrients, though, and can be incorporated in small amounts. If you ferment carrots (and also beetroot), you can eat much larger quantities because the carbohydrate content decreases significantly.

According to the French company Nutriform, which performs its own lab tests to verify the nutrient content of their products, 100g of lacto-fermented carrots contain 1.3g of net carbs. If you ate raw carrots, the net carbohydrate content would be nearly 8g. The same applies to beetroot and other vegetables – once they've gone through the fermentation process, the carbohydrates are reduced, which makes them a lot more keto (and tummy) friendly. Read more about the benefits of fermented foods on page 282.

Pour the vinaigrette over the arugula leaves and carrots and mix well.

PER PORTION (INCLUDING DRESSING)

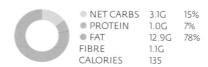

NET CARBS	3.1G	15%
PROTEIN	1.0G	7%
FAT	12.9G	78%
FIBRE	1.1G	
CALORIES	135	

Vinaigrette

1 garlic clove, crushed (3g)
8 tbsp extra virgin olive oil (101g)
4 tbsp cider vinegar (45.6g)
4 tsp lemon juice (20g)
2 tsp wholegrain mustard (20g)
2 tsp ground black pepper (5g)
Pinch of pink rock salt (1g)

Serves 8

It's well worth making a big batch of this vinaigrette and storing it in the fridge for about a week. Make sure you take it out about 15 minutes before using it, though, as the oil can solidify in the fridge.

Put all the ingredients into a blender and whizz at low speed to mix the ingredients and chop the garlic.

PER PORTION

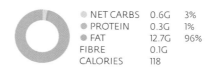

NET CARBS	0.6G	3%
PROTEIN	0.3G	1%
FAT	12.7G	96%
FIBRE	0.1G	
CALORIES	118	

Meal Plan for Week 1 Day 4

RECIPE	QUANTITY		CALORIES	CARBS	PROTEIN	FAT
BREAKFAST						
Greek yoghurt, plain, full fat (no added flavours)	125g		119	5.0g	12.3g	8.8g
Seed mix	25g		146	3.5g	5.6g	11.6g
Keto cacao	302g		398	1.9g	3.9g	41.0g
		Meal total:	663	10.4g	21.8g	61.4g
LUNCH						
Salmon-filled boats	361g		481	10.1g	19.6g	39.0g
Light leafy salad	74g		126	1.1g	0.8g	13.0g
		Meal total:	607	11.2g	20.4g	52.0g
DINNER						
Chicken with red peppers and olives	172g		312	2.7g	25.0g	22.0g
Spiced butternut squash	119g		97	9.2g	1.7g	5.0g
Lemon keto bombs (page 212)	27g		185	0.7g	0.7g	19.3g
		Meal total:	594	12.6g	27.4g	46.3g
PLAN TOTAL:			1,864	34.2g	69.6g	159.7g

Macronutrient Analysis

	CARBOHYDRATE	PROTEIN	FAT	ALCOHOL
INTAKE	34.2g	69.6g	159.7g	0.5g
	7% carbs	**15% protein**	**78% fat**	

Seed mix

1 tbsp pumpkin seeds (12g)
1 tbsp sunflower seeds (10g)
1 tsp flaxseeds (3g)

Serves 1

Yoghurt contains probiotics, which are in foods or supplements containing friendly bacteria that help colonise your gut with health-boosting micro-organisms. Taking care of your gut and the good bacteria in it is one of the most important things you can do to improve your health. Fascinating research is currently going on into the interaction between our microbiome (i.e. all of our microbes' genes), our health and our environment. The genes in our microbiome outnumber the genes in our genome by about 100 to 1! As Dearbhla Reynolds from the Cultured Club said at a fermentation course, 'We're actually bacteria with a human expression.'

If you're looking for a much more potent source of probiotics than yoghurt, you might want to research fermented foods like kefir, kombucha, tempeh, sauerkraut and other lacto-fermented vegetables. Once a food is fermented, its carbohydrate content goes way down because it's 'eaten up' by the bacteria cultures and turned into a food with a greater level of gut-friendly nutrients in a highly bio-available state. This means that your body will be able to absorb it more efficiently. The longer the fermentation process, the more carbohydrates are eaten up by the organisms, which results in a lower carbohydrate count.

Another positive aspect of fermentation is that the process helps break down large proteins into smaller ones, which also means that milk kefir, for instance, typically contains less casein than cheese.

Traditional diets across the world once consisted of about 30% fermented foods. It's time to reintroduce those beneficial foods, even if it's just in small quantities, on a daily basis. It's advisable to only start with very small amounts, and if you're going through treatment or if your immune system is very depressed, I'd hold off on probiotics (both food and supplements) until you feel better.

And as Domini mentioned earlier, don't forget to include the green parts of vegetables, such as leeks and scallions. But equally important, don't throw out the stalks from kale or broccoli. These 'woody' parts are a great way to contribute to a healthy microbiome.

It's a good idea to have some mixed nuts and seeds ready to go. They can be a quick snack or can be sprinkled onto a salad to make it nice and crunchy. If you grind them, make sure you store them in an airtight container in the fridge so they don't go rancid.

There are two ways you can use this seed mix as a topping for your yoghurt – try them out and see what works best for you.

1. Put the seeds into a coffee grinder or food processor and chop them to a coarse or fine flour, whatever you prefer.

2. Roast them in a hot, dry frying pan without oil for a few minutes. Sprinkle on top of the Greek yoghurt.

PER PORTION (SEEDS ONLY)

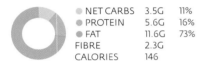

NET CARBS	3.5G	11%
PROTEIN	5.6G	16%
FAT	11.6G	73%
FIBRE	2.3G	
CALORIES	146	

Keto cacao

250ml (1c) unsweetened almond
  milk (250g)
22g (0.8 oz) coconut or MCT oil (22g)
15g (0.5 oz) unsalted goat butter or
  grass-fed butter (15g)
1 tbsp cocoa powder (15g)

Serves 1

Heat the almond milk in a pan until it's hot enough
to ensure the oil and butter will melt, then put into a
blender with all the ingredients and whizz to combine.
Sweeten if necessary with stevia or erythritol.

PER PORTION

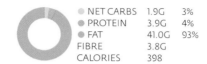

● NET CARBS	1.9G	3%
● PROTEIN	3.9G	4%
● FAT	41.0G	93%
FIBRE	3.8G	
CALORIES	398	

Salmon-filled boats

2 tbsp passata (120g)
6 slices of baked eggplant, sliced
  lengthways (326g)
210g (7.4 oz) salmon pâté (page 285)
  (210g)
1 small onion, finely chopped (60g)
6 tsp chopped fresh chives (6g)
Salt and pepper (3g)

Serves 2

Put some passata on each of the pre-baked eggplant
slices, spread some salmon pâté over it and garnish with
finely chopped onions and chives. If your eggplant slices
are thin enough, you can roll them up. Season to taste.

PER PORTION

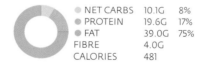

● NET CARBS	10.1G	8%
● PROTEIN	19.6G	17%
● FAT	39.0G	75%
FIBRE	4.0G	
CALORIES	481	

Salmon pâté

This freezes really well and I often save some to make an easy lunch (a bit of pâté on a cracker with a salad), to add to some zucchini 'spaghetti' or to dip celery and cucumber sticks into.

Put all the ingredients into a blender and whizz to combine.

PER PORTION

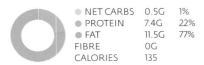

NET CARBS	0.5G	1%
PROTEIN	7.4G	22%
FAT	11.5G	77%
FIBRE	0G	
CALORIES	135	

180g (6.3 oz) red wild salmon canned in brine, drained (180g)
50g (3½tbsp) crème fraîche (50g)
45g (3tbsp) butter (45g)
1 garlic clove, peeled (3g)
1 tsp paprika (2g)
1 tsp dried dill (1g)

Serves 6 (but note that you will need a bigger portion if you make the salmon-filled boats)

Light leafy salad

Wash the leaves well and mix with the vinaigrette on page 280. You can, of course, use any lettuce you like and mix it up.

PER PORTION (INCLUDING DRESSING)

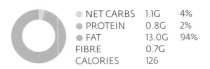

NET CARBS	1.1G	4%
PROTEIN	0.8G	2%
FAT	13.0G	94%
FIBRE	0.7G	
CALORIES	126	

100g (3.5 oz) butterhead lettuce, chopped (100g)
2 portions vinaigrette recipe (page 280) (48g)

Serves 2

Chicken with red peppers and olives

200g (7 oz) roasted red peppers from a jar (200g)

450g (1lb) chicken breast, cut into strips (450g)

110g (3.9 oz) black olives, stones removed (110g)

10 garlic cloves, unpeeled (30g)

125ml (½c) dry white wine (125g)

93ml (⅜c) olive oil (100g)

1 bunch of rosemary (12g)

1 bay leaf (1g)

Serves 6

Preheat the oven to 180°C (350°F).

Drain enough of the red pepper pieces to amount to two whole ones and cut them into thick strips. This is usually about four to six whole pieces of pepper from a jar.

Toss all the ingredients together in the casserole that you will use to cook it in, or if it's easier, in a big bowl and then transfer to a casserole with a tight-fitting lid. Bake it for at least 30 minutes, then remove the lid and give it a little stir, trying to get at some of the juices at the bottom to drizzle onto the top parts, and bake, uncovered, for 15 more minutes. You should have fully cooked, beautifully moist chicken pieces.

PER PORTION

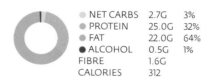

NET CARBS	2.7G	3%
PROTEIN	25.0G	32%
FAT	22.0G	64%
ALCOHOL	0.5G	1%
FIBRE	1.6G	
CALORIES	312	

Preheat the oven to 180°C (350°F).

Cut the butternut squash in half lengthways and remove the seeds and pulp with a spoon. Cut each half into four lengthways so that you have eight long pieces.

Mix the oil, tomato purée and spices together and rub all over the butternut squash until it's evenly coated. Place the squash in a roasting dish and bake for 45–60 minutes, until the flesh is soft, turning the pieces over after 25 minutes.

PER PORTION

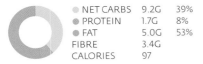

● NET CARBS	9.2G	39%
● PROTEIN	1.7G	8%
● FAT	5.0G	53%
FIBRE	3.4G	
CALORIES	97	

Spiced butternut squash

800g (1.75lbs) butternut squash, washed but unpeeled (800g)
3 tbsp olive oil (39g)
2 tbsp tomato purée (102g)
1½ tsp ground coriander (3g)
1½ tsp ground cumin (3g)
1 tsp salt (5g)
½ tsp ground turmeric (1g)

Serves 8 (or 6 with leftovers)

'Nutritional ketosis, which occurs with carbohydrate restriction and is further enhanced with calorie restriction, forces the physiological shift from a glucose-based metabolism to a fatty acid and ketone metabolism.'
Dr Dominic D'Agostino

Meal Plan for Week 1 Day 5

RECIPE	QUANTITY		CALORIES	CARBS	PROTEIN	FAT
BREAKFAST						
Vegetable muffin, 3 halves	224g		365	10.3g	11.3g	28.0g
3 slices of smoked salmon	60g		85	0g	15.2g	2.7g
3 heaped tsp butter	24g		179	0.1g	0.1g	19.7g
		Meal total:	629	10.4g	26.6g	50.4g
LUNCH						
Portion of detox soup (page 272)	370g		223	5.8g	6.1g	18.2g
3 kale crackers (page 268)	96g		370	5.4g	9.8g	33.0g
		Meal total:	593	11.2g	15.9g	51.2g
DINNER						
Spaghetti squash carbonara	404g		536	8.8g	27.0g	43.0g
Mixed leafy salad	166g		138	2.4g	1.5g	13.2g
		Meal total:	674	11.2g	28.5g	56.2g
PLAN TOTAL:			1,896	32.8g	71.0g	157.8g

Macronutrient Analysis

	CARBOHYDRATE	PROTEIN	FAT	ALCOHOL
INTAKE	32.8g	71.0g	157.8g	0g
	8% carbs	**15% protein**	**77% fat**	

Who said that muffins, bread and pancakes are gone on a low-carb diet?

Preheat the oven to 180°C (350°F). Grease a 12-hole muffin pan.

Mix the coconut flour, chia seeds and baking powder together in a large bowl.

I always just chop all the vegetables in a food processor when I make these muffins, but you could chop and grate them by hand.

In a separate bowl, mix all the wet ingredients together and stir in the vegetables, then add everything to the dry ingredients. Knead until you have a fairly wet but well-formed dough. Form into 12 muffins and put them into the greased muffin pan.

Bake for 20–25 minutes and serve with butter.

Vegetable muffins

180g (6.3 oz) coconut flour (180g)
3 tbsp milled chia seeds (30g)
2 tsp baking powder (8g)
200g (7 oz) carrots, peeled and grated (200g)
200g spinach, chopped (200g)
150g (5.3 oz) red onions, chopped (150g)
1 large zucchini, grated (200g)
1 garlic clove, finely chopped (3g)
180g (12tbsp) butter, melted (180g)
300ml (1¼c) coconut milk in a carton, such as Koko brand (300g)
6 eggs, beaten (342g)
Zest and juice of 1 lemon (2g + 40g)

Makes 12 muffins

PER MUFFIN

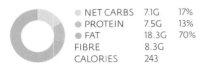

NET CARBS	7.1G	17%
PROTEIN	7.5G	13%
FAT	18.3G	70%
FIBRE	8.3G	
CALORIES	243	

Spaghetti squash carbonara

600g (1.3lbs) spaghetti squash
(save some for leftovers on Day 6)
(600g)

4 tbsp butter or ghee (60g)

200g (7 oz) napa cabbage, cored and
shredded (200g)

4 garlic cloves, crushed (12g)

1 tsp ground turmeric (2g)

1 tsp ground cumin (2g)

Salt and pepper (3g)

2 egg whites (64g)

90g (3.2 oz) grated unpasteurised
Parmesan cheese (90g)

300g (10.6 oz) bacon, cut into small
lardons (300g)

4 egg yolks (72g)

4 tbsp chopped fresh chives (12g)

Serves 4

Spaghetti squash have a relatively short season. Spiralised zucchinis work just as well here.

Preheat the oven to 180°C (350°F).

Cut the spaghetti squash in half lengthwise and remove the seeds. Brush the inside with 2 tablespoons of the melted butter or ghee and place cut side up in a baking dish. Roast for 30–40 minutes, until soft.

In the meantime, melt the remaining 2 tablespoons of butter or ghee in a frying pan and gently fry the cabbage and garlic. Season with the turmeric, cumin and some salt and pepper, then remove from the pan and set aside in a bowl.

Whisk together the egg whites and Parmesan cheese and set aside.

Heat a frying pan and cook the bacon over a medium heat until crisp. Remove the bacon when done, but leave the bacon fat in the pan.

Once the spaghetti squash has cooled down, use a fork to scrape out the squash strands from the skin. Make sure you put some leftovers aside for lunch on Day 6. Add the squash to the pan with the bacon fat along with the fried cabbage and cook over a medium heat for 2–3 minutes. Remove from the heat and pour in the egg white and Parmesan mixture and the bacon, stirring constantly.

Divide the spaghetti/cabbage mix into four bowls and place an egg yolk on top of each bowl, finishing by garnishing with chives. If you prefer having a well-cooked egg yolk, then add it at the same time as you stir in the egg white and Parmesan mix. It does give it a delicious creaminess, though, if you stir it in at the very end. Don't forget to have some leftover spaghetti squash for lunch on Day 6.

PER PORTION

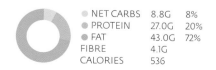

NET CARBS	8.8G	8%
PROTEIN	27.0G	20%
FAT	43.0G	72%
FIBRE	4.1G	
CALORIES	536	

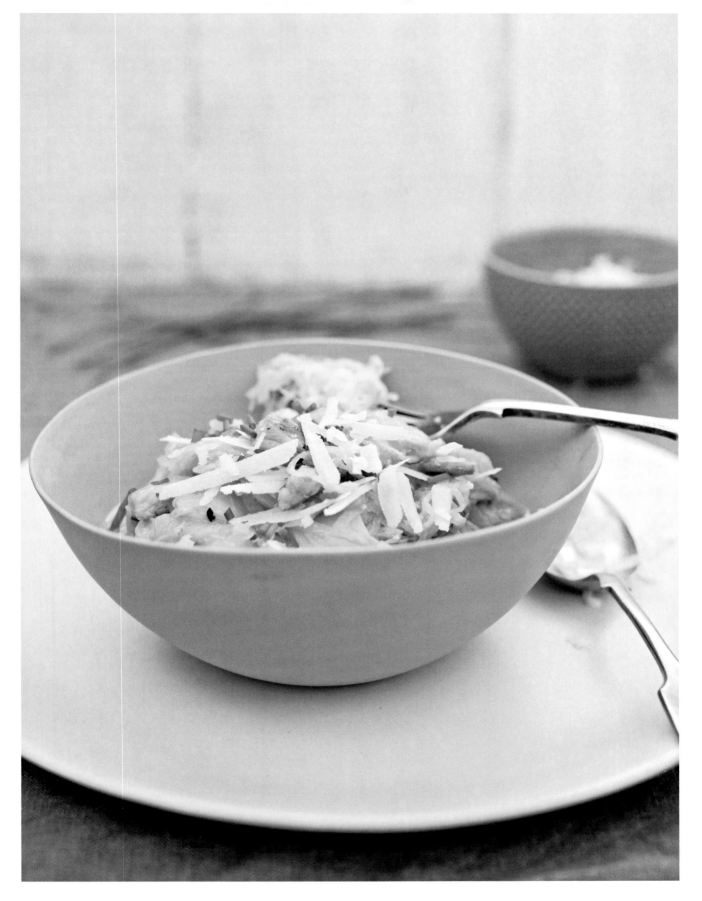

Mixed leafy salad

Wash all the vegetables well and put them into a bowl. Make the vinaigrette as per the recipe on page 280, pour it over the vegetables and mix well.

300g (10.6 oz) butterhead lettuce, washed and shredded (300g)

220g (7.8 oz) cucumber, sliced (220g)

4 cherry tomatoes, halved (48g)

4 portions vinaigrette recipe (page 280) (96g)

Serves 4

PER PORTION (INCLUDING DRESSING)

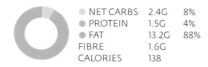

NET CARBS	2.4G	8%
PROTEIN	1.5G	4%
FAT	13.2G	88%
FIBRE	1.6G	
CALORIES	138	

'Confusion about the difference between ketosis and ketoacidosis is a major issue.'
Dr Eric Westman

Meal Plan for Week 1 Day 6

RECIPE	QUANTITY		CALORIES	CARBS	PROTEIN	FAT
BREAKFAST						
Chicken liver brekkie	280g		569	7.6g	24.0g	48.0g
		Meal total:	569	7.6g	24.0g	48.0g
LUNCH						
Squashy lunch	420g		657	12.6g	16.7g	57.0g
		Meal total:	657	12.6g	16.7g	57.0g
DINNER						
Salmon patties	117g		226	1.1g	19.1g	16.0g
Creamy pepper sauce	93g		110	5.7g	3.3g	7.9g
Cauliflower rice	130g		275	3.4g	3.9g	27.0g
		Meal total:	611	10.2g	26.3g	50.9g
PLAN TOTAL:			1,837	30.4g	67.0g	155.9g

Macronutrient Analysis

	CARBOHYDRATE	PROTEIN	FAT	ALCOHOL
INTAKE	30.4g	67.0g	155.9g	0g
	7% carbs	**15% protein**	**78% fat**	

Chicken liver brekkie

55g (1.9 oz) coconut oil (55g)
2 small onions, finely chopped (140g)
2 garlic cloves, crushed (6g)
120g (4.2 oz) chicken liver, chopped (120g)
80g (2.8 oz) bacon, chopped (80g)
1 tbsp capers (9g)
2 tsp wholegrain mustard (20g)
1 tsp salt (5g)
4 zucchini flax crackers (below) (120g)
Handful of parsley, chopped (10g)

Serves 2

I know we've talked about this before, but I need to emphasise it again: offal (organ meat) is awfully good for you. It's just a matter of finding recipes that you like. Try this way of making it in combination with some bacon to help you get used to the taste.

Melt the coconut oil in a frying pan and sauté the onions and garlic for a short while. Fry the chicken liver and bacon in the same pan on medium heat for about 5 minutes.

In a food processor, combine the chicken liver and bacon mix with the capers, mustard and salt and pulse until the texture resembles ground meat. Serve on zucchini flax crackers and garnish with the chopped parsley.

PER PORTION

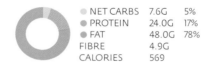

NET CARBS	7.6G	5%
PROTEIN	24.0G	17%
FAT	48.0G	78%
FIBRE	4.9G	
CALORIES	569	

Zucchini flax crackers

2 zuchinnis (500g)
75g (2.6 oz) sun-dried tomatoes preserved in oil, drained (75g)
100g (3.5 oz) soft full-fat goats' cheese (100g)
2 eggs (100g)
120g (4.2 oz) milled flaxseed (120g)
1 tsp ground turmeric (2g)
1 tsp five-spice powder (2g)
1 tsp salt (5g)

Makes 30 crackers

Preheat the oven to 150°C (300°F). Line two baking trays with non-stick baking paper.

Blitz the zucchinis and sun-dried tomatoes in a food processor, then mix with the goats' cheese and eggs. Mix together the milled flaxseeds and spices in a bowl and add to the zucchini mix. Spread the wet dough as thinly as you can on the two lined trays. Bake for about 1 hour, or until your desired consistency is reached. Allow to cool, then break into pieces by hand.

PER CRACKER (30G)

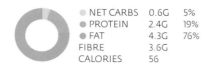

NET CARBS	0.6G	5%
PROTEIN	2.4G	19%
FAT	4.3G	76%
FIBRE	3.6G	
CALORIES	56	

Heat the avocado oil and gently fry the chopped kale, broccoli and scallions for a few minutes. Add the leftover spaghetti squash and the tahini dressing. Mix well and sprinkle with the pistachios and sesame seeds.

PER PORTION (INCLUDING DRESSING)

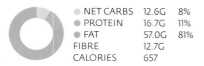

NET CARBS	12.6G	8%
PROTEIN	16.7G	11%
FAT	57.0G	81%
FIBRE	12.7G	
CALORIES	657	

Squashy lunch

2 tbsp avocado oil (28g)

135g (4.8 oz) curly kale, finely chopped (135g)

2 small portions of broccoli, chopped (120g)

2 scallions, bulbs and tops finely chopped (25g)

300g (10.6 oz) spaghetti squash (leftovers from Day 5) (300g)

2 portions tahini dressing (see below) (150g)

60g (2.1 oz) pistachio nuts, roasted and salted (60g)

2 tbsp sesame seeds (22g)

Serves 2

Put all the ingredients into a blender and whizz to combine.

PER PORTION

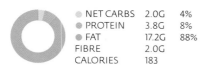

NET CARBS	2.0G	4%
PROTEIN	3.8G	8%
FAT	17.2G	88%
FIBRE	2.0G	
CALORIES	183	

Tahini dressing

70g (2.5 oz) tahini (70g)

1 garlic clove, peeled (3g)

125ml (½c) water (125g)

Juice of 1 lemon (40g)

2 tbsp olive oil (26g)

1 good tbsp cider vinegar (14g)

1½ tsp soy sauce or tamari (9g)

1 tsp coriander seeds, whole or ground (2g)

1 tsp cumin seeds, whole or ground (2g)

1 tsp maple syrup (6g)

Makes 4 portions

Salmon patties

1 large can (12 oz) wild salmon (with bones), drained (325g)
6 whole scallions, finely sliced (60g)
2 eggs (100g)
1 garlic clove, crushed 93g)
1 tbsp wholegrain mustard (30g)
1 tbsp dill, fresh or dried (4g)
1 tbsp parsley, fresh or dried (4g)
1 tsp lemon juice (5g)
2 tsp coconut flour (8g)
2 good tbsp coconut oil (45g)

Makes 5 patties

If you don't tolerate dairy well in any form or if you're reluctant to consume it, there's no need to panic. Bone health is complex, and while dairy certainly is an excellent source of calcium for the bones, there are other factors at play. Doing resistance exercise can help and a good magnesium and vitamin D3 intake is also important.

Other sources of calcium that you can use instead of dairy if you're on a low-carb diet are canned fish (like these salmon patties), kale, bok choy (or napa cabbage), broccoli, sesame seeds (or tahini), almonds, seaweed and, of course, good old bone broth.

These patties are handy if you've run out of fresh ingredients. I have canned wild salmon in my pantry all the time. It's a fabulous source of nutrients, especially calcium, in a highly bio-available form.

Put all the ingredients except the coconut flour and oil into a blender and whizz. Stir in the coconut flour and shape into five patties.

Heat the coconut oil in a frying pan and cook the patties until golden on one side, then flip over and cook the other side for 3–4 minutes. Serve with the creamy pepper sauce on the next page.

PER PORTION

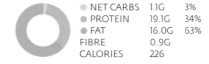

NET CARBS	1.1G	3%
PROTEIN	19.1G	34%
FAT	16.0G	63%
FIBRE	0.9G	
CALORIES	226	

Put all the ingredients into a blender and whizz to combine, then gently heat up in a frying pan. Pour over the salmon patties on page 296 and enjoy.

Creamy pepper sauce

1 red bell pepper, roasted and skin removed (160g)
1 small red onion, roughly chopped (60g)
80g (2.8 oz) cashew nuts (80g)
1 garlic clove (3g)
150ml (⅝c) filtered water (150g)
¾ tbsp lemon juice (12g)

Makes 5 portions

PER PORTION

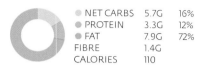

NET CARBS	5.7G	16%
PROTEIN	3.3G	12%
FAT	7.9G	72%
FIBRE	1.4G	
CALORIES	110	

If you're missing rice on a low-carb diet, try this cauliflower version. I find it too bland on its own, but the curry powder turns it from bland to exotic and the tomatoes help to add more flavour too. Don't forget to make a little bit extra for lunch on Day 7.

Blitz the cauliflower in a food processor until it looks similar to small rice grains. Stir in the sun-dried tomatoes, garlic, curry powder and seasoning.

Heat the duck fat in a frying pan and fry the 'rice' on a medium heat for about 10 minutes.

Cauliflower rice

400g (14.1 oz) cauliflower (400g)
4 sun-dried tomatoes, finely chopped (24g)
1 garlic clove, peeled (3g)
1 tsp curry powder (2g)
Salt and pepper (3g)
2 tbsp duck fat (90g)

Serves 4

PER PORTION

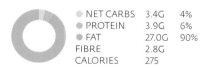

NET CARBS	3.4G	4%
PROTEIN	3.9G	6%
FAT	27.0G	90%
FIBRE	2.8G	
CALORIES	275	

Meal Plan for Week 1 **Day 7**

RECIPE	QUANTITY		CALORIES	CARBS	PROTEIN	FAT
BREAKFAST						
Lemony chia pancakes	407g		784	10.3g	25.0g	66.0g
		Meal total:	784	10.3g	25.0g	66.0g
LUNCH						
Mason jar lunch	430g		629	10.1g	18.1g	55.0g
		Meal total:	629	10.1g	18.1g	55.0g
DINNER						
Creamy lamb burgers	192g		308	2.6g	24.0g	22.0g
Spicy mayo	53g		121	1.6g	2.0g	11.8g
Cucumber salad	136g		127	2.9g	1.8g	11.7g
		Meal total:	556	7.1g	27.8g	45.5g
PLAN TOTAL:			1,969	27.5g	70.9g	166.5g

Macronutrient Analysis

	CARBOHYDRATE	PROTEIN	FAT	ALCOHOL
INTAKE	27.5g	70.9g	166.5g	0g
	6% carbs	**15% protein**	**79% fat**	

These pancakes are light and refreshing because of the lemon juice and zest. Using lemon zest is another way of adding more nutrients to your diet. Not only does it add a nice flavour to various foods, but D-limonene has also been shown to block cancer-forming chemicals and kill cancer cells in preliminary laboratory tests.

Put all the ingredients except the butter into a strong blender. It's best to add liquids first and then dry ingredients. Whizz until you have a smooth batter.

Gently fry the pancakes in butter over a medium heat for 3–4 minutes on each side. Don't overheat, as you might damage the polyunsaturated fats in the chia seeds and almonds.

PER PORTION

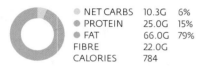

NET CARBS	10.3G	6%
PROTEIN	25.0G	15%
FAT	66.0G	79%
FIBRE	22.0G	
CALORIES	784	

Lemony chia pancakes

75g (2.6 oz) desiccated coconut (75g)
50g (1.8 oz) chia seeds (50g)
4 eggs (200g)
350ml (1½c) coconut milk in a
   carton, such as Koko brand (350g)
Zest of 1 lemon (2g)
4 tbsp lemon juice (60g)
1 heaped tbsp almond butter (40g)
1 tsp baking soda (4g)
½ tsp salt (3g)
2 tbsp butter (30g)

Serves 2

Mason jar lunch

110g (3.9 oz) avocado (110g)
2 tbsp full-fat coconut milk (30g)
2 tbsp lime juice (30g)
120g (4.2 oz) zucchini noodles (120g)
60g (2.1 oz) cauliflower rice (page 297) (60g)
2 tbsp shelled hemp seeds (18g)
2 tbsp chopped fresh cilantro (8g)
3 slices of red pepper, chopped (24g)
50g (1.8 oz) feta cheese, diced (50g)

Serves 1

This recipe serves as inspiration for anybody who has to take packed lunches to the office every day. The principle is simple: make a nice dressing, add leftovers, seeds and a protein source on top and place in the fridge until you're leaving the house. Shake well and enjoy! Simple, isn't it?

Whizz the avocado, coconut milk and lime juice in a blender to make a smooth dressing. Add enough water to reach your desired consistency. Pour it into the bottom of a mason jar, then add the zucchini noodles.

In a separate bowl, mix together the cauliflower rice, hemp seeds and chopped cilantro and toss to combine, then add on top of the zucchini noodles. Place the chopped peppers and feta on top. Put the lid on the mason jar and refrigerate. When you're ready to eat, turn the jar upside down to mix all the ingredients with the dressing, shake it a little bit and enjoy.

PER PORTION

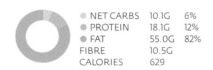

NET CARBS	10.1G	6%
PROTEIN	18.1G	12%
FAT	55.0G	82%
FIBRE	10.5G	
CALORIES	629	

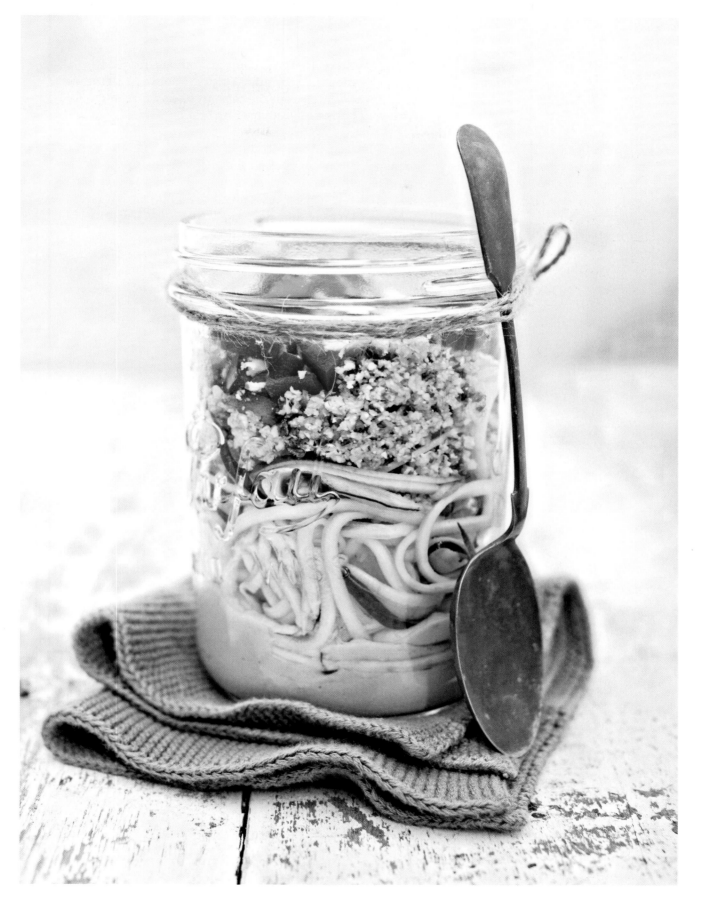

Creamy lamb burgers

100g (3.5 oz) broccoli (100g)
100g (3.5 oz) mushrooms (100g)
80g (2.8 oz) onions (80g)
450g (1lb) minced lamb (450g)
3 garlic cloves, crushed (9g)
1 tsp dried oregano (2g)
Salt and pepper (3g)
1 good tbsp coconut oil (27g)

Makes 4 burgers

Whizz the broccoli, mushrooms and onions in a food processor until they resemble a coarse flour. Add all the other ingredients except the coconut oil and mix well with your hands, then shape into four burgers.

Fry the burgers in the coconut oil on a medium heat for about 6 minutes on each side. After frying the lamb burgers, add some sliced yellow pepper to the pan so that you can just gently fry it for lunch the following day (see the recipe on page 306). Serve with a dollop of the spicy mayo below.

PER PORTION

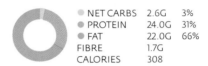

NET CARBS	2.6G	3%
PROTEIN	24.0G	31%
FAT	22.0G	66%
FIBRE	1.7G	
CALORIES	308	

Spicy mayo

150g (5.3 oz) silken tofu (150g)
3 tbsp avocado oil (42g)
3 tsp wasabi paste or 1 tsp wasabi powder (12g)
1 tsp lemon juice (5g)
⅛ tsp matcha green tea powder (1g)

Serves 4

You won't find many soy-based recipes in this book, but this one can come in handy if you want to make a mayonnaise but don't have eggs to hand, or indeed have a sensitivity to eggs. Because tofu is very bland but has a nice texture, combining it with wasabi paste works really well.

Put all the ingredients into a blender and whizz until you have a smooth paste.

PER PORTION

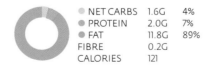

NET CARBS	1.6G	4%
PROTEIN	2.0G	7%
FAT	11.8G	89%
FIBRE	0.2G	
CALORIES	121	

Cucumber salad

Prepare some more cucumber ribbons so that you can make this salad again for lunch on Day 8. Don't mix the vinaigrette with the cucumber until the last minute, though, as it will go too watery.

Using a spiraliser or julienne peeler, cut the cucumber into long ribbons. Whisk together the olive oil, lime juice, sour cream and soy sauce, then stir in the chopped red onion and dill. Toss with the cucumber noodles and sprinkle the nori flakes over the salad.

PER PORTION

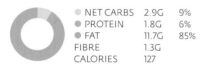

NET CARBS	2.9G	9%
PROTEIN	1.8G	6%
FAT	11.7G	85%
FIBRE	1.3G	
CALORIES	127	

1 cucumber (360g)

2 tbsp olive oil (26g)

2 tbsp lime juice (30g)

2 tbsp sour cream (or soy yoghurt for dairy-free) (84g)

1 tsp soy sauce (6g)

1 small red onion, finely chopped (30g)

1 tbsp chopped fresh dill (4g)

2 tbsp nori flakes (5g)

Serves 4

Meal Plan for Week 2 **Day 8**

RECIPE	QUANTITY		CALORIES	CARBS	PROTEIN	FAT
BREAKFAST						
Keto cornflakes	275g		704	9.3g	19.3g	63.0g
		Meal total:	704	9.3g	19.3g	63.0g
LUNCH						
Egg-free sandwich	156g		580	4.6g	17.3g	51.0g
Cucumber salad (page 303)	136g		127	2.9g	1.8g	11.7g
		Meal total:	707	7.5g	19.1g	62.7g
DINNER						
Sea bass with celeriac and chorizo purée	471g		541	9.4g	26.0g	42.0g
		Meal total:	541	9.4g	26.0g	42.0g
PLAN TOTAL:			1,952	26.2g	64.4g	167.7g

Macronutrient Analysis

	CARBOHYDRATE	PROTEIN	FAT	ALCOHOL
INTAKE	26.2g	64.4g	167.7g	0g
	6% carbs	**14% protein**	**80% fat**	

Put the toasted coconut flakes, almonds and cinnamon into a bowl and toss well. Pour over as much protein shake as you like and have the rest as a drink.

Keto cornflakes

PER PORTION

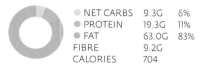

NET CARBS	9.3G	6%
PROTEIN	19.3G	11%
FAT	63.0G	83%
FIBRE	9.2G	
CALORIES	704	

30g (1.1 oz) toasted coconut flakes (30g)
25g (0.9 oz) flaked almonds (25g)
1 tsp ground cinnamon (2g)
1 portion protein coconut shake (see below) (218g)

Serves 1

Put all the ingredients into a blender and whizz. Pour some over the cornflakes and drink the rest if you don't feel like drowning your cereal.

Protein coconut shake

PER PORTION

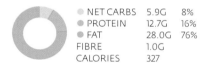

NET CARBS	5.9G	8%
PROTEIN	12.7G	16%
FAT	28.0G	76%
FIBRE	1.0G	
CALORIES	327	

250ml (1c) coconut milk in a carton, such as Koko brand (250g)
125ml (½c) full-fat coconut milk (125g)
1½ scoops protein powder (32g)
1 good tbsp coconut oil (27g)
1 tsp ground cinnamon (2g)

Serves 1

Egg-free bread

250g (8.8 oz) milled flaxseed (250g)

80g (2.8 oz) macadamia nuts, ground to a fine flour (80g)

Zest of 1 lemon (8g)

1 tsp baking soda (4g)

1 tsp dried oregano (1.8g)

1 tsp dried thyme (1g)

½ tsp salt (3g)

50g (3½tbsp) coconut oil or butter, melted (50g)

100ml (⅜c) water (100g)

2 tbsp apple cider vinegar (23g)

Serves 8

There are quite a lot of people – me included – who are sensitive to eggs, which is why I've created a number of egg-free recipes. I cut them out completely for about three months after noticing a lot of digestive discomfort whenever I ate them. During that time, I used an egg replacer to make breads and crackers. As with any so-called allergenic foods (i.e. those that most commonly cause serious allergic reactions), it's not a good idea to eat them every single day, but rather to take a break. I have eggs about three times a week now and often rotate between duck, quail and hen's eggs, and I have no more symptoms.

Preheat the oven to 150°C (300°F). Line a baking tray with non-stick baking paper.

Put all the dry ingredients into a bowl and mix well, then add the butter, water and apple cider vinegar. Knead to a firm dough and spread onto the lined tray until it's about 2cm (¾in) thick. Bake for about 1 hour, depending on how crunchy you like it. Allow to cool slightly before you slice it, otherwise it could fall apart.

PER PORTION

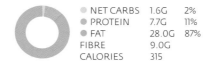

NET CARBS	1.6G	2%
PROTEIN	7.7G	11%
FAT	28.0G	87%
FIBRE	9.0G	
CALORIES	315	

Egg-free sandwich

1 portion of egg-free bread (see above) (65g)

40g (1.4 oz) goats' cheese, sliced (40g)

4 sun-dried tomatoes (24g)

3 slices of yellow bell pepper, lightly fried (24g)

5 fresh basil leaves (3g)

Serves 1

Slice the bread lengthways to create two thin slices. Top with the goats' cheese, tomatoes, pepper and basil.

PER PORTION

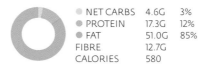

NET CARBS	4.6G	3%
PROTEIN	17.3G	12%
FAT	51.0G	85%
FIBRE	12.7G	
CALORIES	580	

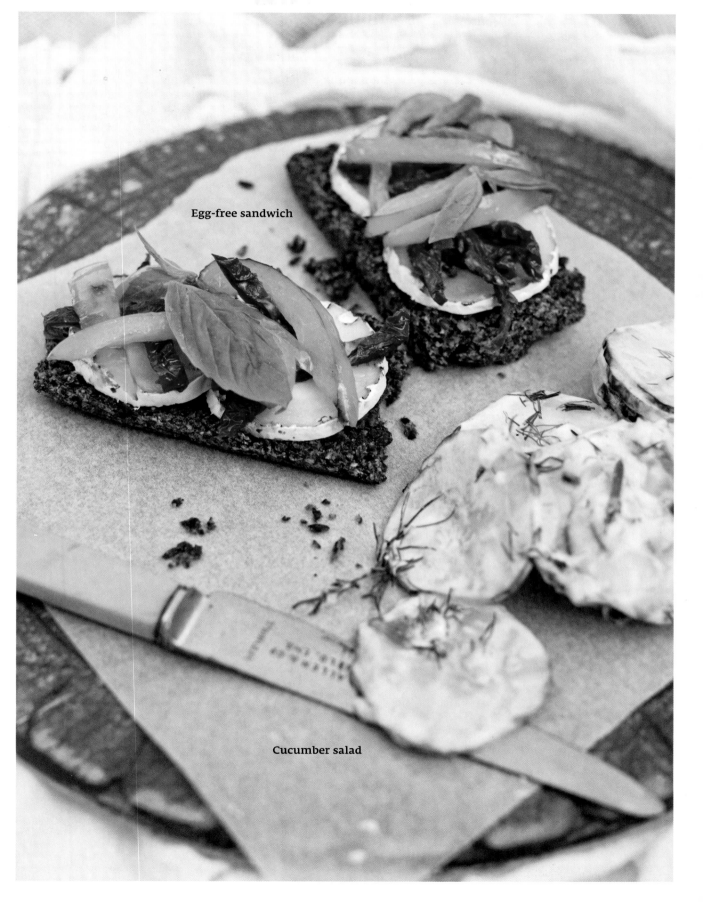

Egg-free sandwich

Cucumber salad

Sea bass with celeriac and chorizo purée

We talked about the downsides of processed meat earlier (see page 246), so please only use chorizo that comes from happy pigs and doesn't contain any additives or preservatives. It can be really hard to find, so use some other good-quality meat that adds a bit of spicy flavour to this dish instead – the celeriac mash can be a bit boring otherwise.

800g (1.75lbs) celeriac, peeled and chopped into small cubes (800g)
4 small fillets of sea bass (320g)
Juice of 1 lemon (40g)
1 good tbsp coconut oil, melted (27g)
1½ tbsp duck fat (68g)
1 leek, cut into slices (300g)
6 garlic cloves, chopped (18g)
60g (2.1 oz) fresh chorizo, chopped (60g)
250ml (1c) full-fat coconut milk (250g)

Serves 4

Preheat the oven to 180°C (350°F).

Steam the celeriac for about 20 minutes.

Put the sea bass fillets on a baking tray and drizzle with the lemon juice and melted coconut oil. You could add herbs as well, such as dill, rosemary or marjoram. Bake for 15 minutes.

Meanwhile, melt the duck fat in a large pan. Add the leek, garlic and chorizo. Lightly fry until the leek is soft and the chorizo is well cooked. Add the steamed celeriac to the chorizo mixture, then add the coconut milk (you might not need all of it depending on your preference for consistency) and blend everything together in a food processor. Serve the purée with the sea bass.

Make sure you have 100g sea bass baked in coconut oil and lemon left over for lunch on Day 9.

PER PORTION

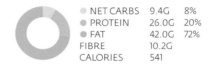

● NET CARBS	9.4G	8%
● PROTEIN	26.0G	20%
● FAT	42.0G	72%
FIBRE	10.2G	
CALORIES	541	

Meal Plan for Week 2 **Day 9**

RECIPE	QUANTITY		CALORIES	CARBS	PROTEIN	FAT
BREAKFAST						
Blackberry pancakes	210g		671	6.7g	15.6g	63.0g
		Meal total:	671	6.7g	15.6g	63.0g
LUNCH						
Sea bass (leftovers)	100g		161	0.2g	19.6g	9.1g
40g pesto (page 262)	40g		252	1.2g	3.1g	26.1g
Tomato salad (page 176)	200g		161	6.7g	1.4g	17.3g
		Meal total:	574	8.1g	24.1g	52.5g
DINNER						
Zucchini 'spaghetti'	236g		142	3.9g	4.9g	10.3g
Bolognese sauce	319g		437	4.8g	24.0g	35.0g
		Meal total:	579	8.7g	28.9g	45.3g
PLAN TOTAL:			1,829	24.6g	68.6g	160.8g

Macronutrient Analysis

	CARBOHYDRATE	PROTEIN	FAT	ALCOHOL
INTAKE	24.6g	68.6g	160.8g	0.5g
	6% carbs	**15% protein**	**79% fat**	

Blackberry pancakes

55g (3⅔ tbsp) coconut oil (55g)

2 eggs (100g)

1 tbsp vanilla essence, no alcohol (15g)

3 scant tbsp coconut flour (18g)

1 tsp gluten-free baking powder (4g)

30g (1.1 oz) blackberries (30g)

Serves 1

Melt 1 tablespoon of coconut oil in a frying pan over a medium heat. Melt the rest of the coconut oil in a separate pan and add it to a mixing bowl with the eggs and vanilla essence. Mix well, then add the coconut flour and baking powder and whisk together. You should have a smooth batter – you might have to add some more coconut milk or water. Ladle some batter into the frying pan and cook for about 3 minutes on each side, until golden brown. The smaller the pancakes, the easier they will be to turn. Top with the blackberries before serving.

PER PORTION

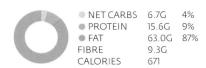

NET CARBS	6.7G	4%
PROTEIN	15.6G	9%
FAT	63.0G	87%
FIBRE	9.3G	
CALORIES	671	

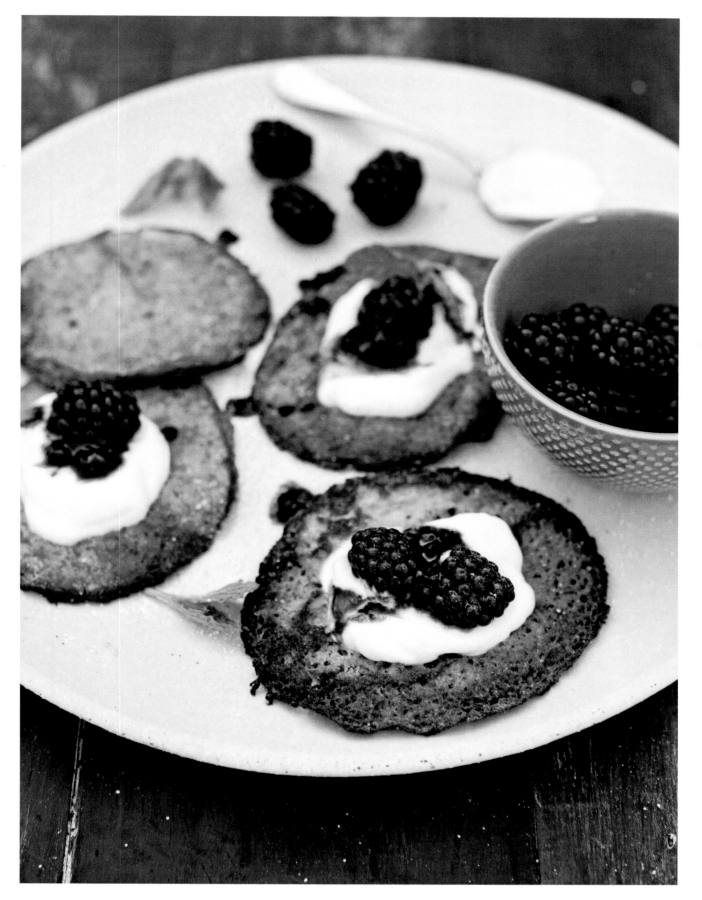

Zucchini spaghetti

65g (4⅓tbsp) butter (65g)
900g (2lbs) zucchinis, cut into
  spirals (900g)
450g (1lb) spinach (450g)
Salt and pepper (3g)

Serves 6

If you're anything like me and ate a lot of spaghetti before you switched to a low-carb regime, this might be for you. I usually make spelt, brown rice or buckwheat spaghetti for my family and mix some of the zucchini spirals in too. It's a great way to get your kids to eat vegetables, that's for sure.

Heat the butter in a frying pan over a medium heat. Add the zucchini spirals (you can make spirals with a julienne peeler or with a spiraliser) and fry them for 2–3 minutes, then add the spinach and fry just until it's wilted. Season with salt and pepper.

PER PORTION

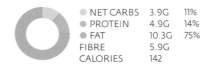

NET CARBS	3.9G	11%
PROTEIN	4.9G	14%
FAT	10.3G	75%
FIBRE	5.9G	
CALORIES	142	

I don't just use this Bolognese sauce with spaghetti. You can also try making a lasagne with it by slicing zucchinis or eggplants lengthways into very thin slices. You then layer the sauce with the vegetables and maybe also some cheese and bake it in the oven until cooked through.

Tomatoes are part of the so-called nightshade family, which includes white potatoes, eggplants and peppers (sweet peppers and chillies) as well as spices like paprika, red chilli flakes and cayenne pepper (but not black pepper). Nightshades are often talked about in the context of rheumatoid arthritis or any autoimmune condition. They can cause flare-ups in sensitive people and evoke an inflammatory response. Because inflammation tends to be a problem in cancer patients too, I would definitely not overdo it with them. Peppers and tomatoes are rather high in carbohydrates anyway compared to other non-starchy vegetables, so just have them in small amounts.

Heat the oil in a large frying pan. When it's hot enough, add the lamb and fry at a high temperature for 2–3 minutes. Turn down the heat and add all the vegetables, the chopped anchovies and the tomato purée. Cook for a little while, until they soften. Add the red wine and cook for 2 minutes, then add the chicken stock. Add the herbs, smoked paprika and salt and pepper to taste, then simmer for another 15 minutes.

PER PORTION

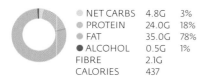

NET CARBS	4.8G	3%
PROTEIN	24.0G	18%
FAT	35.0G	78%
ALCOHOL	0.5G	1%
FIBRE	2.1G	
CALORIES	437	

Bolognese sauce

120g (4.2 oz) coconut or olive oil (120g)

600g (1.3lbs) minced lamb (600g)

140g (4.9 oz) mushrooms, thinly sliced (140g)

60g (2.1 oz) spinach (60g)

3 average-sized ripe tomatoes, chopped (255g)

3 stalks of celery, chopped (180g)

2 scallions, bulbs and tops chopped (20g)

3 garlic cloves, crushed (9g)

1 × 50g can (1.7 oz) anchovies, drained and finely chopped (50g)

2 tbsp tomato purée (102g)

125ml (½c) red wine (125g)

250ml (1c) homemade chicken stock (see the note on page 340) (250g)

1 tsp dried rosemary (1g)

1 tsp dried thyme (1g)

1 tsp dried oregano (1g)

1 tsp smoked paprika (2g)

Salt and pepper (3g)

Serves 6

Meal Plan for Week 2 Day 10

RECIPE	QUANTITY		CALORIES	CARBS	PROTEIN	FAT
BREAKFAST						
Budwig cream	170g		274	6.8g	21.0g	16.8g
Keto coffee	324g		384	1.3g	1.1g	42.0g
		Meal total:	658	8.1g	22.1g	58.8g
LUNCH						
Mushroom and leek omelette	338.5g		636	4.5g	21.0g	57.0g
		Meal total:	636	4.5g	21.0g	57.0g
DINNER						
Mediterranean vegetables with chicken legs	236g		585	9.3g	22.0g	50.0g
		Meal total:	585	9.3g	22.0g	50.0g
PLAN TOTAL:			1,879	21.9g	65.1g	165.8g

Macronutrient Analysis

	CARBOHYDRATE	PROTEIN	FAT	ALCOHOL
INTAKE	21.9g	65.1g	165.8g	0g
	5% carbs	**15% protein**	**80% fat**	

The Budwig diet is another well-known cancer diet. It was designed in 1951 by Dr Johanna Budwig, a renowned German biochemist and expert on fats and oils. The rationale of her approach is that fatty acids are deficient in most diets (which we totally agree on!) and that they are used more efficiently when they are combined with sulphur-rich amino acids of dairy proteins – hence the mixing of flax oil (which is rich in alpha-linolenic acid) with quark or cottage cheese, for instance. There are some elements of the Budwig approach that are very compatible with a ketogenic diet. Full-fat quark can be hard to get, but you can also use cottage cheese, preferably organic, instead.

Mill the flaxseed in a food processor (if shop bought, make sure they are stored in the fridge). Add the quark, blueberries and flax oil and whizz again to combine.

Budwig cream

1 heaped tbsp milled flaxseeds (15g)
120g (4.2 oz) full-fat quark (120g)
25g (0.9 oz) blueberries (25g)
1 scant tbsp flaxseed oil (10g)

Serves 1

PER PORTION

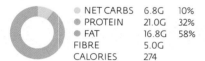

NET CARBS	6.8G	10%
PROTEIN	21.0G	32%
FAT	16.8G	58%
FIBRE	5.0G	
CALORIES	274	

Coffee is an incredibly antioxidant-rich beverage and can be part of a ketogenic diet unless it raises your blood sugar levels. Unfortunately, this can be the case. The only way to find out if this applies to you is by testing your blood glucose levels.

Put all the ingredients into a blender and whizz to combine.

Keto coffee

250ml (1c) hot coffee or organic chaga tea (250g)
2 tbsp full-fat coconut milk (30g)
2 tbsp liquid coconut oil (24g)
1 tbsp butter or ghee (15g)
1 tsp vanilla essence (5g)

Serves 1

PER PORTION

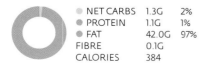

NET CARBS	1.3G	2%
PROTEIN	1.1G	1%
FAT	42.0G	97%
FIBRE	0.1G	
CALORIES	384	

Mushroom and leek omelette

1 tbsp duck fat (45g)

125g (4.4 oz) Portobello mushrooms, sliced (125g)

1 small leek, cut into small pieces (75g)

2 bacon, diced (40g)

3 large eggs (171g)

½ tsp dried thyme (1g)

Salt and pepper (3g)

1 avocado, sliced (220g)

Serves 2

Heat the duck fat in a frying pan over a medium heat. Fry the mushrooms, leek and bacon for 5–10 minutes, until the leek has softened. Whisk together the eggs and thyme and some salt and pepper. Pour the egg mix over the vegetables, cover the pan with a lid and cook for about 15 minutes, until the egg is set. Cover with the sliced avocado.

PER PORTION

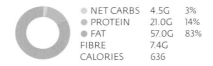

NET CARBS	4.5G	3%
PROTEIN	21.0G	14%
FAT	57.0G	83%
FIBRE	7.4G	
CALORIES	636	

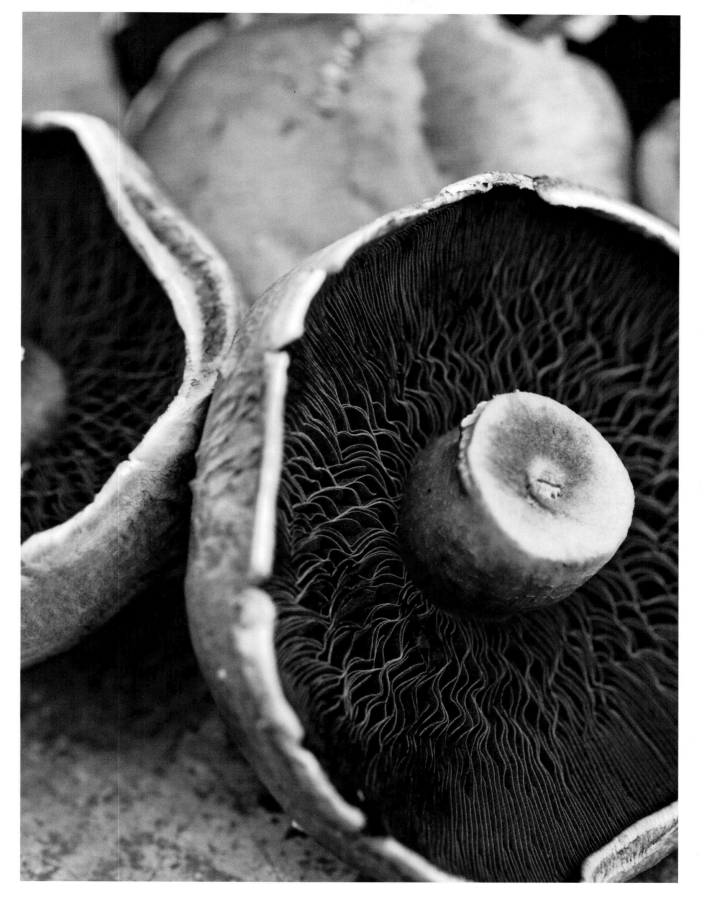

Mediterranean vegetables with chicken legs

1 tsp wholegrain mustard (16g)

1 tsp mixed paprika (2g)

Salt and pepper (5g)

4 organic chicken legs, skin on and bone in (720g)

2 sprigs of rosemary (5g)

2 red or yellow bell peppers, roughly chopped (320g)

2 zucchinis, roughly chopped (200g)

2 small onions, cut into wedges (120g)

4 garlic cloves, unpeeled (12g)

6 good tbsp coconut oil (135g)

Serves 4

Preheat the oven to 180°C (350°F).

Mix together the mustard, paprika, salt and pepper and rub it onto the chicken legs. Place the chicken in a roasting pan and put the rosemary sprigs on top.

Place all the vegetables in a separate roasting pan (you can squeeze out the softened garlic cloves after cooking). Put the coconut oil on top of the vegetables and place both pans in the oven. Stir the vegetables after about 5 minutes, when the coconut oil has melted.

Bake for 45–60 minutes, stirring halfway through to turn the vegetables. When the chicken is ready (the juices should run clear), take both trays out of the oven and serve.

Make sure you cook some extra chicken so that you have leftovers for lunch on Day 11 and Day 14. Keep the bones because you can make bone broth out of them – we discuss the benefits of this in more detail on page 340.

PER PORTION

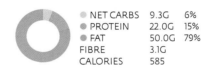

NET CARBS	9.3G	6%
PROTEIN	22.0G	15%
FAT	50.0G	79%
FIBRE	3.1G	
CALORIES	585	

Meal Plan for Week 2 Day 11

RECIPE	QUANTITY		CALORIES	CARBS	PROTEIN	FAT
BREAKFAST						
Keto start-up	466g		652	6.9g	21.0g	56.0g
		Meal total:	652	6.9g	21.0g	56.0g
LUNCH						
Quick chicken salad	424g		664	7.8g	23.0g	59.0g
		Meal total:	664	7.8g	23.0g	59.0g
DINNER						
3 lamb liver heaps	114g		213	1.5g	18.6g	14.4g
Cauliflower purée	178g		197	3.4g	5.7g	17.2g
Light leafy salad	74g		126	1.1g	0.8g	13.0g
		Meal total:	536	6.0g	25.1g	44.6g
PLAN TOTAL:			1,855	20.7g	69.1g	159.6g

Macronutrient Analysis

	CARBOHYDRATE	PROTEIN	FAT	ALCOHOL
INTAKE	20.7g	69.1g	159.6g	0g
	5% carbs	**15% protein**	**80% fat**	

Keto start-up

250ml (1c) unsweetened almond
   milk (250g)
55ml (3¾tbsp) full-fat coconut milk
   (55g)
½ avocado (110g)
15g (0.5 oz) protein powder (15g)
2 tbsp chia seeds (20g)
1 tbsp cocoa butter (14g)
1 tsp ground cinnamon (2g)

Serves 1

This breakfast is something between a smoothie and a thick
pudding. It could be a nice recipe to try when you're going
through treatment and you don't feel like chewing or eating
spicy foods.

Put all the ingredients into a blender and whizz.

PER PORTION

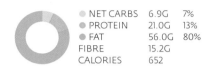

NET CARBS	6.9G	7%
PROTEIN	21.0G	13%
FAT	56.0G	80%
FIBRE	15.2G	
CALORIES	652	

Quick chicken salad

1 garlic clove, crushed (3g)
2 tbsp homemade turmeric mayo
   (page 321) (30g)
1 tbsp lemon juice (15g)
1 portion leftover chicken legs (150g)
2 stalks of celery, chopped (120g)
½ small red onion, finely chopped
   (30g)
30g (1.1 oz) iceberg lettuce, shredded
   (30g)
10 whole pecan nuts, finely chopped
   (36g)
Salt and pepper (3g)

Serves 1

**Put the garlic, mayonnaise and lemon juice in a large
bowl and whisk well. Add all the other ingredients and
mix together. Season with salt and pepper if needed.**

PER PORTION

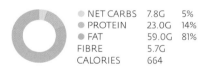

NET CARBS	7.8G	5%
PROTEIN	23.0G	14%
FAT	59.0G	81%
FIBRE	5.7G	
CALORIES	664	

I'm not quite sure why so many recipes make mayonnaise so complicated, especially when it comes to the emulsification process. Many instructions get you to very slowly drizzle the oil into the egg mix and the whole process takes forever. After trying (and failing) many times with this method, I read somewhere that I can just use a hand-held stick blender – *et voilà!* Now the whole process takes me about 20 seconds and the result is fabulous.

There's more and more interest in how different foods interact with each other and enhance each other's benefits (known as food synergy). Here are the most important combinations that will help you get more out of your foods:

Turmeric + black pepper: The anti-cancer activity of curcumin (the main phytochemical in the spice turmeric) is increased by a factor of 1,000 (!) in the presence of piperine (in black pepper). Olive or fish oil may further enhance the effect.

Green tea + citrus: Citrus fruits help preserve the catechins (a type of disease-fighting flavonoid and antioxidant) in green tea.

Turmeric + green tea: Synergistic (enhanced) effect on cancer cells.

Chopped garlic + time: The anti-cancer compound diallyl disulphide is made when garlic is left to sit for 10 minutes after being crushed or chopped.

The turmeric in this recipe gives the mayonnaise a vibrant colour. Just make sure you also add black pepper.

Place everything in a narrow glass jar (like a wide-mouth mason jar) and let the oil rise to the top. The eggs can come straight out of a fridge. Place a hand-held stick/immersion blender at the bottom of the jar and turn it on. Stay at the bottom of the jar for 10–20 seconds, until the mayo starts to emulsify, i.e. turn white. Then slowly raise the blender out of the jar and pulse a few times until the whole mixture is thick and creamy.

Homemade turmeric mayo

250ml (1c) mild olive oil (232g)
1 large egg (57g)
½ garlic clove (2g)
2 tsp cider vinegar (8g)
1 tsp wholegrain mustard (10g)
½ tsp ground turmeric (1g)
Salt and pepper (3g)

Makes 300g

PER TABLESPOON (15G)

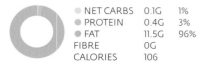

● NET CARBS	0.1G	1%
● PROTEIN	0.4G	3%
● FAT	11.5G	96%
FIBRE	0G	
CALORIES	106	

Lamb liver heaps

450g (1lb) lamb liver (450g)

2 garlic cloves, peeled (6g)

2 good tbsp coconut oil (54g)

1 tbsp dried rosemary (3g)

1 tsp dried sage (1g)

1 tsp dried thyme (1g)

2 tsp wholegrain mustard (20g)

Salt and pepper (3g)

450g (1lb) minced lamb (450g)

1 medium onion, finely diced (150g)

1 tbsp nutritional yeast flakes with
   B12 (11g)

Makes 30 heaps

Here's another sneaky attempt to get some liver into you. You can even lower the liver content initially and then slowly increase it once your palate adapts and gets used to the taste. I'm not giving up!

Preheat the oven to 180°C (350°F). Line a baking tray with non-stick baking paper.

Grind the liver, garlic, coconut oil, spices, mustard and some salt and pepper in a food processor to a smooth paste. Add to a large bowl along with the minced lamb, finely diced onion and yeast flakes and mix well to combine.

Using a large spoon, place small portions of the meat mixture onto the lined tray. Bake in the oven for about 20 minutes.

If you haven't already baked the flax and coconut focaccia on page 328, this is a good opportunity to do that while the oven is already on. Otherwise, don't forget to take some out of the freezer for the following day.

PER PORTION (1 'HEAP')

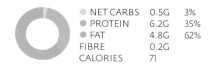

NET CARBS	0.5G	3%
PROTEIN	6.2G	35%
FAT	4.8G	62%
FIBRE	0.2G	
CALORIES	71	

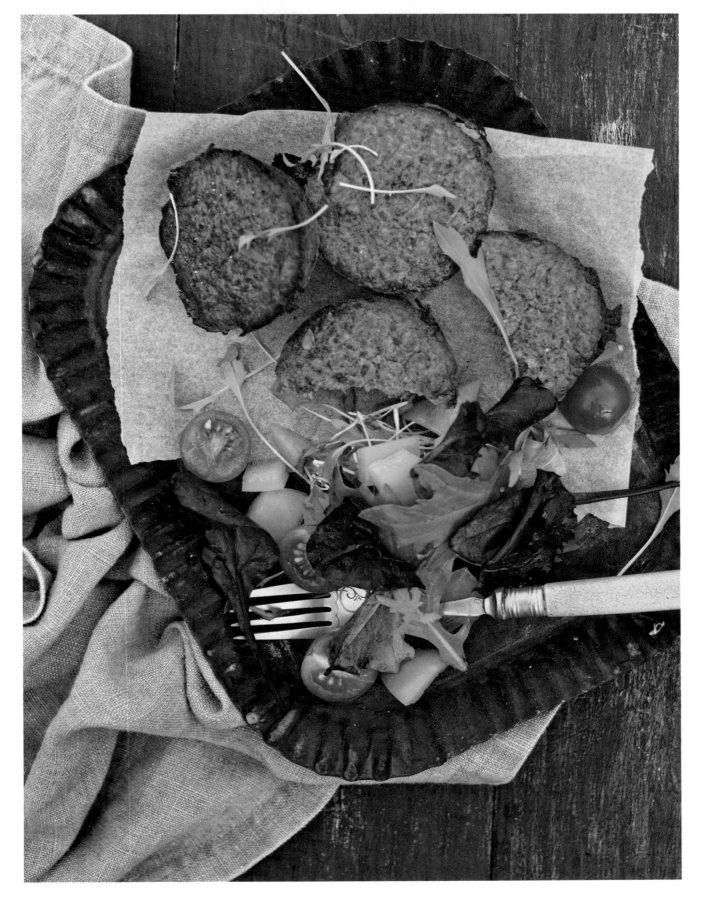

Cauliflower purée

Mashed potatoes are another typical comfort food that we unfortunately have to remove from our meal plans on a ketogenic diet. But we've come up with a nice alternative – cauliflower purée!

1 head of cauliflower, broken into florets (600g)

100g (3.5 oz) homemade turmeric mayo (page 321) (100g)

2 garlic cloves, roasted (6g)

Serves 4

Lightly steam or boil the cauliflower. Mix with the mayonnaise and roasted garlic (just squeeze it out) and then purée with a hand-held stick blender.

PER PORTION

NET CARBS	3.4G	7%
PROTEIN	5.7G	12%
FAT	17.2G	81%
FIBRE	2.5G	
CALORIES	197	

Light leafy salad

Wash the leaves well and mix with the vinaigrette.

4 cups butterhead lettuce, chopped (200g)

4 portions vinaigrette (page 280) (96g)

Serves 4

PER PORTION (INCLUDING DRESSING)

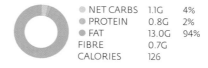

NET CARBS	1.1G	4%
PROTEIN	0.8G	2%
FAT	13.0G	94%
FIBRE	0.7G	
CALORIES	126	

Meal Plan for Week 2 Day 12

RECIPE	QUANTITY		CALORIES	CARBS	PROTEIN	FAT
BREAKFAST						
Scrambled duck eggs	241g		603	6.3g	21.0g	54.0g
		Meal total:	603	6.3g	21.0g	54.0g
LUNCH						
Spinach salad	284g		387	4.5g	14.4g	34.0g
Flax and coconut focaccia	80g		302	2.6g	8.9g	26.0g
		Meal total:	689	7.1g	23.3g	60.0g
DINNER						
Manchego pizza	189g		612	4.4g	21.0g	55.0g
		Meal total:	612	4.4g	21.0g	55.0g
PLAN TOTAL:			1,904	17.8g	65.3g	169.0g

Macronutrient Analysis

	CARBOHYDRATE	PROTEIN	FAT	ALCOHOL
INTAKE	17.8g	65.3g	169.0g	0g
	4% carbs	**14% protein**	**82% fat**	

Scrambled duck eggs

1 tbsp duck fat (45g)

35g (1.2 oz) curly kale, finely chopped (35g)

3 fresh shiitake mushrooms (84g)

4 cherry tomatoes, quartered (48g)

1 good tbsp coconut oil (27g)

3 duck eggs (225g)

2 tbsp shelled hemp seeds (18g)

Serves 2

Duck eggs are fabulous and bring more variety into your diet. Did you know that they have almost twice the nutritional value of a chicken egg? They're also higher in fat and albumin, which can make cakes fluffier and richer. And most importantly, many people who can't tolerate eggs from chickens are fine with duck eggs.

Melt the duck fat in a frying pan and add the curly kale, shiitake mushrooms and tomatoes. Cover with a lid and fry on a medium heat for 4–5 minutes.

In a separate pan, heat the coconut oil and scramble the duck eggs. Serve with the vegetables and sprinkle with hemp seeds. You can also scramble the eggs in the same pan as the vegetables if that's your preference.

PER PORTION

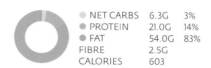

● NET CARBS	6.3G	3%
● PROTEIN	21.0G	14%
● FAT	54.0G	83%
FIBRE	2.5G	
CALORIES	603	

Smoking fish and meats is one of the earliest preservation techniques developed by humans. But do the smoke and heat damage the delicate omega-3 fatty acids? A study* examined just that, and surprisingly, it found that smoking salmon at 95°C (200°F) made the fragile polyunsaturated fish fats more stable than in fresh fish. It looks like smoke-processing provides the extracted oils with antioxidant potential. Although this is encouraging, I'd still limit smoked fish consumption and go for top quality, like organic or wild smoked salmon. It's more expensive, but a lot of commercially produced smoked salmon is smoked by using sawdust instead of actual wood like hickory, oak or alderwood. At the risk of repeating myself, quality matters, and it's important to know where the produce you eat comes from.

Melt the coconut oil in a frying pan, then fry the mushrooms over a medium heat. Once the mushrooms have softened, add the smoked salmon to gently heat it.

Whisk together the olive oil, vinegar, passata and some salt and pepper.

Place the spinach and celery in a large bowl, then pour over the dressing and toss well. Top the salad with the sliced mushrooms and smoked salmon.

PER PORTION

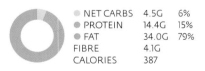

● NET CARBS	4.5G	6%
● PROTEIN	14.4G	15%
● FAT	34.0G	79%
FIBRE	4.1G	
CALORIES	387	

Spinach salad

2 good tsp coconut oil (28g)

125g (4.4 oz) Portobello mushrooms, sliced (125g)

80g (2.8 oz) smoked salmon (80g)

8 tsp extra virgin olive oil (34g)

8 tsp apple cider vinegar (30g)

2 tbsp plain tomato passata (60g)

Salt and pepper (3g)

90g (3.2 oz) spinach (90g)

2 stalks of celery, finely chopped (120g)

Serves 2

* Bower, C.K. et al (2009) 'Stabilizing oils from smoked pink salmon (Oncorhynchus gorbuscha)', *Journal of Food Science*, 73(3), pp. C248–275.

Flax and coconut focaccia

120g (4.2 oz) milled flaxseeds (120g)
85g (3 oz) desiccated coconut (85g)
2 tbsp chia seeds (20g)
¾ tsp cream of tartar (5g)
½ tsp baking soda (3g)
½ tsp rock salt (3g)
3 eggs (150g)
2 tbsp liquid coconut oil (24g)
1 tsp blackstrap molasses (8g)
55ml (3¾tbsp) warm water (55g)

Makes 6 slices

When I want to make an egg-free bread, this works brilliantly with egg replacer (e.g. Orgran). It freezes really well and is very versatile.

Preheat the oven to 180°C (350°F). Oil a square baking dish.

Mix all the dry ingredients together and stir well.

In a different bowl, combine the eggs and coconut oil. Dissolve the molasses in the warm water and mix with the other wet ingredients. Stir the wet ingredients into the dry and allow the batter to sit for 1–2 minutes to thicken.

Put the dough into the oiled baking dish, spread it out until it's about 2cm (¾in) thick and bake for 25–30 minutes, until the bread is firm and cooked through.

You will need more of this focaccia for lunch on Day 17. You can freeze it in handy portions until then.

PER PORTION

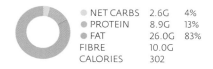

NET CARBS	2.6G	4%
PROTEIN	8.9G	13%
FAT	26.0G	83%
FIBRE	10.0G	
CALORIES	302	

Preheat the oven to 160°C (320°F). Oil a large 30cm (11in) cake pan or springform pan.

Make the base by mixing all the dry ingredients together, then adding the egg and water to form a dough. Use your hands to press it into the oiled pan. Bake for 15–20 minutes and let it cool down slightly before adding the toppings.

You will need this pizza base for lunch on Day 19, so freeze the amount you need for that day after baking it.

PER PORTION

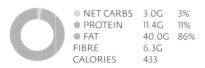

NET CARBS	3.0G	3%
PROTEIN	11.4G	11%
FAT	40.0G	86%
FIBRE	6.3G	
CALORIES	433	

Nutty pizza base

150g (5.3 oz) ground almonds (150g)
120g (4.2 oz) ground Brazil nuts (120g)
35g (1.2 oz) cold butter, diced into cubes (35g)
1 tbsp coconut flour (7g)
½ tsp salt (3g)
1 egg, beaten (50g)
70ml (4¾ tbsp) filtered water (70g)

Serves 5

'A high-fat diet in the presence of carbohydrate is different than a high-fat diet in the presence of low carbohydrate.'
Dr Richard Feinman

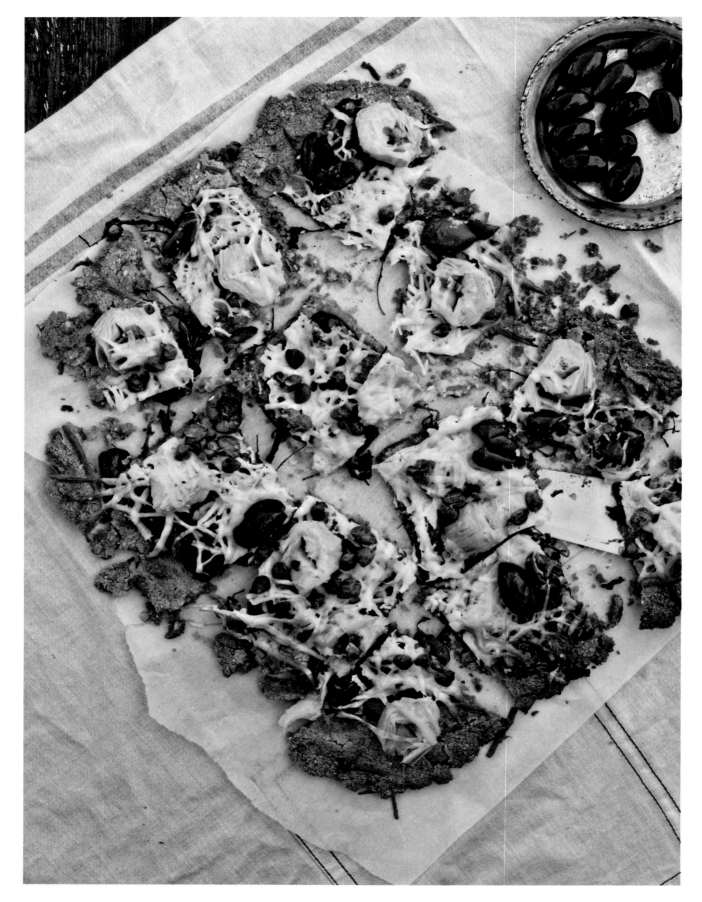

Preheat the oven to 200°C (400°F).

Gently fry the garlic and arugula in the olive oil. Place on the pre-baked base and spread the artichoke hearts, anchovies, olives and capers over the arugula, then sprinkle over the cheese, making sure it covers all the ingredients. Bake the pizza for 10 minutes, until the cheese is melted.

When baking the Manchego pizza, you can also roast the peppers for about 20 minutes for lunch on Day 13.

PER PORTION

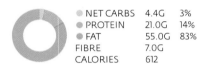

● NET CARBS	4.4G	3%
● PROTEIN	21.0G	14%
● FAT	55.0G	83%
FIBRE	7.0G	
CALORIES	612	

Manchego pizza

3 garlic cloves, crushed (9g)

60g (2.1 oz) arugula (60g)

2 tbsp extra virgin olive oil (26g)

1 × nutty pizza base (see page 329) (435g)

6 artichoke hearts, chopped (120g)

18 anchovies canned in oil, drained and chopped (54g)

12 olives in brine (24g)

2 tbsp capers, drained (17g)

200g (7 oz) Manchego cheese, grated (200g)

Serves 5

Meal Plan for Week 2 Day 13

RECIPE	QUANTITY		CALORIES	CARBS	PROTEIN	FAT
BREAKFAST						
Bacon with veg	253g		586	3.6g	22.0g	53.0g
		Meal total:	586	3.6g	22.0g	53.0g
LUNCH						
Kipper sandwich	235g		630	4.8g	22.0g	54.0g
		Meal total:	630	4.8g	22.0g	54.0g
DINNER						
Baked lamb	202g		466	4.8g	21.0g	40.0g
Broccoli purée	145g		154	3.4g	3.1g	13.3g
		Meal total:	620	8.2g	24.1g	53.3g
PLAN TOTAL:			1,836	16.6g	68.1g	160.3g

Macronutrient Analysis

	CARBOHYDRATE	PROTEIN	FAT	ALCOHOL
INTAKE	16.6g	68.1g	160.3g	0g
	4% carbs	**15% protein**	**81% fat**	

What form of dairy should you choose? When I use dairy, I go for the best quality I can find. Here in Ireland we're blessed with a lot of organic grass-fed dairy, but I know that this can be more challenging to find in other parts of the world. Maybe it's because I'm Swiss, but I also love all the unpasteurised types of cheese, like Gruyère and Emmental, as well as Brie and queso fresco. When milk isn't pasteurised, it tends to be more nutrient dense and better tolerated and it may reduce the risk of developing childhood asthma, allergies and other immune-diseases.*

Although consuming unpasteurised dairy products has several positive health benefits, raw milk can be contaminated with bacteria or other pathogens. It's definitely not recommended for anybody with a compromised immune system, such as cancer patients undergoing treatment.

Heat the avocado oil in a frying pan. When the oil is hot enough, add the rashers and vegetables and fry for about 5 minutes, turning occasionally. Top with the grated Gruyère cheese, season to taste with salt and pepper and serve.

PER PORTION

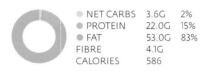

● NET CARBS	3.6G	2%
● PROTEIN	22.0G	15%
● FAT	53.0G	83%
FIBRE	4.1G	
CALORIES	586	

Bacon with veg

2 tbsp avocado oil (28g)
200g (7 oz) bacon, chopped (200g)
30g (1.1 oz) spinach (30g)
2 small ripe tomatoes, halved (100g)
½ avocado, sliced (110g)
4 garlic cloves, crushed (12g)
25g (0.9 oz) Gruyère cheese, grated (25g)
Salt and pepper (3g)

Serves 2

* Waser, M. et al (2007) 'Inverse association of farm milk consumption with asthma and allergy in rural and suburban populations across Europe', *Clinical & Experimental Allergy*, 37(5), pp. 661–670.

Kipper sandwich

1 leaf of butterhead lettuce (25g)

1 thick slice of egg-free bread (page 306) (85g)

50g (1.8 oz) kipper fillets in brine, e.g. John West (50g)

1 slice of roasted red bell pepper (20g)

55g (1.9 oz) avocado, sliced (55g)

Salt and pepper (3g)

Serves 1

Put the lettuce leaf on the bread, then add the kippers and roasted red pepper. Top with sliced avocado and some salt and pepper and try to eat without making a mess.

PER PORTION

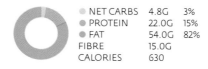

NET CARBS	4.8G	3%
PROTEIN	22.0G	15%
FAT	54.0G	82%
FIBRE	15.0G	
CALORIES	630	

'The FDA may see ketones as a drug. I see them as a fourth macronutrient. You have fats, proteins, and carbs. Ketones are an energy-containing molecule.'
Dr Dominic D'Agostino

Baked lamb

This recipe is adapted from one of the Avoca Café cookbooks. Avoca is an Irish-run family business with wonderful food markets and shops across the country. It's always easy for me to make ketogenic choices in their restaurants, as many of their lovely salads and hearty main dishes can easily be made keto-friendly by omitting the potatoes or other sources of carbohydrates.

Preheat the oven to 180°C (350°F).

Melt some of the butter in a frying pan and brown the lamb in batches.

Heat the rest of the butter in a casserole and gently sauté the onion until soft. Add the garlic, chilli, ginger, ground almonds and all the spices and cook for 5 minutes while stirring well. Transfer the lamb to the casserole, add the coconut milk and chicken stock and bring to the boil. Cover with a lid and bake in the oven for 1 hour, or you can stew the lamb longer if you feel it isn't tender enough.

If you haven't baked the breakfast buns yet, this would be a good opportunity to do so while the oven is on. Otherwise, take one out of the freezer for breakfast on Day 14.

75g (5tbsp) butter (75g)

350g (12.3 oz) stewing lamb, diced (350g)

1 medium onion, chopped (50g)

1 garlic clove, crushed (3g)

1 green chilli, deseeded and finely chopped (20g)

2cm (¾in) thumb of ginger, peeled and grated (5g)

50g (1.8 oz) ground almonds (50g)

1 tsp cardamom pods (2g)

½ tsp chilli powder (1g)

½ tsp ground cumin (1g)

½ tsp ground black pepper (1g)

200ml (⅞c) full-fat coconut milk (200g)

150ml (⅝c) homemade chicken stock (see the note on page 340) (150g)

Serves 5

PER PORTION

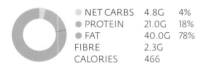

NET CARBS	4.8G	4%
PROTEIN	21.0G	18%
FAT	40.0G	78%
FIBRE	2.3G	
CALORIES	466	

Broccoli purée

62g (2.2 oz) coconut oil (62g)

1 leek, sliced (190g)

1 small onion, chopped (95g)

1 garlic clove, chopped (3g)

1 tsp ground turmeric (2g)

Salt and pepper (3g)

310g (10.9 oz) broccoli, chopped (stem and florets) (310g)

50ml (3⅓tbsp) homemade chicken stock
    (see the note on page 340) (50g)

1 tbsp lemon juice (15g)

Serves 4

Heat the coconut oil in a saucepan and fry the leek, onion and garlic for 5 minutes. Add the turmeric, salt and pepper and cook for another minute while stirring. Add the broccoli and stir everything well so that the vegetables are evenly coated with the spices. Add the stock, cover and cook for 12–15 minutes, until the broccoli is soft.

Purée the vegetables with a blender to the desired consistency. Season with salt, pepper and the lemon juice.

PER PORTION

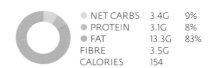

NET CARBS	3.4G	9%
PROTEIN	3.1G	8%
FAT	13.3G	83%
FIBRE	3.5G	
CALORIES	154	

Meal Plan for Week 2 Day 14

RECIPE	QUANTITY		CALORIES	CARBS	PROTEIN	FAT
BREAKFAST						
1 breakfast bun	93g		423	3.7g	8.4g	41.0g
3 slices of Parma ham	51g		114	0g	13.9g	6.5g
1 tbsp butter	15g		112	0.1g	0.1g	12.3g
		Meal total:	649	3.8g	22.4g	59.8g
LUNCH						
Creamy chicken soup	447g		562	4.8g	22.0g	50.0g
		Meal total:	562	4.8g	22.0g	50.0g
DINNER						
Sardine omelette	223g		440	1.3g	21.0g	38.0g
Stir-fried bok choy	137g		138	3.6g	1.7g	12.4g
		Meal total:	578	4.9g	22.7g	50.4g
PLAN TOTAL:			1,789	13.5g	67.1g	160.2g

Macronutrient Analysis

	CARBOHYDRATE	PROTEIN	FAT	ALCOHOL
INTAKE	13.5g	67.1g	160.2g	0g
	4% carbs	**15% protein**	**81% fat**	

Breakfast buns

200g (7 oz) unsalted macadamia
    nuts (200g)
60g (4tbsp) butter (60g)
3 eggs (150g)
60ml (4tbsp) coconut milk in a
    carton, such as Koko brand (60g)
1 tsp cider vinegar (4g)
40g (1.4 oz) coconut flour (40g)
35g (1.2 oz) almond flour (35g)
1 tsp baking soda (4g)
1 tsp salt (5g)

Makes 6 buns

Preheat the oven to 160°C (320°F). Line a baking tray with non-stick baking paper.

Grind the macadamia nuts to a coarse flour in a strong food processor. Add the butter, eggs, coconut milk and vinegar and blend again until you have a smooth paste.

Put all the remaining dry ingredients into a bowl and stir well. Add the wet ingredients and mix until you have a wet dough. Form into six buns, place on the lined tray and bake for 25 minutes. Eat on the same day or freeze.

On Day 14, cut one bun in half, spread each half with ½ tbsp butter and top with three slices of Parma ham.

PER PORTION

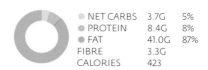

NET CARBS	3.7G	5%
PROTEIN	8.4G	8%
FAT	41.0G	87%
FIBRE	3.3G	
CALORIES	423	

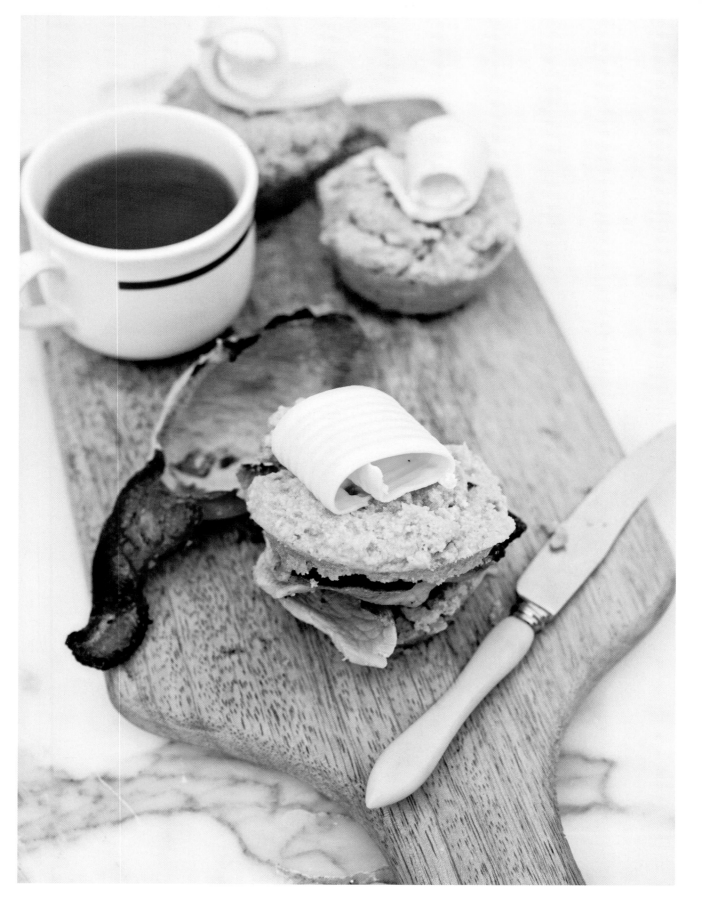

Creamy chicken soup

70g (2.5 oz) coconut oil (70g)

4 tsp curry powder (8g)

620g (1.3lbs) leftover chicken legs from Day 10, thawed (620g)

4 broccoli florets (180g)

2 garlic cloves, crushed (6g)

500ml (2⅛c) homemade chicken stock (see the intro) (500g)

375ml (1½c) full-fat coconut milk (380g)

Salt and pepper (3g)

4 handfuls of fresh parsley, chopped (16g)

Makes 4

We talk a lot about homemade chicken stock or broth in this book. Maybe you remember your mum or granny making it for you when you were sick. This isn't a coincidence – bone broth can be an incredibly useful tool when you're feeling unwell. A study* conducted by the University of Nebraska Medical Center found that the amino acids that were produced when chicken stock is prepared reduced inflammation in the respiratory system and resulted in improved digestion.

Bone broth contains nutrients like calcium, magnesium, phosphorous, silicon, sulphur, chondroitin sulphates, glucosamine and many others in a very bio-available form. Collagen seems to be the source of the main immune-boosting properties. Collagen is a protein found in the connective tissue of vertebrates (animals with an internal skeleton made of bones) and produces gelatin. Gelatin has been shown to soothe and heal the lining of the digestive tract, promote probiotic balance and growth and prevent bone loss, to name just a few benefits.

I use a slow cooker to make my stock and I use any kind of bones – often a carcass of a roast chicken, but also body parts that aren't commonly found in a supermarket, like the feet or neck. Ask your local butcher for them and inquire about the quality and origin of the animals. After browning any part that hasn't been cooked, transfer the bones to a large pan or a slow cooker and cover everything with filtered water and add about 50ml apple cider vinegar (depending on how big your pot is), which helps pull out important nutrients from the bones. Bring to a quick boil, then reduce the heat to a simmer for at least 6 hours, but ideally a lot longer (two to three days is best).

Melt the coconut oil over a low heat. Stir in the curry powder and mix well, then add the defrosted leftover chicken, broccoli, garlic, chicken stock and coconut milk. Bring to a quick boil, then reduce the heat and let the soup simmer for 5 minutes. Season with salt and pepper and garnish with chopped fresh parsley.

PER PORTION

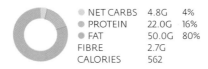

NET CARBS	4.8G	4%
PROTEIN	22.0G	16%
FAT	50.0G	80%
FIBRE	2.7G	
CALORIES	562	

* Rennard, B.O. et al (2000) 'Chicken soup inhibits neutrophil chemotaxis in vitro', *Chest*, 118(4), pp. 1,150–1,157.

Heat 2 tablespoons of coconut oil in a pan and gently fry the scallions and garlic for a few minutes. Add the mushrooms and spinach and fry for 2 minutes, until the mushrooms are lightly browned and the spinach is wilted. Set the vegetables aside.

Blend the drained sardines in a blender or food processor to make sure all the bones are removed or ground up. Whisk the eggs in a large bowl and add the turmeric, salt and pepper, then mix in the puréed sardines and the vegetables.

Heat the remaining 2 tablespoons of coconut oil in a frying pan. Pour the egg mixture into the pan and leave to cook, covered with a lid, over a low heat until the eggs are set. Slide the omelette onto a plate and cut into four slices.

Sardine omelette

4 good tbsp coconut oil (108g)
4 scallions, bulbs and tops chopped (40g)
2 garlic cloves, finely chopped (6g)
180g (6.3 oz) mushrooms, chopped (180g)
60g (2.1 oz) spinach (60g)
6 sardines canned in brine, drained (150g)
6 large eggs (342g)
1 tsp ground turmeric (2g)
Salt and pepper (3g)

Serves 4

PER PORTION

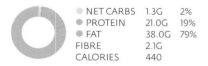

NET CARBS	1.3G	2%
PROTEIN	21.0G	19%
FAT	38.0G	79%
FIBRE	2.1G	
CALORIES	440	

Melt the butter in a frying pan over a medium heat. Add the finely chopped mushroom, garlic and ginger and sauté for about 1 minute. Add the bok choy and cook for about 3 minutes, stirring occasionally. Add the fish sauce, then cover and steam the bok choy for 2–3 minutes, until the leaves are wilted. Drizzle with sesame oil before serving.

Stir-fried bok choy

3 tbsp butter or ghee (44g)
1 large shiitake mushroom, finely chopped (56g)
2 garlic cloves, crushed (6g)
1 tsp freshly grated root ginger (10g)
400g (14.1 oz) bok choy, roughly chopped (400g)
1 tbsp fish sauce (18g)
1 tbsp sesame oil (12g)

Serves 4

PER PORTION

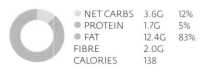

NET CARBS	3.6G	12%
PROTEIN	1.7G	5%
FAT	12.4G	83%
FIBRE	2.0G	
CALORIES	138	

Meal Plan for Week 3 Day 15

RECIPE	QUANTITY		CALORIES	CARBS	PROTEIN	FAT
BREAKFAST						
Keto granola bars	54g		374	2.7g	6.3g	37.0g
Light protein shake	141g		202	2.0g	6.9g	18.4g
		Meal total:	576	4.7g	13.2g	55.4g
LUNCH						
Temaki	169g		614	1.5g	24.0g	56.0g
		Meal total:	614	1.5g	24.0g	56.0g
DINNER						
Asian baked salmon	148g		417	2.1g	24.0g	35.0g
Cauliflower rice (page 297)	130g		275	3.4g	3.9g	27.0g
		Meal total:	692	5.5g	27.9g	62.0g
PLAN TOTAL:			1,882	11.7g	65.1g	173.4g

Macronutrient Analysis

	CARBOHYDRATE	PROTEIN	FAT	ALCOHOL
INTAKE	11.8g	65.1g	173.4g	0g
	3% carbs	**14% protein**	**83% fat**	

My kids love granola bars, but I'm obviously not a fan of the sugar-laden commercial ones. This is a good alternative and I always make a batch for myself and then a separate one for my kids, to which I add some honey or other sweetener. They freeze well too.

Place the macadamia nuts, walnuts and chocolate in a food processor and grind to a coarse flour. Add the desiccated coconut and ground almonds and pulse a few times to mix well.

In a separate bowl, mix together the hazelnut butter, coconut oil and vanilla. Combine with the dry ingredients and put into a small loaf pan. Put in the fridge or freezer to set, then cut into 12 bars. Store in the fridge.

PER PORTION

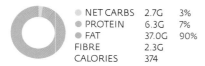

● NET CARBS	2.7G	3%
● PROTEIN	6.3G	7%
● FAT	37.0G	90%
FIBRE	2.3G	
CALORIES	374	

Keto granola bars

100g (3.5 oz) unsalted macadamia nuts (100g)

90g (3.2 oz) walnut halves (90g)

50g (1.8 oz) dark chocolate, e.g. Lindt 90% cocoa solids, chopped (50g)

65g (2.3 oz) desiccated coconut (65g)

45g (1.6 oz) ground almonds (45g)

240g (8.5 oz) hazelnut butter (240g)

50g (3½tbsp) coconut oil, melted (50g)

1 tsp vanilla essence (5g)

Makes 12 bars

Put all the ingredients into a blender and whizz to combine.

PER PORTION

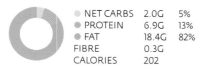

● NET CARBS	2.0G	5%
● PROTEIN	6.9G	13%
● FAT	18.4G	82%
FIBRE	0.3G	
CALORIES	202	

Light protein shake

125ml (½c) filtered water (125g)

125ml (½c) full-fat coconut milk (125g)

1 scant scoop protein powder (17g)

½ good tbsp coconut oil (14g)

Serves 2

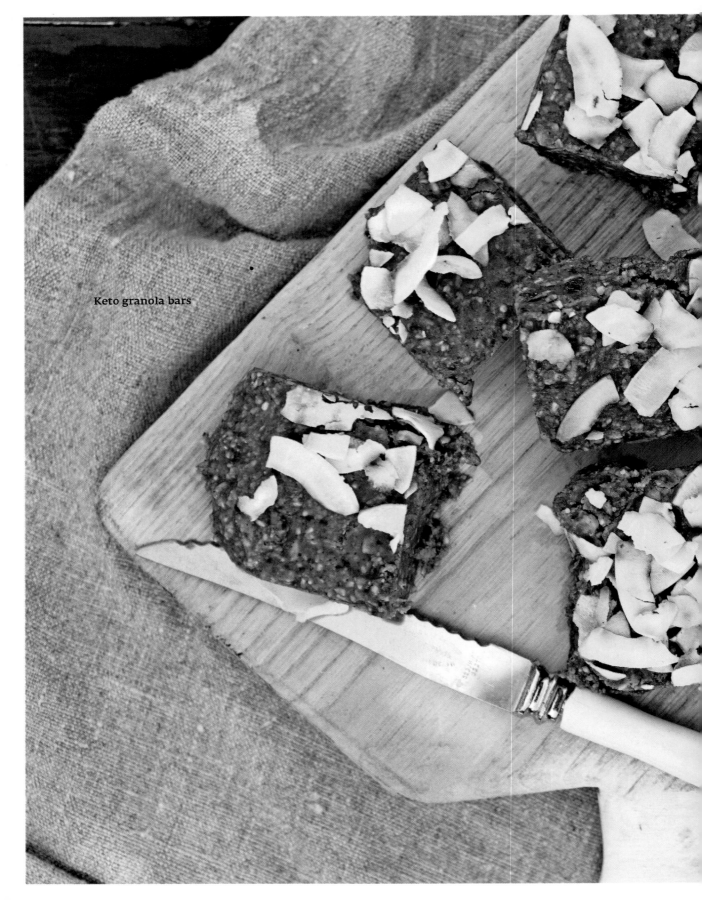

Keto granola bars

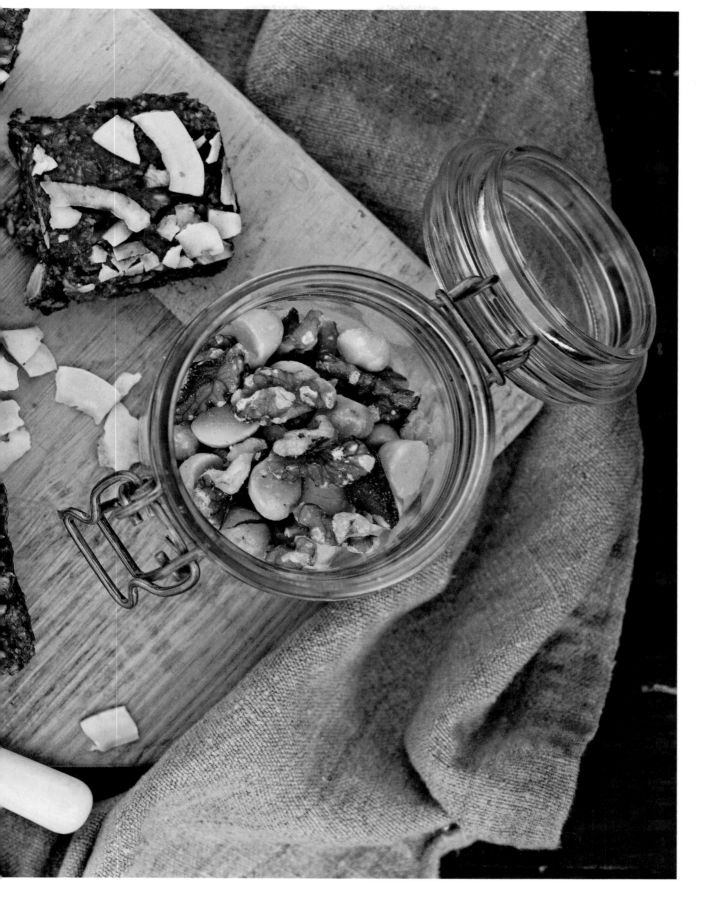

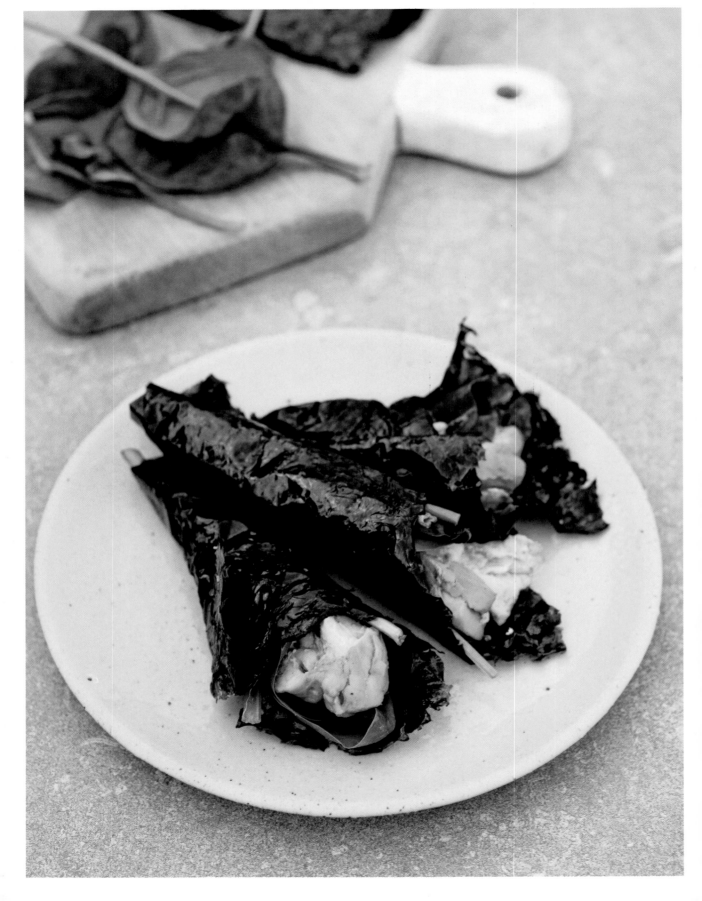

Seaweed is another often overlooked food full of nutrients. We all know about the benefits of (oily) fish and are always told to increase our intake. But many people seem to forget that the sea also hosts a massive amount of plant foods, seaweed included. In many cases, they are even more nutritious than vegetables growing on land and are particularly high in iodine (which is essential to make thyroid hormones), calcium, iron, magnesium, manganese and various other bioactive components that promote optimal health.

Apart from using nori sheets to make temaki, you can also use other types of seaweed to add to soups, salads, sauces and stir-fries.

Gently warm the chicken in the coconut oil over a medium heat.

Meanwhile, cut the nori sheets in half so that you have four sheets. Put one-quarter of the chicken, some spinach and one-quarter of the pesto in the top third of the sheet and roll into cones (temaki).

Temaki

80g (2.8 oz) roast chicken, dark
   meat only (80g)
1 good tbsp coconut oil (27g)
2 sheets of nori seaweed (2g)
30g (1.1 oz) spinach (30g)
40g (1.4 oz) pesto (page 262) (40g)

Makes 4

PER PORTION

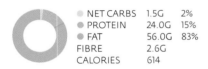

	NET CARBS	1.5G	2%
	PROTEIN	24.0G	15%
	FAT	56.0G	83%
	FIBRE	2.6G	
	CALORIES	614	

Asian baked salmon

90g (3.2 oz) coconut oil (90g)

4 garlic cloves, crushed (12g)

4cm (1.5in) piece of ginger, peeled and grated (10g)

4 tbsp soy sauce or tamari (72g)

2 tsp five-spice powder (4g)

1 tsp ground cinnamon (2g)

4 × 100g (3.5 oz) salmon fillets (400g)

Serves 4

Preheat the oven to 180°C (350°F).

Place the salmon fillets in an ovenproof glass baking dish. Melt the coconut oil in a small pan, then add the garlic, ginger, soy sauce and spices. Pour the sauce over the salmon fillets and bake for 15 minutes. Serve with the cauliflower rice on page 297.

Don't forget to make an extra portion to have for lunch on Day 16.

PER PORTION

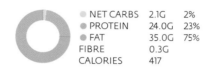

● NET CARBS	2.1G	2%
● PROTEIN	24.0G	23%
● FAT	35.0G	75%
FIBRE	0.3G	
CALORIES	417	

Meal Plan for Week 3 Day 16

RECIPE	QUANTITY		CALORIES	CARBS	PROTEIN	FAT
BREAKFAST						
Iced egg coffee	385g		484	2.6g	21.0g	43.0g
1 kale cracker (page 268)	32g		123	1.8g	3.3g	11.1g
1 tsp butter	5g		37	0g	0g	4.1g
		Meal total:	644	4.4g	24.3g	58.2g
LUNCH						
125g Asian baked salmon (leftovers)	125g		352	1.7g	20.0g	29.0g
Lettuce with turmeric dressing	105g		212	2.1g	1.2g	21.0g
		Meal total:	564	3.8g	21.2g	50.0g
DINNER						
4 lamb meatballs	120g		307	0.8g	19.7g	25.0g
Roast asparagus	75g		115	1.5g	1.9g	10.8g
Hollandaise sauce	38g		250	0.2g	0.9g	27.0g
		Meal total:	672	2.5g	22.5g	62.8g
PLAN TOTAL:			1,880	10.7g	68.0g	171.0g

Macronutrient Analysis

	CARBOHYDRATE	PROTEIN	FAT	ALCOHOL
INTAKE	10.7g	68.0g	171.0g	0g
	2% carbs	**15% protein**	**83% fat**	

Iced egg coffee

250ml (1c) strong, cold coffee (espresso, instant or decaf) (180g)

60ml (¼c) cream (60g)

1 egg, pasteurised if necessary (50g)

½ scoop chocolate protein powder (15g)

1 good tbsp coconut oil (27g)

1 tsp vanilla essence (5g)

4 ice cubes (48g)

Serves 1

I was super sceptical when I first read about adding egg to a coffee. It just sounded wrong! But I had to try it and was pleasantly surprised by the creamy texture and lovely taste. You can buy pasteurised eggs if you're concerned about using a raw egg.

Put all the ingredients into a blender and whizz to combine. Enjoy with a kale cracker with butter.

PER PORTION

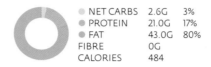

NET CARBS	2.6G	3%
PROTEIN	21.0G	17%
FAT	43.0G	80%
FIBRE	0G	
CALORIES	484	

Turmeric pops up over and over in our book. This isn't because of a lack of imagination, but to show you how incredibly versatile and easy to use this spice is.

Turmeric is a real powerhouse of nutrition – more than 1,000 research studies have explored the benefits of this spice. In the context of cancer, it has been shown to have the potential to:
- Inhibit the activation of genes that trigger cancer
- Inhibit the spread of tumour cells
- Inhibit the transformation of a normal cell into a cancer cell
- Kill cells that mutate into cancer
- Shrink tumour cells
- Enhance the cancer-destroying effects of some chemotherapy drugs and radiation

You can buy turmeric as a powdered, ground spice, which is more concentrated than the fresh root. However, I use a mix of the two to make sure I can get the most benefit out of it. In India, the average person eats about 1 teaspoon of turmeric daily spread out over three meals.

Foods you can add turmeric to include oils, salts, sprinkles, chicken salads, pestos, eggs, stir-fries, sautéed vegetables . . . the options are endless. The absorption of curcumin (one of the active components of turmeric) is enhanced with black pepper or dairy.

Put all the ingredients except the lettuce into a blender and whizz to a creamy dressing. Pour over the shredded butterhead lettuce. Serve the salad with leftover Asian baked salmon from Day 15.

Lettuce with turmeric dressing

110g (3.9 oz) avocado (110g)
1 garlic clove (3g)
Juice of 1 lemon (40g)
70ml (¼c) olive oil (65g)
2 tsp ground turmeric (4g)
200g (7 oz)butterhead lettuce, shredded (200g)

Serves 4

PER PORTION

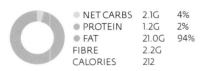

NET CARBS	2.1G	4%
PROTEIN	1.2G	2%
FAT	21.0G	94%
FIBRE	2.2G	
CALORIES	212	

Lamb
meatballs

400g (14.1 oz) minced lamb (400g)

4 garlic cloves, crushed (12g)

2 tbsp chopped parsley (8g)

1 heaped tsp wholegrain mustard (10g)

½ tsp ground black pepper (1g)

½ tsp pink rock salt (3g)

2 tbsp coconut oil (45g)

Serves 4 (makes 16 meatballs)

Don't worry, this time I didn't sneak any liver in!

Mix together all the ingredients except the coconut oil using your hands. Shape into 16 round meatballs and fry them in the coconut oil until cooked through.

PER PORTION (4 MEATBALLS AT 30G)

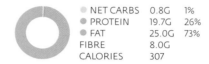

NET CARBS	0.8G	1%
PROTEIN	19.7G	26%
FAT	25.0G	73%
FIBRE	8.0G	
CALORIES	307	

Roast
asparagus

1 bunch of asparagus (250g)

3 tbsp avocado oil (42g)

1 garlic clove, chopped (3g)

1 tsp salt (5g)

½ tsp ground black pepper (1g)

Serves 4

Preheat the oven to 180°C (350°F).

After snapping off the woody ends, place the asparagus on a baking tray and drizzle with the avocado oil. Toss well to make sure the spears are well coated, then sprinkle with the garlic, salt and pepper. Arrange the asparagus in a single layer and bake for 12–15 minutes, until just tender, which will depend on how thick the spears are.

You will need some extra asparagus for the vegetable frittata on Day 17.

PER PORTION

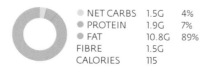

NET CARBS	1.5G	4%
PROTEIN	1.9G	7%
FAT	10.8G	89%
FIBRE	1.5G	
CALORIES	115	

Whisk the egg yolks, water and cider vinegar in the saucepan for a few moments, until thick and pale. Set the pan over a very low heat and continue to whisk at a reasonable speed, reaching all over the bottom and insides of the pan, where the eggs tend to overcook. If the eggs seem to be cooking too fast, set the pan in a bowl of cold water to cool the bottom, then continue. As they cook, the eggs will become frothy and increase in volume and then thicken. When you can see the bottom of the pan through the streaks of the whisk and the eggs are thick and smooth, remove the pan from the heat.

Add the soft butter one spoonful at a time, whisking constantly to incorporate each addition. As the emulsion forms, you can add the butter in slightly larger amounts, always whisking until it is fully absorbed. Continue incorporating the butter until the sauce has thickened to the consistency you want. Season lightly with salt and pepper, whisking in well. Taste and adjust the seasoning. Serve lukewarm.

After dinner, be sure to take a half portion of the flax coconut focaccia out of the freezer for lunch on Day 17.

Hollandaise sauce

2 egg yolks (36g)
1 tbsp water (11g)
1 tsp cider vinegar (4g)
250g (1c) butter, softened (250g)
Salt and pepper (3g)

Makes 8 servings

PER PORTION

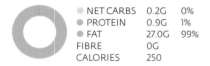

NET CARBS	0.2G	0%
PROTEIN	0.9G	1%
FAT	27.0G	99%
FIBRE	0G	
CALORIES	250	

Meal Plan for Week 3 Day 17

RECIPE	QUANTITY		CALORIES	CARBS	PROTEIN	FAT
BREAKFAST						
Salmon-wrapped avocado	265g		626	2.7g	22.0g	57.0g
		Meal total:	626	2.7g	22.0g	57.0g
LUNCH						
Coleslaw	99g		195	2.5g	2.2g	19.0g
Mackerel on flax coconut focaccia	120g		434	1.3g	19.6g	38.0g
		Meal total:	629	3.8g	21.8g	57.0g
DINNER						
Vegetable frittata	294g		410	3.6g	21.0g	34.0g
Broccoli with creamy green dressing	117g		145	1.9g	3.6g	12.9g
		Meal total:	555	5.5g	24.6g	46.9g
PLAN TOTAL:			1,851	12.0g	68.4g	160.9g

Macronutrient Analysis

	CARBOHYDRATE	PROTEIN	FAT	ALCOHOL
INTAKE	12.0g	68.4g	160.9g	0g
	3% carbs	**15% protein**	**82% fat**	

Spread some mayonnaise onto the salmon and wrap it around the sliced avocado. If this is too messy, just dip the wraps into the mayo.

PER PORTION

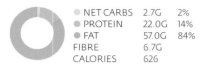

● NET CARBS	2.7G	2%
● PROTEIN	22.0G	14%
● FAT	57.0G	84%
FIBRE	6.7G	
CALORIES	626	

Salmon-wrapped avocado

3 tbsp homemade turmeric mayo (page 321) (180g)

70g (2.5 oz) smoked salmon, cut into 3 slices (70g)

150g (5.3 oz) avocado, cut into 3 slices (150g)

Serves 1

Mix together the mayonnaise and apple cider vinegar in a large bowl, then add the shredded cabbage and toss well.

PER PORTION

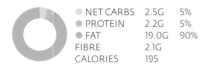

● NET CARBS	2.5G	5%
● PROTEIN	2.2G	5%
● FAT	19.0G	90%
FIBRE	2.1G	
CALORIES	195	

Coleslaw

12 tbsp homemade turmeric mayo (page 321) (180g)

4 tsp cider vinegar (15g)

400g (14.1 oz) red cabbage, shredded (400g)

Serves 4

Mackerel on flax coconut focaccia

½ portion flax and coconut focaccia
(leftovers from Day 12) (40g)
80g (2.8 oz)smoked mackerel (80g)

Serves 1

Mackerel is an oily fish, and as we've already mentioned numerous times throughout the book, it's rich in omega-3 fatty acids. Both omega-3s and 6s are essential fatty acids, meaning that the body can't actually produce them, so they need to be added via diet.

Omega-3s are found in oily fish, grass-fed meat, flaxseeds, chia seeds, hemp seeds and walnuts. DHA (docosahexaenoic acid) and EPA (eicosapentaenoic acid) are functionally important, which are found in oily fish and grass-fed meat. If we eat ALA (alpha-linolenic acid) from flaxseed, for instance, we need to convert it first into DHA and EPA, which is a delicate process. Conversion into DHA is particularly problematic, with less than 1% being converted.

Omega-6s are in most nuts (except macadamia nuts) and seeds, vegetable oils, processed meat and grains. Linoleic acid is converted into arachidonic acid, which is the precursor to a different group of molecules that are pro-inflammatory and prothromotic.

One of the challenges is that omega-3 and omega-6 fatty acids compete for the same enzymes for conversion into longer-chain, more functional fats. In today's Western diet, the ratio of omega-6 to omega-3 ranges from 10:1 to 25:1 instead of the preindustrial range of 1:1 to 2:1. High omega-6 intake is associated with thrombosis, inflammatory conditions and poor cellular health.

The best thing to do is to avoid vegetable oils (corn, safflower, sunflower, cottonseed, etc.), limit nuts/seeds to every other day and to have oily fish and pâté about four times a week. Blood tests are available to establish tissue levels, and in some cases I use fish oil supplements to quickly increase the ratio.

Top the flax coconut focaccia with the mackerel. You can toast the bread beforehand if you prefer.

PER PORTION

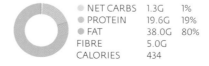

NET CARBS	1.3G	1%
PROTEIN	19.6G	19%
FAT	38.0G	80%
FIBRE	5.0G	
CALORIES	434	

Preheat the oven to 180°C (350°F).

Sweat the leek in the coconut oil in a large frying pan and season well. Add the garlic and gently fry, then add the spinach and let it wilt slightly. Take off the heat.

Scatter the asparagus on top along with the feta. Finally, add the beaten eggs with the spices mixed in. Poke the mixture to make sure everything is well mixed. Bake in the oven for 25–30 minutes, until firm. You can also bake the broccoli needed for the side dish on page 352 at the same time.

PER PORTION

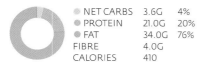

NET CARBS	3.6G	4%
PROTEIN	21.0G	20%
FAT	34.0G	76%
FIBRE	4.0G	
CALORIES	410	

Vegetable frittata

1 leek, thinly sliced (150g)
80g (5⅓tbsp) coconut oil (80g)
½ tsp salt (3g)
½ tsp pepper (3g)
3 garlic cloves, crushed (9g)
200g (7 oz) baby spinach (200g)
250g (8.8 oz) asparagus (leftover from Day 16), cut into pieces (250g)
80g (2.8 oz) feta cheese, diced (80g)
8 eggs, beaten (400g)
1 tsp ground turmeric (1g)
1 tsp ground cumin (1g)

Serves 4

Broccoli with creamy green dressing

Put all the ingredients except the broccoli into a food processor and blend to a smooth paste. Dip the baked broccoli florets into the green dressing.

You'll need some extra broccoli for lunch on Day 18.

180g (6.3 oz) crème fraîche (180g)

3 scallions, bulbs and tops (30g)

3 anchovy fillets, drained (9g)

2 tbsp chopped fresh parsley (8g)

2 tbsp chopped fresh chives (6g)

1 tbsp dried tarragon (2g)

1 tbsp lemon juice (15g)

Salt and pepper (3g)

450g (1lb) broccoli florets, baked in a hot oven for 7 minutes (450g)

Serves 6

PER PORTION

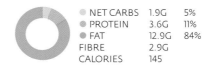

NET CARBS	1.9G	5%
PROTEIN	3.6G	11%
FAT	12.9G	84%
FIBRE	2.9G	
CALORIES	145	

Meal Plan for Week 3 Day 18

RECIPE	QUANTITY		CALORIES	CARBS	PROTEIN	FAT
BREAKFAST						
Ketogenic porridge	225g		572	3.7g	22.0g	51.0g
		Meal total:	572	3.7g	22.0g	51.0g
LUNCH						
100g roasted duck leg	100g		423	0g	20.0g	38.0g
Broccoli with dressing	111g		148	2.4g	4.2g	12.8g
		Meal total:	571	2.4g	24.2g	50.8g
DINNER						
2 portions of liver mousse	156g		363	2.5g	16.6g	32.0g
Mixed salad topped with hemp	189g		345	3.2g	4.6g	34.0g
		Meal total:	708	5.7g	21.2g	66.0g
PLAN TOTAL:			1,855	11.8g	67.4g	167.8g

Macronutrient Analysis

	CARBOHYDRATE	PROTEIN	FAT	ALCOHOL
INTAKE	11.8g	67.4g	167.8g	0g
	2% carbs	**15% protein**	**83% fat**	

Ketogenic porridge

60g (2.1 oz) whole walnuts (60g)

4 tbsp desiccated coconut (16g)

2 tbsp milled flaxseeds (18g)

2 tbsp liquid coconut oil (24g)

2 pinches of rock salt (2g)

200ml (⅞c) boiling water (200g)

90ml (⅜c) full-fat coconut milk (90g)

2 scoops chocolate or vanilla protein powder (40g)

Serves 2

Put the walnuts, desiccated coconut, flaxseeds, coconut oil and salt into a food processor. Add the boiling water and process until it reaches your desired consistency. Some people prefer it smooth like a chia pudding, while others prefer a coarse texture, similar to an oat-based porridge (you might want to add a little bit less water if this is the case). Let it sit for a minute or two, then add the coconut milk mixed with the protein powder and pulse again in the food processor to combine.

PER PORTION

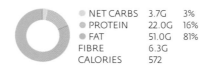

NET CARBS	3.7G	3%
PROTEIN	22.0G	16%
FAT	51.0G	81%
FIBRE	6.3G	
CALORIES	572	

Broccoli with dressing

1 garlic clove, crushed (6g)

2 tbsp sesame oil (24g)

1 tbsp grated fresh ginger (5g)

1 tbsp lime juice (15g)

1 tbsp soy sauce or tamari (9g)

½ tsp finely chopped fresh red chilli (3g)

160g (5.6 oz) broccoli, leftover from dinner on Day 17 (160g)

Serves 2

Mix together the garlic, sesame oil, ginger, lime juice, soy sauce and chilli and pour it over the broccoli. Serve this with 100g roasted duck legs. Duck is a perfect ketogenic food that is high in fat, moderate in protein and has no carbs. It's incredibly easy to make, too: just bake it in the oven at 180°C (350°F) for 20 minutes. That's it!

Make an extra portion of duck so that you can use the leftovers for lunch on Day 20.

PER PORTION (BROCCOLI WITH DRESSING ONLY – FOR NUTRIENT DETAILS ON THE DUCK, CHECK THE DAILY OVERVIEW ON PAGE 359)

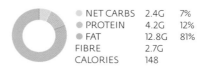

NET CARBS	2.4G	7%
PROTEIN	4.2G	12%
FAT	12.8G	81%
FIBRE	2.7G	
CALORIES	148	

This recipe was inspired by the Hemsley sisters and has been such a big hit with my family that it's become our favourite way of eating liver – my kids call them 'meat cakes'. I've also made them with kidney instead of liver, which works well too. They freeze very well, which is handy as you'll need two of them for breakfast on Day 26.

Preheat the oven to 130°C (260°F). Grease a 12-hole muffin pan.

Put all the ingredients into a strong blender and pulse until you have a smooth paste. Divide the paste between the cups of the greased muffin pan and bake for 20–25 minutes.

Liver mousse

400g (14.1 oz) chicken liver (400g)
200g (7 oz) butter, at room
   temperature (200g)
4 eggs (200g)
1 small apple, cored (67g)
1 small onion (60g)
1 tsp ground allspice (2g)
1 tsp ground black pepper (2g)

Makes 12 portions

PER PORTION (2 LIVER MOUSSE 'CAKES')

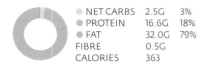

●	NET CARBS	2.5G	3%
●	PROTEIN	16.6G	18%
●	FAT	32.0G	79%
	FIBRE	0.5G	
	CALORIES	363	

Mixed salad topped with hemp

200g (7 oz) butterhead lettuce, washed and shredded (200g)

220g (7.8 oz) cucumber, sliced (220g)

8 cherry tomatoes, lightly steamed (96g)

1 portion of avocado dressing (see below) (200g)

4 tbsp shelled hemp seeds (39g)

Serves 4

Wash all the vegetables and put them into a bowl. If possible, steam or fry the tomatoes lightly to make the nutrients more available. Toss with the avocado dressing and mix well, then sprinkle the hemp seeds on top.

PER PORTION (INCLUDING DRESSING)

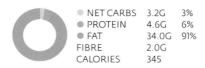

NET CARBS	3.2G	3%
PROTEIN	4.6G	6%
FAT	34.0G	91%
FIBRE	2.0G	
CALORIES	345	

Avocado dressing

125ml (½c) avocado oil (116g)

80ml (⅓c) white wine vinegar (80g)

3 garlic cloves, peeled (9g)

Salt and pepper (3g)

Serves 4

Put everything into a blender and pulse until the garlic cloves are chopped up.

If you want to get ahead for lunch on Day 19, make sure you prepare the pizza dough now or else take a portion out of the freezer.

PER PORTION

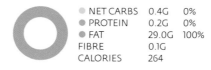

NET CARBS	0.4G	0%
PROTEIN	0.2G	0%
FAT	29.0G	100%
FIBRE	0.1G	
CALORIES	264	

Meal Plan for Week 3 Day 19

RECIPE	QUANTITY		CALORIES	CARBS	PROTEIN	FAT
BREAKFAST						
Filled coconut crêpes	178g		543	3.3g	20.0g	49.0g
		Meal total:	543	3.3g	20.0g	49.0g
LUNCH						
Quick pizza	205g		629	4.4g	26.0g	54.0g
		Meal total:	629	4.4g	26.0g	54.0g
DINNER						
Prawn veggie broth	400g		455	2.8g	17.6g	41.0g
2 cheesy flax crackers	68g		198	1.4g	8.6g	15.6g
		Meal total:	653	4.2g	26.2g	56.6g
PLAN TOTAL:			1,828	11.9g	72.2g	159.6g

Macronutrient Analysis

	CARBOHYDRATE	PROTEIN	FAT	ALCOHOL
INTAKE	11.9g	72.2g	159.6g	0g
	3% carbs	**16% protein**	**81% fat**	

Filled coconut crêpes

2 eggs (100g)

80ml (⅓c) full-fat coconut milk (80g)

2 tbsp liquid coconut oil (24g)

30g (2tbsp) butter, softened (30g)

½ tsp ground turmeric (1g)

Sea salt and pepper (1g)

2 tbsp coconut flour (15g)

3 pieces bacon, cut into strips (75g)

30g (1.1 oz) goats' cheese, cubed
  (30g)

Serves 2

Mix together the eggs, coconut milk, coconut oil, 1 tablespoon of the butter and the turmeric, salt and pepper. Add the coconut flour and mix well.

To make the filling, fry the rashers for a few minutes. Add the goats' cheese towards the end so that it melts. Keep the filling warm until the crêpes are ready.

Melt the remaining butter in a frying pan. Depending on the pan you're using, you might need more so that the crêpe doesn't stick to the pan. Pour in half of the batter and cook for a few minutes on one side with the lid on. Turning might be tricky because the crêpe is so thin. Put half of the bacon and cheese filling onto one side of the batter and gently fold the crêpe over. You can then take it out of the pan and put it onto a plate.

Repeat with the remaining batter and filling and serve.

PER PORTION

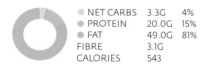

NET CARBS	3.3G	4%
PROTEIN	20.0G	15%
FAT	49.0G	81%
FIBRE	3.1G	
CALORIES	543	

Quick pizza

1 portion nutty pizza base
  (page 329) (87g)

2 tsp red hemp pesto (page 262) (5g)

20g (0.7 oz) mozzarella cheese,
  shredded (20g)

8 thin slices of zucchini (40g)

½ small can (1.4 oz) tuna in brine,
  drained (40g)

5 fresh basil leaves (3g)

Serves 1

Preheat the oven to 180°C (350°F).

Top the defrosted or freshly baked pizza base first with the red pesto, then the shredded mozzarella, zucchini slices and tuna. Scatter the basil leaves on top and bake for 10 minutes.

PER PORTION

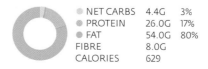

NET CARBS	4.4G	3%
PROTEIN	26.0G	17%
FAT	54.0G	80%
FIBRE	8.0G	
CALORIES	629	

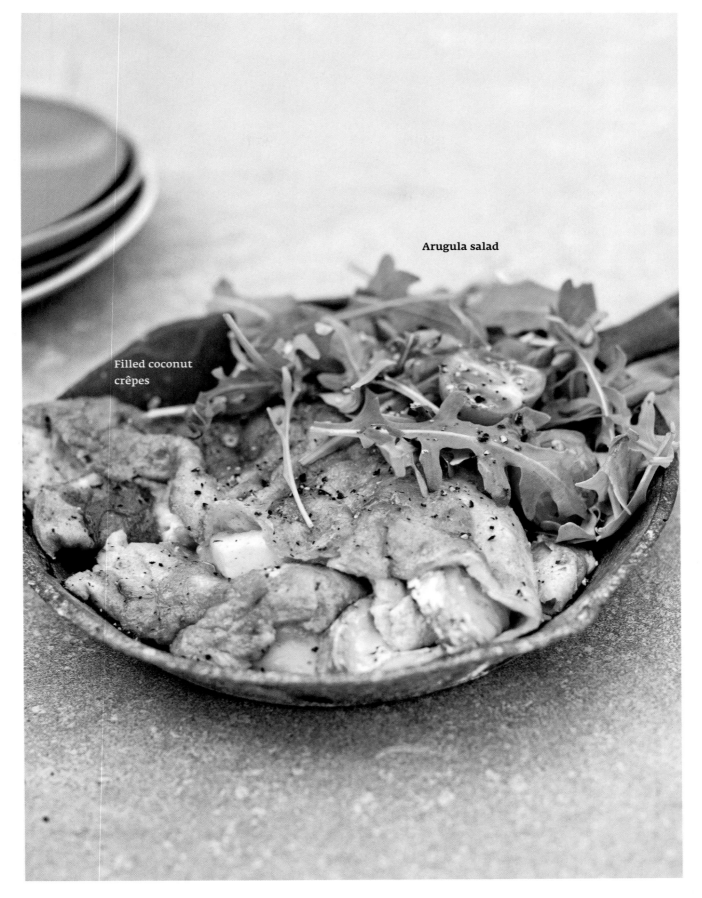

Arugula salad

Filled coconut
crêpes

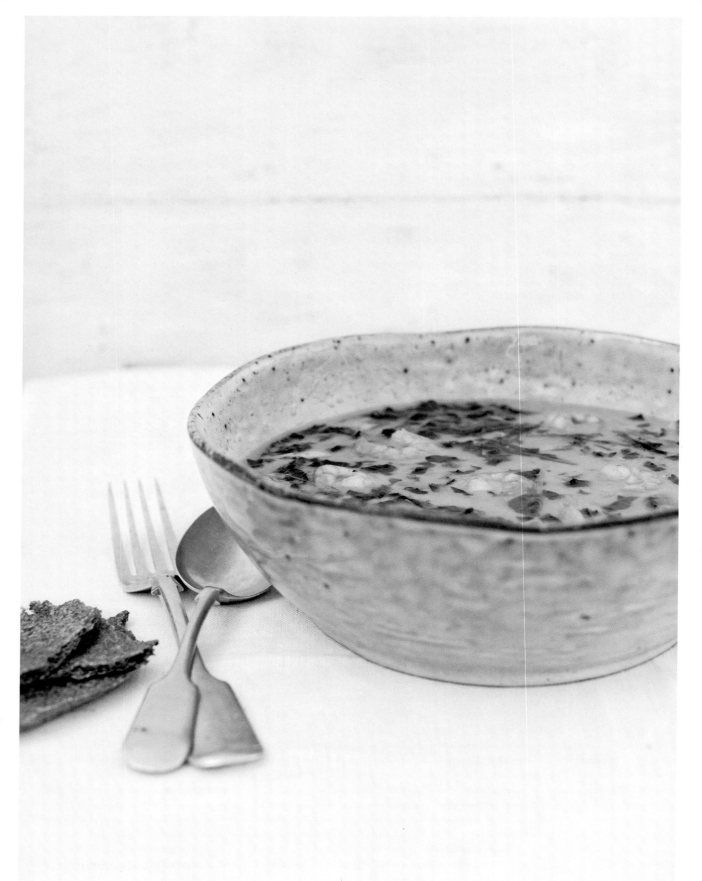

Many people are concerned about going low-carb or ketogenic because they assume their food bills will go up tremendously. My colleague Marty Kendall from optimisingnutrition. wordpress.com recently did a useful analysis using the USDA Cost of Food at Home database. Surprisingly, it showed that protein is the most expensive macronutrient per calorie, with the most expensive high-protein foods being seafood. We often hear the term 'cheap carbohydrates', but according to Marty's analysis, the data suggests that a higher-carbohydrate diet is actually more expensive overall. So increasing the proportion of fat in your diet while lowering carbohydrates will not only be gentler on your blood sugar levels, but also on your budget. The reason for this could be that many people typically consume fewer calories when lowering their carbohydrate intake. Also, we mustn't forget that it's probably also due to the fact that 1 gram of fat has more than double the amount of calories than carbohydrates or protein.

A whole food-based, low-carbohydrate, high-fat approach that combines moderate protein, lower carbohydrates and high fat seems to have a lot of potential, not just in terms of health, but budget-wise too.

Melt the coconut oil in a saucepan, then add the ginger and all the vegetables and stir-fry for a few minutes. Add the chicken stock, coconut milk and nori and let it simmer for about 10 minutes, until the vegetables reach your desired tenderness. At the very end, add the prawns just to warm them through. Season well with turmeric, cardamom, salt and pepper – you could also add some green curry paste if you like it spicy.

Prawn veggie broth

4 good tbsp coconut oil (108g)
1 tsp grated fresh ginger (5g)
110g (3.9 oz) celery, chopped (110g)
70g (2.5 oz) curly kale, chopped (70g)
70g (2.5 oz) mushrooms, chopped (70g)
30g (1.1 oz) spinach (30g)
750ml (3⅛c) homemade chicken stock (see the note on page 340) (750g)
250ml (1c) full-fat coconut milk (250g)
4 sheets of nori seaweed, torn into pieces (4g)
200g (7 oz) prawns, boiled (200g)
1 tsp ground turmeric (1g)
1 tsp ground cardamom (1g)
Salt and pepper (3g)

Serves 4

PER PORTION

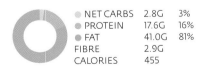

NET CARBS	2.8G	3%
PROTEIN	17.6G	16%
FAT	41.0G	81%
FIBRE	2.9G	
CALORIES	455	

Cheesy flax crackers

50g (1.8 oz) Gruyère cheese (50g)
130g (4.6 oz) milled flaxseeds (130g)
2 tsp dried oregano (4g)
1 tsp chilli flakes (2g)
½ tsp salt (3g)
½ tsp ground black pepper (1g)
150ml (⅝c) filtered water (150g)

Makes 10 crackers

Another super easy and tasty cracker recipe that also makes for great party food.

Preheat the oven to 130°C (260°F). Line a baking tray with non-stick baking paper.

Grate the cheese in a food processor and mix it well with the milled flaxseeds, spices, salt and pepper. Pour in the water and mix everything into a wet dough. Using your hands, spread the dough as thinly as you can onto the lined tray.

Bake for 40 minutes, then raise the oven temperature to 200°C (400°F) and bake for another 10 minutes. Remove from the oven and allow to cool for a little bit before breaking into crackers.

PER PORTION (1 CRACKER)

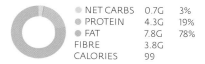

NET CARBS	0.7G	3%
PROTEIN	4.3G	19%
FAT	7.8G	78%
FIBRE	3.8G	
CALORIES	99	

'Patience and persistence are an absolute must as you pursue ketosis.'
Dr Eric Westman

Meal Plan for Week 3 Day 20

RECIPE	QUANTITY		CALORIES	CARBS	PROTEIN	FAT
BREAKFAST						
Kale shake	308g		586	3.4g	22.0g	53.0g
		Meal total:	586	3.4g	22.0g	53.0g
LUNCH						
Wrapped duck	251g		597	4.8g	21.0g	54.0g
		Meal total:	597	4.8g	21.0g	54.0g
DINNER						
Chicken with walnut sauce	179g		350	2.6g	22.0g	27.0g
Mushroom and celery salad	217g		276	1.3g	6.1g	26.0g
		Meal total:	626	3.9g	281.1g	53.0g
PLAN TOTAL:			1,809	12.1g	71.1g	160.0g

Macronutrient Analysis

	CARBOHYDRATE	PROTEIN	FAT	ALCOHOL
INTAKE	12.1g	71.1g	160.0g	0g
	3% carbs	**16% protein**	**81% fat**	

Kale shake

It's incredibly challenging to create ketogenic shakes that are actually drinkable, but this one is. You can modify it a bit as required and also add some sweetener if you prefer.

50g (1.8 oz) curly kale, lightly steamed (50g)
1 scoop protein powder (25g)
150ml (⅝c) filtered water (150g)
2 tbsp butter or goat butter (30g)
2 tbsp cider vinegar (23g)
1 good tbsp coconut oil (27g)
1 tsp ground cinnamon (2g)
1 pinch of pink rock salt (1g)

Serves 1

Put all the ingredients into a blender and whizz to combine. If the smoothie is too dense, just add some water.

NOTE: It's important to lightly steam the kale to reduce the goitrogen load.

PER PORTION

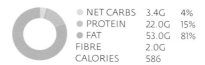

NET CARBS	3.4G	4%
PROTEIN	22.0G	15%
FAT	53.0G	81%
FIBRE	2.0G	
CALORIES	586	

Wrapped duck

Put some duck onto each lettuce leaf. Add a slice of red bell pepper and ½ tablespoon of mayo. Sprinkle over some spices, season to taste with salt and pepper and wrap up.

180g (6.3 oz) duck leg leftover from Day 18, shredded (180g)
8 large lettuce leaves (192g)
8 slices of red bell pepper (64g)
4 tbsp homemade turmeric mayo (page 321) (60g)
1 tsp ground turmeric (2g)
1 tsp paprika (2g)
Salt and pepper (3g)

Serves 2

PER PORTION

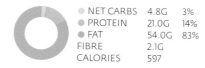

NET CARBS	4.8G	3%
PROTEIN	21.0G	14%
FAT	54.0G	83%
FIBRE	2.1G	
CALORIES	597	

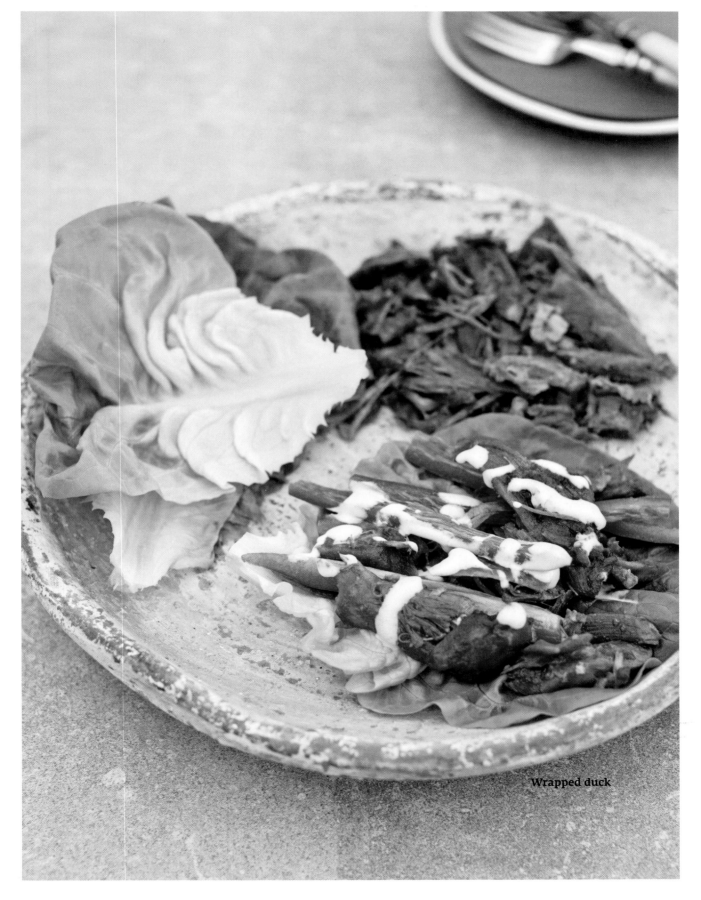

Wrapped duck

Chicken with walnut sauce

160g (5.6 oz) walnuts (160g)
1 medium onion, chopped (100g)
110ml (½c) olive oil (100g)
2 garlic cloves, crushed (6g)
3 tsp paprika (7g)
½ tsp cayenne pepper (1g)
Salt and pepper (3g)
80g (2.8 oz) ground almonds (80g)
120ml (½c) lemon juice (120g)
Big bunch of parsley, finely chopped
   (15g)
1 tbsp full-fat Greek yoghurt (45g)
6 small chicken fillets, cut into
   chunks (plus extra for lunch on
   Day 22) (540g)
600ml (2½c) homemade chicken
   stock (see the note on page 340)
   (600g)

Serves 10

A recipe by Domini and 'keto-fied' by me, this makes for ideal party food because it's delicious even if it's only at room temperature.

Preheat the oven to 160°C (320°F).

Cook the walnuts in the oven on a baking tray for about 10 minutes, until lightly toasted.

Meanwhile, sweat the onion in plenty of olive oil until soft, then add the garlic, paprika and cayenne pepper. Season well. Add the ground almonds and a bit more olive oil, then take off the heat and cool slightly while you blitz the walnuts in a food processor. Add the onion mixture, some lemon juice, the parsley and a bit of yoghurt to the food processor. Blitz again, adding in the rest of the lemon juice and yoghurt to taste. Adjust the seasoning and set aside.

Heat a little more olive oil in the same pan you cooked the onion in and fry the chicken over a high heat to get some colour on it. Season well and turn the chunks over. When you have a good colour, gradually add the stock so that you are deglazing and also poaching the chicken.

Cook gently until most of the stock has evaporated and the chicken is fully cooked. Remove some of the chicken and keep it in the fridge to use it for lunch on Day 22.

Add the chicken to the walnut sauce and mix well. The walnut sauce should be thick enough to coat the chicken, but not so thick that you feel like you are eating poached chicken smothered in peanut butter (or rather, walnut butter). It should be loose enough to be pleasant in the mouth. It then becomes unbelievably moreish.

PER PORTION

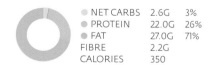

NET CARBS	2.6G	3%
PROTEIN	22.0G	26%
FAT	27.0G	71%
FIBRE	2.2G	
CALORIES	350	

Heat 3 tablespoons of the olive oil in a frying pan over a medium heat. When the oil is hot, add the sliced mushrooms and sauté until golden brown. Season with a little salt and pepper, then set aside to cool.

In a large serving bowl, whisk the remaining 4 tablespoons of olive oil with the lemon juice and a little salt and pepper. Add the cooled mushrooms along with the celery, cheese and parsley and toss to combine. Season with salt and pepper and serve.

PER PORTION

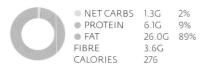

NET CARBS	1.3G	2%
PROTEIN	6.1G	9%
FAT	26.0G	89%
FIBRE	3.6G	
CALORIES	276	

Mushroom and celery salad

7 tbsp olive oil (91g)
450g (1lb) mushrooms, sliced (450g)
Salt and pepper (3g)
2 tbsp lemon juice (30g)
4 stalks of celery, finely chopped (240g)
40g (1.4 oz) Parmesan cheese, grated (40g)
4 tbsp chopped parsley (16g)

Serves 4

Meal Plan for Week 3 **Day 21**

RECIPE	QUANTITY		CALORIES	CARBS	PROTEIN	FAT
BREAKFAST						
Protein almond shake	252g		372	2.3g	15.5g	33.0g
Hazelnut bread	50g		177	2.8g	5.8g	15.6g
Butter	15g		112	0.1g	0.1g	12.3g
		Meal total:	661	5.2g	21.4g	60.9g
LUNCH						
Prawn veggie broth (page 367)	399g		455	2.8g	17.6g	41.0g
1 cheesy flax cracker (page 368)	34g		99	0.7g	4.3g	7.8g
		Meal total:	554	3.5g	21.9g	48.8g
DINNER						
Salmon niçoise	362g		603	4.2g	27.0g	52.0g
		Meal total:	603	4.2g	27.0g	52.0g
PLAN TOTAL:			1,801	12.9g	70.3g	161.7g

Macronutrient Analysis

	CARBOHYDRATE	PROTEIN	FAT	ALCOHOL
INTAKE	12.9g	70.3g	161.7g	0g
	3% carbs	**16% protein**	**81% fat**	

Put all the ingredients into a blender and whizz to combine.

PER PORTION

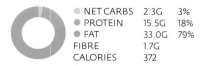

● NET CARBS	2.3G	3%
● PROTEIN	15.5G	18%
● FAT	33.0G	79%
FIBRE	1.7G	
CALORIES	372	

Protein almond shake

250ml (1c) unsweetened almond
    milk (250g)
1 scant scoop protein powder (20g)
30g (2tbsp) coconut oil (30g)
1 tsp ground cinnamon (2g)

Serves 1

Hazelnut bread

Butter for greasing the pan
4 eggs, separated (228g)
60ml (¼c) coconut milk from a
  carton, such as Koko brand (60g)
1 tbsp blackstrap molasses (20g)
240g (8.5 oz) hazelnut butter (240g)
1 tbsp cider vinegar (12g)
30g (1.1 oz) coconut flour (30g)
1 tsp baking soda (4g)
½ tsp rock or sea salt (3g)

Makes 12 slices

I love this bread because it reminds me more of a cake once I add a good layer of butter to it! It's incredibly filling and you would struggle to eat more than one slice. It freezes really well, though, and I often bake two at once so that I'm stocked up for a while.

Preheat the oven to 150°C (300°F). Grease a 1lb loaf pan with butter or line it with non-stick baking paper.

Place the egg whites in a bowl and mix with a hand-held immersion blender until soft peaks form.

Heat the coconut milk in a small pan and add the molasses to melt it in the milk. In a large bowl, mix together the egg yolks, hazelnut butter, vinegar and the warmed milk mixture. Sift the coconut flour, baking soda and salt into the nut butter mixture and beat until well combined. Gently stir in the whipped egg whites, but be careful not to overmix the batter. Pour into the prepared loaf pan and put in the oven straight away.

Bake for 45 minutes, then remove and let it cool on a wire rack for 15 minutes. Free the sides from the pan with a knife and flip the pan upside down to release the loaf. Cool on a rack before serving. Serve with butter on top.

PER PORTION (WITHOUT BUTTER)

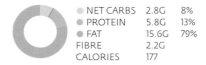

● NET CARBS	2.8G	8%
● PROTEIN	5.8G	13%
● FAT	15.6G	79%
FIBRE	2.2G	
CALORIES	177	

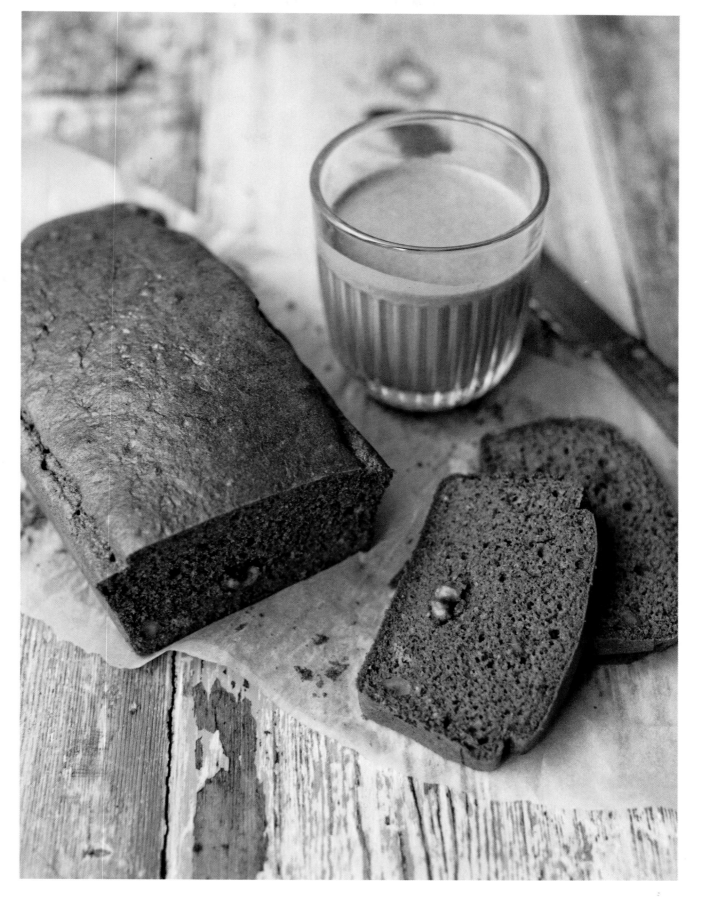

Salmon niçoise

2 tbsp + 85ml (⅓c) extra virgin olive oil (110g in total)

1 tbsp + 40ml (2½tbsp) lemon juice (55g in total)

4 small salmon fillets, skin on (320g)

Salt and pepper (3g)

200g (7 oz) green beans (200g)

200g (7 oz) cauliflower (200g)

3 tbsp butter (44g)

8 ripe cherry tomatoes, halved (96g)

1 small head of cos lettuce, torn (160g)

4 eggs, hard boiled and sliced (200g)

24 black olives (48g)

4 anchovies, drained (12g)

1 garlic clove, peeled (3g)

Serves 4

This could also be a good party dish because you can prepare a lot in advance and keep it warm.

Preheat the oven to 180°C (350°F).

Drizzle 2 tablespoons of olive oil and 1 tablespoon of lemon juice over the salmon fillets and season with salt and pepper.

Lightly steam the green beans and cauliflower until tender, then put them in a frying pan and sauté them in the butter. Transfer the cauliflower to a small roasting pan along with the cherry tomatoes.

Fry the salmon skin side down in the same frying pan for about 4 minutes. Add to the roasting pan with the cauliflower and tomatoes and place in the hot oven for about 8 minutes.

In the meantime, arrange the lettuce, steamed green beans, sliced eggs and olives on four plates. Leave some space in the middle of the plates.

Put 85ml (⅓c) of olive oil, 40ml (2½tbsp) of lemon juice, the anchovies, garlic and some pepper into a blender and whizz to combine.

Place the salmon, cauliflower and cherry tomatoes in the middle of each plate, then drizzle everything with the dressing and serve.

You will need some red pesto for the meat pizza on Day 22, so take some out of your freezer now.

PER PORTION

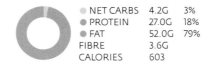

NET CARBS	4.2G	3%
PROTEIN	27.0G	18%
FAT	52.0G	79%
FIBRE	3.6G	
CALORIES	603	

Meal Plan for Week 4 **Day 22**

RECIPE	QUANTITY		CALORIES	CARBS	PROTEIN	FAT
BREAKFAST						
Zucchini bread	97g		242	2.8g	8.7g	21.0g
2 tbsp tahini paste	36g		219	0.3g	6.7g	21.0g
½ portion keto coffee (page 315)	162g		192	0.7g	0.6g	21.0g
		Meal total:	653	3.8g	16.0g	63.0g
LUNCH						
Watercress and avocado salad	308g		593	2.6g	25.0g	52.0g
		Meal total:	593	2.6g	25.0g	52.0g
DINNER						
Meat pizza	245g		422	2.0g	27.0g	33.0g
Refreshing salad	152g		254	2.1g	0.9g	26.0g
		Meal total:	676g	4.1g	27.9g	59.0g
PLAN TOTAL:			1,922	10.5g	68.9g	174.0g

Macronutrient Analysis

	CARBOHYDRATE	PROTEIN	FAT	ALCOHOL
INTAKE	10.5g	68.9g	174.0g	0g
	2% carbs	**15% protein**	**83% fat**	

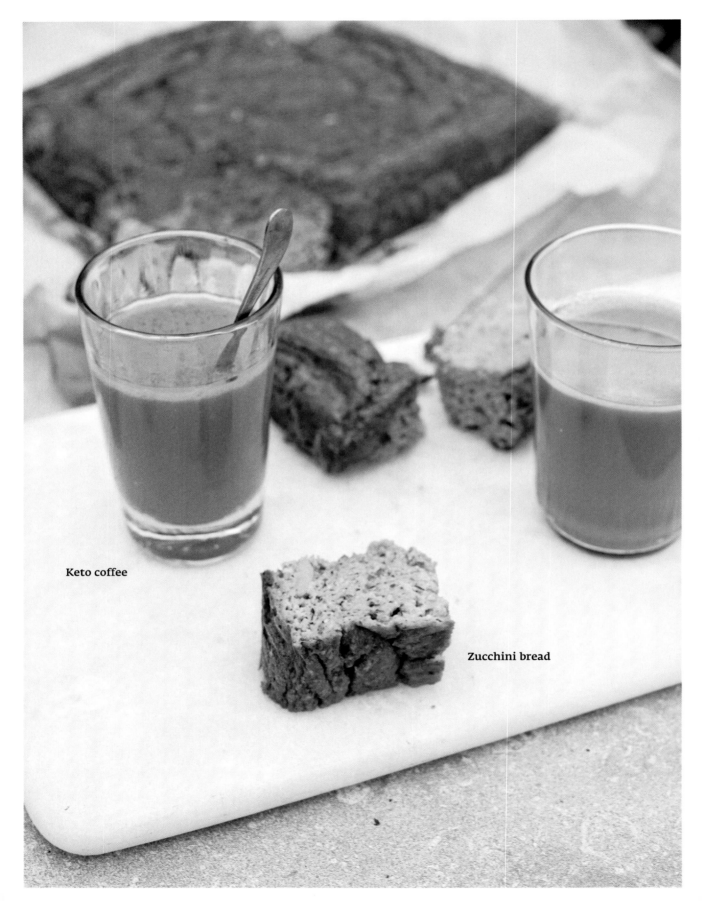

Keto coffee

Zucchini bread

I like this bread because it doesn't have any nuts. While nuts are very nutrient dense and keto friendly, they can be harsh on your digestive system, which is why I definitely recommend not having them on a daily basis. Serve this with tahini (sesame paste).

Preheat the oven to 160°C (320°F). Line a 1lb loaf pan with non-stick baking paper.

Grind the sesame and pumpkin seeds in a good food processor to a fine flour. Add the baking soda and salt and pulse briefly just to combine.

Heat the almond milk lightly, then add the molasses and stir well. Add to all the remaining ingredients, including the seed mixture. Mix well and form a wet dough with the dry ingredients. Put into the lined loaf pan and bake for 50–60 minutes. Allow to cool on a wire rack before slicing.

Zucchini bread

145g (5.1 oz) sesame seeds (145g)
70g (2.5 oz) pumpkin seeds (70g)
1 tsp baking soda (3g)
½ tsp salt (3g)
125ml (½c) unsweetened almond milk (125g)
1 tsp blackstrap molasses (8g)
3 eggs (150g)
180g (6.3 oz) avocado, mashed (180g)
80g (2.8 oz) zucchini, finely chopped in a food processor (80g)
1 tbsp cider vinegar (12g)

Makes 8 slices

PER PORTION

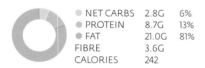

	NET CARBS	2.8G	6%
	PROTEIN	8.7G	13%
	FAT	21.0G	81%
	FIBRE	3.6G	
	CALORIES	242	

Watercress and avocado salad

1 large bunch of watercress (160g)
220g (7.8 oz) avocado, cubed (220g)
140g (4.9 oz) chicken breast, sliced
   (leftovers from Day 20) (140g)
3 tbsp lemon juice (45g)
46ml (3tbsp) olive oil (50g)
Salt and pepper (3g)

Serves 2

Surely you've noticed by now that avocados, the so-called alligator pear (because it's pear-shaped and has bumpy green skin), are a staple food of a ketogenic lifestyle. They're low in carbs (2g of net carbs per 100g), high in fat (15g per 100g) and packed with nutrients like folate, potassium, vitamin C, vitamin K, B vitamins and vitamin E, for instance. And they have more potassium than bananas! They also contain valuable antioxidants. Because of their creamy texture, they can be a great substitute for dairy in desserts and other recipes.

Divide the watercress between two plates, then top with the avocado cubes and chicken.

Mix the lemon juice and olive oil in a small bowl, season with salt and pepper and drizzle over the salads.

PER PORTION

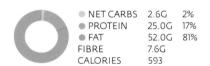

● NET CARBS	2.6G	2%
● PROTEIN	25.0G	17%
● FAT	52.0G	81%
FIBRE	7.6G	
CALORIES	593	

Meat pizza

If you miss pizza but you don't like a nut or cauliflower crust, you can try this meat base.

Preheat the oven to 180°C (350°F). Line a baking tray with non-stick baking paper.

Mix the minced lamb with the garlic, rosemary, mustard, salt and pepper. With your hands, press the mixture as thinly as you can onto the lined tray. Bake in the oven for about 15 minutes, until lightly browned.

In the meantime, heat the coconut oil in a frying pan and gently cook the mushrooms and spinach. When the meat base is cooked, top it with the pesto, mushroom and spinach mixture and the artichokes. Sprinkle evenly with Parmesan cheese and put it back in the oven for a few minutes to melt the cheese.

450g (1lb) minced lamb (450g)
2 garlic cloves, crushed (6g)
2 sprigs of fresh rosemary, finely chopped (8g)
1 tsp wholegrain mustard (10g)
Salt and pepper (3g)
1 good tbsp coconut oil (27g)
160g (5.6 oz) mushrooms, sliced (160g)
30g (1.1 oz) spinach (30g)
50g (1.8 oz) red hemp pesto (page 262) (50g)
200g (7 oz) jarred artichokes, drained and finely chopped (200g)
40g (1.4 oz) Parmesan cheese, grated (40g)

Serves 4

PER PORTION

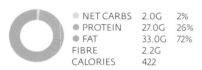

NET CARBS	2.0G	2%
PROTEIN	27.0G	26%
FAT	33.0G	72%
FIBRE	2.2G	
CALORIES	422	

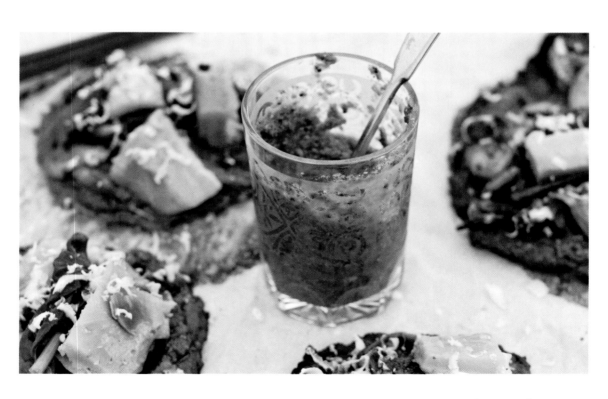

Refreshing salad

8 tbsp extra virgin olive oil (104g)

4 tbsp lemon juice (60g)

1 tsp paprika (2g)

Salt and pepper (3g)

200g (7 oz) iceberg lettuce, cut into thin strips (200g)

120g (4.3 oz) fennel, thinly sliced (120g)

2–3 stalks of celery, finely chopped (120g)

Serves 4

Whisk together the olive oil, lemon juice, paprika, salt and pepper in a large bowl. Add the lettuce, fennel and celery and toss to combine.

PER PORTION

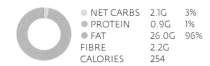

NET CARBS	2.1G	3%
PROTEIN	0.9G	1%
FAT	26.0G	96%
FIBRE	2.2G	
CALORIES	254	

Meal Plan for Week 4 Day 23

RECIPE	QUANTITY	CALORIES	CARBS	PROTEIN	FAT
BREAKFAST					
Bulletproof-ish coffee	236g	465	0.7g	0.1g	53.0g
2 duck eggs, boiled or fried	132g	261	0g	19.0g	20.0g
	Meal total:	726	0.7g	19.1g	73.0g
LUNCH					
Chicken liver pâté	142g	236	1.5g	15.3g	18.6g
Seaweed and cucumber salad	159g	223	2.4g	3.1g	22.0g
2 zucchini flax crackers (page 294)	60g	111	1.3g	4.8g	8.7g
	Meal total:	570	5.2g	23.2g	49.3g
DINNER					
Pork belly with cabbage	287g	547	4.3g	26.0g	46.0g
	Meal total:	547	4.3g	26.0g	46.0g
PLAN TOTAL:		1,843	10.2g	68.3g	168.3g

Macronutrient Analysis

	CARBOHYDRATE	PROTEIN	FAT	ALCOHOL
INTAKE	10.2g	68.3g	168.3g	2.0g
	2% carbs	**16% protein**	**81% fat**	**1% alcohol**

Bulletproof-ish coffee

180ml (¾c) hot coffee (regular or decaf) or chaga tea (180g)
25g (0.9 oz) coconut oil (25g)
1 tbsp butter (15g)
1 tbsp cocoa butter (14g)

Serves 1

The term 'bulletproof coffee' was coined by Dave Asprey, who recommends having this type of coffee instead of breakfast to enhance physical and mental performance. He uses 'upgraded' coffee that doesn't contain any mycotoxins (mould toxins) and mixes this with grass-fed butter and MCT (medium-chain triglycerides) oil. It is often used on a ketogenic diet because it can be metabolised into ketone bodies as quickly as glucose. The chemical structure of MCTs allows them to pass from the intestinal tract straight to the liver. In the liver, they're immediately broken down into ketone bodies.

While some people thrive on MCT oils and successfully manage to increase their ketone bodies, I observe that many cancer patients struggle to digest this type of fat. A large number of my clients – including myself, by the way – complain about nausea, bloating or lack of appetite for a long time after consuming this type of coffee. Another tricky thing about having a 'butter coffee'-only breakfast is that there is a clear lack of protein and other essential nutrients. My conclusion: it can be fabulous for somebody who needs to lose weight and enhance performance, but in the case of a chronically ill patient, it might not be the best choice. It's wiser to have it only on occasion and in combination with eggs or some other nutritious food, as suggested in our recipes.

Put all the ingredients into a blender and whizz to combine.

PER PORTION

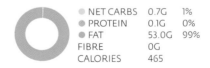

NET CARBS	0.7G	1%
PROTEIN	0.1G	0%
FAT	53.0G	99%
FIBRE	0G	
CALORIES	465	

No ketogenic cookbook focusing on optimising nutrient content by eating organ meat would be complete without a liver pâté recipe, so here you go. This one is made with chicken livers, but I've also tried it with lamb or beef liver.

Sauté the liver and onion in a couple tablespoons of the butter until the livers are browned and the onions are tender. Add the garlic, herbs, wine, lemon juice and mustard. Cook, uncovered, until most of the liquid has gone. Transfer the mixture to a food processor along with the rest of the butter and blend until smooth. Add salt and pepper to taste.

PER PORTION

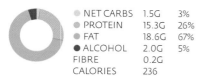

● NET CARBS	1.5G	3%
● PROTEIN	15.3G	26%
● FAT	18.6G	67%
● ALCOHOL	2.0G	5%
FIBRE	0.2G	
CALORIES	236	

Chicken liver pâté

500g (1.1lbs) chicken liver (500g)
1 small onion, chopped (60g)
120g (4.2 oz) butter (goat butter works too) (120g)
3 garlic cloves, crushed (9g)
2 sprigs of fresh thyme (8g)
1 sprig of fresh rosemary (5g)
125ml (½c) red wine (125g)
1 tbsp lemon juice (15g)
1 tsp Dijon mustard (10g)
Salt and pepper (3g)

Makes 6 portions

Soak the sea vegetables in water for 5 minutes, then drain. Mix the scallion, ginger, oil, lime juice and zest and tamari together. Combine the seaweed, cucumber and spinach, then drizzle over the dressing. Toss well and serve.

PER PORTION

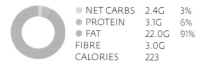

● NET CARBS	2.4G	3%
● PROTEIN	3.1G	6%
● FAT	22.0G	91%
FIBRE	3.0G	
CALORIES	223	

Seaweed and cucumber salad

5g (0.2 oz) mixed seaweed, e.g. nori, dulse, kelp, arame (5g)
1 scallion, bulb and top thinly sliced (10g)
1cm (0.4in) piece of ginger, peeled and grated (2g)
3 tbsp olive or avocado oil (42g)
2 tbsp lime juice + zest of 2 limes (30g + 4g)
1 tbsp tamari (18g)
½ cucumber, cut into long strips (150g)
60g (2.1 oz) spinach (60g)

Serves 2

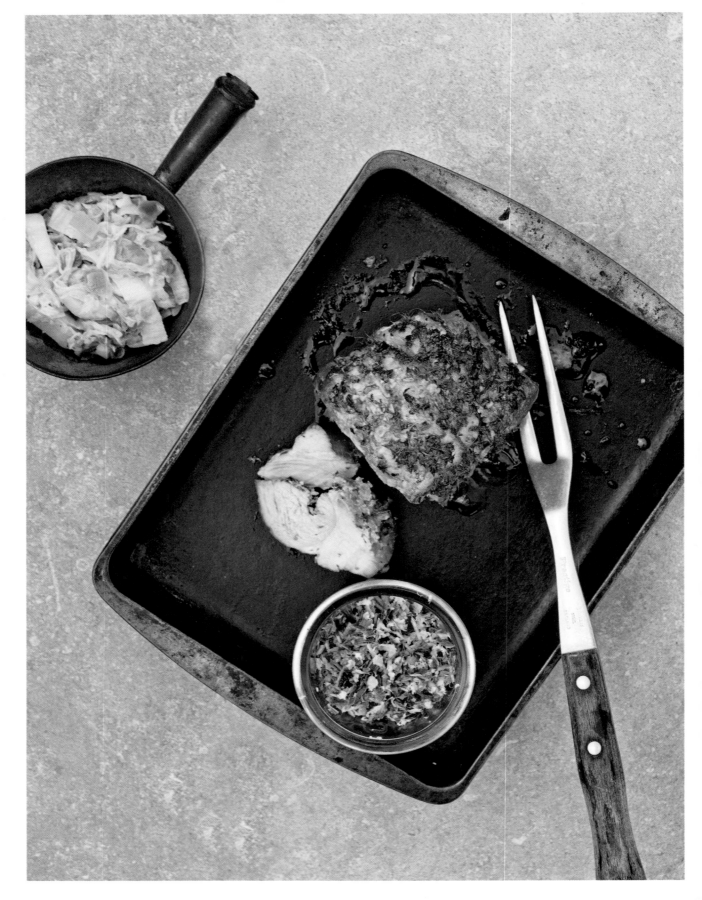

Preheat the oven to 225°C (440°F).

Blend the lemon zest, four crushed garlic cloves and the parsley together to make a gremolata. Season the pork belly with salt and pepper, then cover with a layer of the gremolata. Roll the belly up like a Swiss roll and tie it tightly with string in three places to secure it. Roast it in the oven for 45 minutes, then turn the heat down to 140°C (280°F) and roast for 2 hours more of slow cooking.

Heat the duck fat in a frying pan and gently fry the chopped onion, the remaining clove of garlic and the ginger. Chop the cabbage into finely shredded 'noodles', add to the pan and cook for 30 minutes. Add the coconut milk (crème fraîche is nice too) and simmer for another 30 minutes (or put in the oven with the pork). Season with the soy sauce and sprinkle with sesame seeds.

You can roast the eggplants in the oven at the same time as the pork belly for the baba ganoush on Day 24, which will be made in no time then. You will also need some roast eggplant cubes for lunch on Day 25.

Pork belly with cabbage

Zest of 4 lemons (8g)

5 garlic cloves, crushed (15g)

Handful of fresh parsley, finely chopped (8g)

480g (1.1lbs) pork belly (plus more for leftovers for Day 27) (480g)

Salt and pepper (3g)

2 tbsp duck fat (90g)

1 small red onion, chopped (60g)

1 tsp grated fresh ginger (5g)

700g (1.5lbs) napa cabbage (700g)

250ml (1c) full-fat coconut milk (250g)

2 tbsp soy sauce, tamari or coconut aminos (36g)

4 tbsp sesame seeds (44g)

Serves 6

PER PORTION

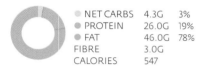

NET CARBS	4.3G	3%
PROTEIN	26.0G	19%
FAT	46.0G	78%
FIBRE	3.0G	
CALORIES	547	

Meal Plan for Week 4 **Day 24**

RECIPE	QUANTITY		CALORIES	CARBS	PROTEIN	FAT
BREAKFAST						
Chia chocolate pudding	345g		684	3.5g	19.1g	63.0g
		Meal total:	684	3.5g	19.1g	63.0g
LUNCH						
Goats' cheese salad	161g		625	2.6	21.0g	58.0g
Baba ganoush	63g		101	1.2g	2.0g	9.3g
		Meal total:	726	3.8g	23.0g	67.3g
DINNER						
Ham-wrapped fish	293g		458	4.0g	26.0g	37.0g
		Meal total:	458	4.0g	26.0g	37.0g
PLAN TOTAL:			1,868	11.3g	68.1g	167.3g

Macronutrient Analysis

	CARBOHYDRATE	PROTEIN	FAT	ALCOHOL
INTAKE	11.3g	68.1g	167.3g	1.4g
	3% carbs	**15% protein**	**81% fat**	**1% alcohol**

This recipe can be really handy for people struggling with constipation, as chia seeds can help with bowel movements. Instead of using dark chocolate, I sometimes substitute it with 1 or 2 teaspoons of raw organic cacao powder.

Put all the ingredients into a strong blender and whizz until very smooth.

PER PORTION

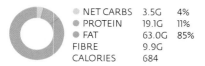

● NET CARBS	3.5G	4%
● PROTEIN	19.1G	11%
● FAT	63.0G	85%
FIBRE	9.9G	
CALORIES	684	

Chia chocolate pudding

500ml (2⅛c) unsweetened fortified almond milk (500g)

40g (1.4 oz) chia seeds (40g)

30g (2tbsp) hazelnut butter (30g)

1 heaped scoop chocolate protein powder (30g)

2 squares of dark chocolate, such as Lindt 90% cocoa solids (4g)

2 good tbsp coconut oil (85g)

Serves 2

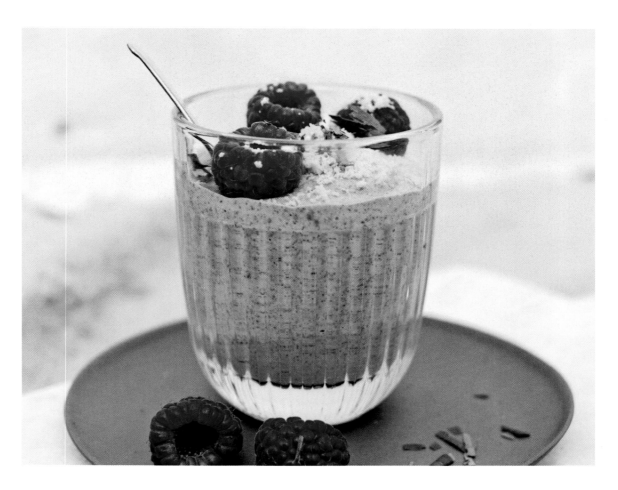

Goats' cheese salad

60g (2.1 oz) walnuts (60g)
3 tbsp walnut oil (36g)
1 tbsp white wine vinegar (11g)
1 tbsp finely chopped red onions (15g)
Salt and pepper (3g)
50g (1.8 oz) baby spinach (50g)
120g (4.2 oz) full-fat goats' cheese, cubed (120g)

Serves 2

Toast the walnuts in a dry frying pan without any oil over a medium heat for about 10 minutes, stirring now and then. Allow to cool, then roughly chop.

Make the dressing by mixing together the walnut oil, vinegar and chopped onions with some salt and pepper. Put the spinach in a bowl and top with the lightly toasted walnuts and goats' cheese. Pour the dressing over the salad and mix well.

PER PORTION

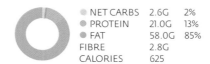

NET CARBS	2.6G	2%
PROTEIN	21.0G	13%
FAT	58.0G	85%
FIBRE	2.8G	
CALORIES	625	

Baba ganoush

1 eggplant, sliced (250g)
2 garlic cloves, peeled (6g)
50g (1.8 oz) tahini (50g)
3 tbsp lemon juice (45g)
2 tbsp extra virgin olive oil (26g)
½ tsp pink rock salt (3g)
½ tsp smoked paprika (3g)

Makes 6 portions

Preheat the oven to 140°C (280°F).

Place the sliced eggplants on a baking tray and cook in the oven for 30–40 minutes, until soft. Make sure you don't skip this step – the taste of the baba ganoush really changes if the eggplants are well cooked! Once they've cooled down you can take off the skin, but I usually don't bother with this. Put everything into a food processor and whizz to combine. Drizzle with some more olive oil after you've put the baba ganoush into a bowl.

PER PORTION

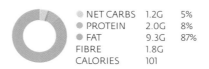

NET CARBS	1.2G	5%
PROTEIN	2.0G	8%
FAT	9.3G	87%
FIBRE	1.8G	
CALORIES	101	

You've probably noticed that we use alcohol for various dishes, but we haven't mentioned anything about alcohol consumption in general yet. As you certainly know, alcohol content drastically reduces when it's cooked, but it still has calories, which is why we have to include it in our nutritional information charts. But what about having the odd glass of wine – is that suitable on a ketogenic diet?

In the initial stages, before you're fully keto adapted, I recommend staying off alcohol. Once you are in well-established ketosis with a GKI of between 1 and 2 on a consistent basis, you can see if and how alcohol/wine affects your ketone levels. Moderation and self-experimentation are essential because alcohol can have a greater and faster effect for somebody following a ketogenic diet. I'd definitely recommend that you strongly limit your alcohol intake, but there is no research confirming that two to three small glasses of wine a week can be harmful for cancer patients – unless you're undergoing treatment or if it doesn't agree with you, of course. Definitely have your alcohol with food, though. My approach is that I hardly have any alcohol when I'm at home but I always have a glass of dry wine when I'm out socialising, which is usually once a week.

The carbohydrate content of alcohol is as follows:
- Dry red wine (e.g. Syrah, Pinot Noir, Cabernet Sauvignon): About 3.5 to 4g per 150ml (⅝c).
- Dry white wine (e.g. Sauvignon Blanc, Chardonnay): About 3g per 150ml (⅝c).
- Distilled spirits (e.g. vodka, rum, whiskey): Zero carbs, but mixers are sugary! You can make your own mixer by adding club soda, a bit of lemon juice and a sweetener (e.g. stevia).
- Another thing worth mentioning is that being in ketosis can give false-positive breath-alcohol tests.[*]

[*] Jones, A.W. and Rössner, S. (2007) 'False-positive breath-alcohol test after a ketogenic diet', *International Journal of Obesity*, 31(3), pp. 559–561.

Ham-wrapped fish

4 mackerel fillets, halved (800g)
8 slices of Parma ham (136g)
75g (5tbsp) butter or ghee (75g)
Salt and pepper (3g)
4 leeks, thinly sliced (800g)
1 glass of white wine, dry (125g)
200g (7 oz) mushrooms, sliced (200g)
200g (7 oz) crème fraîche (200g)
1 tsp ground turmeric (2g)
2 tsp chopped fresh parsley (4g)

Serves 8

Preheat the oven to 180°C (350°F).

Wrap each halved mackerel fillet in a slice of Parma ham. Make sure you buy Parma ham (or any other ham, for that matter) with an ingredient list that reads 'pork and salt' and nothing else! Place on a baking tray, dot generously with half of the butter or ghee, season well and bake for 15 minutes.

Meanwhile, sweat the leeks in the other half of the butter/ghee in a large saucepan for about 5 minutes. Add the wine and let it cook off by turning up the heat, then add the mushrooms, crème fraîche and turmeric. Let it cook for another 5 minutes, until the mushrooms are soft. Season well and serve with the fish sprinkled with some chopped parsley.

Make sure you have one portion of mackerel and ham (without the vegetables) left over for lunch on Day 26.

PER PORTION

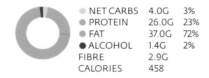

● NET CARBS	4.0G	3%
● PROTEIN	26.0G	23%
● FAT	37.0G	72%
● ALCOHOL	1.4G	2%
FIBRE	2.9G	
CALORIES	458	

Meal Plan for Week 4 Day 25

RECIPE	QUANTITY		CALORIES	CARBS	PROTEIN	FAT
BREAKFAST						
Keto granola	72g		495	3.9g	6.5g	48.0g
½ portion protein almond shake (page 375)	126g		186g	1.1g	7.7g	16.5g
		Meal total:	681	5.0g	14.2g	64.5g
LUNCH						
Sardine salad	329g		572	3.1g	22.0g	52.0g
		Meal total:	572	3.1g	22.0g	52.0g
DINNER						
Shepherd's pie	328g		509	3.0g	27.0g	41.0g
Light leafy salad (page 318)	74g		126	1.1g	0.8g	13.0g
		Meal total:	635	4.1g	27.8g	54.0g
PLAN TOTAL:			1,888	12.2g	64.0g	170.5g

Macronutrient Analysis

	CARBOHYDRATE	PROTEIN	FAT	ALCOHOL
INTAKE	12.2g	64.0g	170.5g	0g
	3% carbs	**14% protein**	**83% fat**	

Keto granola

100g (6⅔ tbsp) coconut oil, melted (100g)
½ tsp vanilla essence (3g)
255g (9 oz) coconut flakes (255g)
90g (3.2 oz) flaked almonds (90g)
60g (2.1 oz) hazelnuts, chopped (60g)
45g (1.6 oz) walnuts, chopped (45g)
2 tbsp chia seeds (20g)
2 tsp ground cinnamon (5g)
½ tsp ground cardamom (1g)
Pinch of salt (1g)

Serves 8

Preheat the oven to 140°C (280°F). Line a baking tray with non-stick baking paper.

Melt the coconut oil in a small saucepan and add the vanilla extract. Add all the other ingredients to a large bowl and mix well. You can also add some stevia or erythritol if you need to sweeten it a bit. Pour the melted coconut oil over the dry ingredients and stir gently, making sure everything is evenly coated with oil.

Transfer to the lined tray and bake for 20–25 minutes, stirring occasionally to prevent burning.

When the mix has cooled down, you can add coconut or almond milk or coconut yoghurt to serve. Make sure you add some more protein if your requirements for breakfast aren't met, like the protein almond shake on page 375. Store the granola in an airtight container for up to one week.

PER PORTION

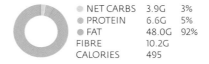

NET CARBS	3.9G	3%
PROTEIN	6.6G	5%
FAT	48.0G	92%
FIBRE	10.2G	
CALORIES	495	

Sardine salad

Mix the cubed eggplant (that you roasted on Day 23), sardines and lettuce together in a large bowl. Sprinkle the chopped artichokes and capers on top. Whisk together the oil and vinegar, season with salt and pepper and pour over the salad. Mix well.

PER PORTION

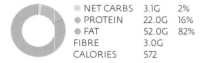

● NET CARBS	3.1G	2%
● PROTEIN	22.0G	16%
● FAT	52.0G	82%
FIBRE	3.0G	
CALORIES	572	

180g (6.3 oz) roasted eggplant, cut into cubes (180g)

2 small cans (6 oz) sardines in olive oil or brine, drained (170g)

100g (3.5 oz) butterhead lettuce, chopped (100g)

90g (3.2 oz) jarred artichokes, drained and chopped (90g)

2 tbsp capers (17g)

6 tbsp extra virgin olive oil (76g)

2 tbsp cider vinegar (23g)

Salt and pepper (3g)

Serves 2

Shepherd's pie

3 good tbsp coconut oil (81g)

700g (1.5lbs) minced lamb (700g)

230g (8.1 oz) mushrooms, quartered (230g)

6 stalks of celery, finely chopped (360g)

3 scallions, bulbs and tops chopped (30g)

1 tbsp passata (30g)

1 tsp dried thyme (1g)

Salt and pepper (3g)

800g (1.75lbs) celeriac, peeled and cut into chunks (800g)

230g (8.1 oz) raw milk Gruyère cheese, grated (230g)

4 tbsp butter (60g)

2 tbsp fresh cream (48g)

1 egg (50g)

1 tsp smoked paprika (2g)

Serves 8

Melt the coconut oil in a large frying pan, add the minced lamb and cook over a high heat until it loses its raw red colour. After turning down the heat, stir in the mushrooms, celery, scallions, passata and thyme. Season with salt and pepper and let it simmer for about 20 minutes, until the vegetables are soft.

In the meantime, preheat the oven to 180°C (350°F). Grease a 23cm (9in) square baking dish.

Steam the celeriac for about 20 minutes, then blend well in a food processor. Remove about 1 cup of the purée and stir it into the lamb. Add the cheese, butter and cream to the remaining celeriac and blend well, then add the egg and blend again until smooth. Stir in the smoked paprika at the end.

Spread the lamb mixture into the greased baking dish and cover with the celeriac purée. Bake for about 45 minutes, until bubbly and browned.

PER PORTION

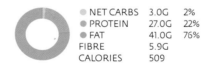

● NET CARBS	3.0G	2%
● PROTEIN	27.0G	22%
● FAT	41.0G	76%
FIBRE	5.9G	
CALORIES	509	

Meal Plan for Week 4 Day 26

RECIPE	QUANTITY		CALORIES	CARBS	PROTEIN	FAT
BREAKFAST						
Morning broth	601g		758	4.5g	18.1g	72.0g
		Meal total:	758	4.5g	18.1g	72.0g
LUNCH						
1 portion ham-wrapped fish without veg (leftovers from Day 24)	121g		284	0.4g	23.0g	21.0g
Nutty beetroot arugula	95g		251	3.4g	1.5g	25.0g
		Meal total:	535	3.8g	24.5g	46.0g
DINNER						
Duck breast	114g		432	1.0g	20.0g	38.0g
Brussels sprouts with chorizo	126g		166	3.0g	5.4g	14.1g
		Meal total:	598	4.0g	25.4g	52.1g
PLAN TOTAL:			1,891	12.3g	68.0g	170.1g

Macronutrient Analysis

	CARBOHYDRATE	PROTEIN	FAT	ALCOHOL
INTAKE	12.3g	68.0g	170.1g	0.7g
	3% carbs	**15% protein**	**82% fat**	

Morning broth

40g (2½ good tbsp) coconut oil (40g)

2 scallions, bulbs and tops finely
chopped (20g)

2 slices of red pepper (16g)

1 garlic clove, crushed (3g)

350ml (½c) homemade chicken
stock (see the note on page 340)
(350g)

2 portions of liver mousse (page 361),
cut into small pieces (156g)

Handful of dried kombu seaweed
(10g)

½ tsp ground turmeric (1g)

½ tsp ground cumin (1g)

Salt and pepper (3g)

Serves 1

Melt the coconut oil in a pan and gently fry the scallions, peppers and garlic. Add the chicken stock and bring everything to a quick boil. Throw in the chopped-up liver mousse and the kombu (or any other good seaweed). Simmer for about 5 minutes and season well with turmeric, cumin and some salt and pepper.

PER PORTION

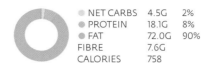

NET CARBS	4.5G	2%
PROTEIN	18.1G	8%
FAT	72.0G	90%
FIBRE	7.6G	
CALORIES	758	

Nutty beetroot arugula

2 tbsp hazelnut oil (25g)

40g (1.4 oz) beetroot, peeled and
grated (40g)

30g (1.1 oz) arugula (30g)

Salt and pepper (3g)

Serves 1

Sprinkle the oil over the beetroot and arugula. Toss well and season with some salt and pepper. Serve with some leftover mackerel from Day 24.

PER PORTION

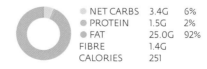

NET CARBS	3.4G	6%
PROTEIN	1.5G	2%
FAT	25.0G	92%
FIBRE	1.4G	
CALORIES	251	

Melt the coconut oil in a frying pan. When it's hot, start frying the duck breasts skin side down to let the fat render down; this helps make the skin crisp. When the skin is crisp and brown, remove the duck from the pan. Add the passata, garlic, red wine and seasoning to deglaze the pan of all the lovely juices (stand back for this). Turn the heat down and let the juices reduce by about half before adding the duck breasts back to cook them until done. Serve with the Brussels sprouts on page 402.

Keep some leftovers for lunch on Day 28.

Duck breast

1 tsp coconut oil (4g)
4 duck breasts, including fat and
    skin, halved (800g)
100g (3.5 oz) tomato passata (100g)
4 garlic cloves, crushed (15g)
½ glass of red wine (63g)
Salt and pepper (3g)

Serves 4

PER PORTION

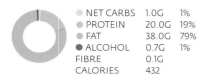

NET CARBS	1.0G	1%
PROTEIN	20.0G	19%
FAT	38.0G	79%
ALCOHOL	0.7G	1%
FIBRE	0.1G	
CALORIES	432	

Brussels sprouts with chorizo

100g (3.5 oz) chorizo, finely diced
  (100g)
3 good tbsp coconut oil (81g)
500g (1.1lbs) Brussels sprouts,
  shredded (500g)
145g (5.1 oz) broccoli, processed into
  'rice' (145g)
1 garlic clove, crushed (3g)
180ml (¾c) homemade chicken
  stock (see the note on page 340)
  (180g)
1 tsp ground turmeric (2g)
Salt and pepper (3g)

Serves 8

Cook the chorizo in the coconut oil in a large frying pan over a medium heat until crisp. Remove the chorizo from the pan and set aside, but leave the oil in the pan. Add the shredded Brussels sprouts, broccoli and garlic to the pan and sauté in the remaining oil for 5 minutes. Add the chicken broth, turmeric, salt and pepper, cover and steam for 5–10 minutes.

PER PORTION

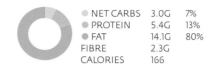

NET CARBS	3.0G	7%
PROTEIN	5.4G	13%
FAT	14.1G	80%
FIBRE	2.3G	
CALORIES	166	

Meal Plan for Week 4 Day 27

RECIPE	QUANTITY		CALORIES	CARBS	PROTEIN	FAT
BREAKFAST						
Green kedgeree	294g		684	5.7g	23.0g	62.0g
		Meal total:	684	5.7g	23.0g	62.0g
LUNCH						
Konjac noodles	325g		618	2.8g	21.0g	54.0g
		Meal total:	618	2.8g	21.0g	54.0g
DINNER						
Fish fingers	166g		445	1.4g	24.0g	38.0g
½ portion mixed salad topped with hemp (page 362)	94g		173	1.6g	2.3g	17.0g
		Meal total:	618	3.0g	26.3g	55.0g
PLAN TOTAL:			1,920	11.5g	70.3g	171.0g

Macronutrient Analysis

	CARBOHYDRATE	PROTEIN	FAT	ALCOHOL
INTAKE	11.5g	70.3g	171.0g	0g
	3% carbs	**15% protein**	**82% fat**	

Green kedgeree

1 tbsp duck fat (45g)

⅓ small onion, finely chopped (20g)

2 slices red bell pepper, finely chopped (16g)

80g (2.8 oz) broccoli, processed into 'rice' (80g)

1 red chilli, deseeded and thinly sliced (20g)

1 tsp curry powder

½ tsp ground turmeric (1g)

Salt and pepper (3g)

60g (2.1 oz) grilled kipper, flaked (60g)

1 egg, hard boiled and quartered (50g)

Serves 1

Heat the duck fat in a frying pan over a medium heat and add the onion and red pepper. Cook for about 5 minutes, until soft. Add the broccoli 'rice', chilli, curry powder and turmeric. Season with salt and pepper and stir-fry for 5 minutes before adding the flaked kipper. Serve with the egg wedges on top.

PER PORTION

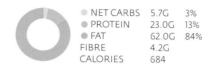

NET CARBS	5.7G	3%
PROTEIN	23.0G	13%
FAT	62.0G	84%
FIBRE	4.2G	
CALORIES	684	

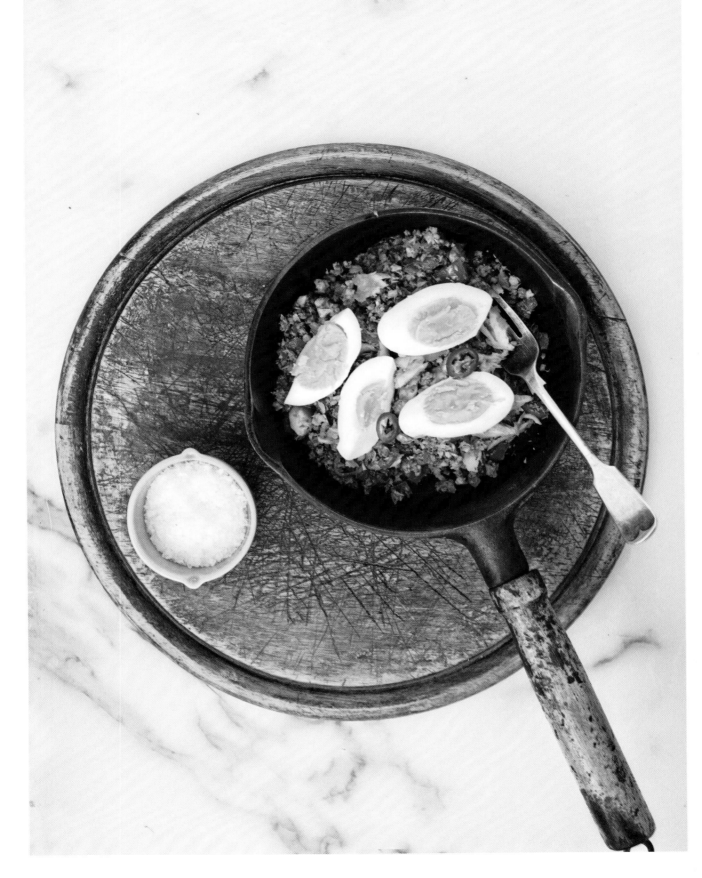

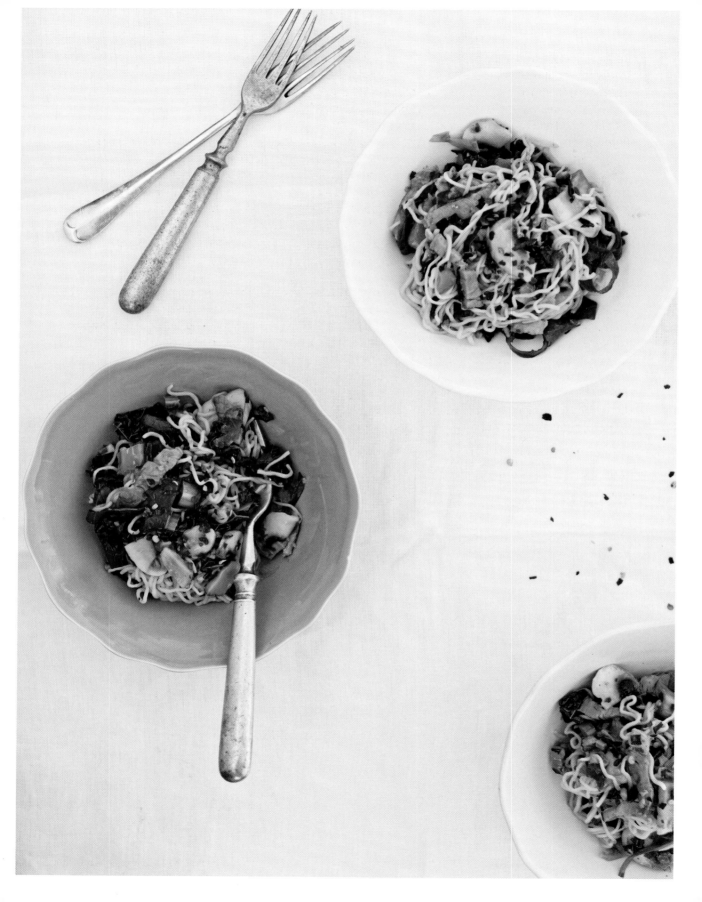

Konjac noodles are also called shirataki noodles, made from the root of the konjac plant that is widely cultivated in China and Japan. The main component of the konjac root is glucomannan, a water-soluble dietary fibre consisting of mannose and glucose sugars. Noodles made from konjac fibre are thin, translucent and gelatinous. Their carbohydrate content is virtually zero and they're also very low in calories. They have an 'eggy' smell, which is why it's a good idea to rinse them for a while before using them in a stir-fry, for instance. Konjac has numerous health benefits and the Japanese regard it as a high-quality food that benefits intestinal function. It's certainly not a highly nutritious food, but it can be a welcome substitute for grain-based noodles on an occasional basis.

Soak the sea spaghetti in warm water for 10 minutes. Gently heat the coconut oil in a frying pan and add the sliced pork belly, scallion, garlic and ginger and cook for 5 minutes while stirring. Add the vinegar, coconut aminos, salt and chilli flakes and stir-fry for 1 minute. Reduce the heat to a simmer, then add the konjac noodles, mushrooms, kale and soaked sea spaghetti. Cook for 10 minutes, until the vegetables are soft. Finally, pour the sesame oil over and mix well.

Konjac noodles

¼ pack sea spaghetti, soaked for 10 minutes (12g)

1 good tbsp coconut oil (27g)

60g (2.1 oz) pork belly (leftover from Day 23), sliced into thin strips (60g)

1 scallion, bulb and top chopped (10g)

1 garlic clove, crushed (3g)

1 tsp freshly grated ginger (2g)

1 tbsp cider vinegar (11g)

1 tbsp coconut aminos, soy sauce or tamari (18g)

½ tsp salt (3g)

¼ tsp chilli flakes (1g)

100g (3.5 oz) konjac noodles, rinsed for about a minute (100g)

35g (1.2 oz) mushrooms, sliced (35g)

35g (1.2 oz) curly kale, chopped (35g)

1 tbsp sesame oil (12g)

Serves 1

PER PORTION

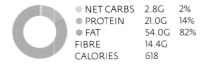

NET CARBS	2.8G	2%
PROTEIN	21.0G	14%
FAT	54.0G	82%
FIBRE	14.4G	
CALORIES	618	

Fish fingers

2 eggs, beaten (100g)
800g (1.75lbs) cod, cut into fish
    finger-sized pieces (800g)
120g (4.2 oz) ground almonds (120g)
½ tsp ground coriander (1g)
½ tsp ground cumin (1g)
½ tsp ground turmeric (1g)
Salt and pepper (3g)
1 batch of hollandaise sauce
    (page 353) (304g)

Serves 8

Whenever you make white fish, make sure you don't 'overdose' on protein and always make a nice sauce or mayonnaise to increase your fat intake. These fish fingers are a good example of how to do this. The batter works very well with chicken too.

Preheat the oven to 180°C (350°F). Line a baking tray with non-stick baking paper.

Crack the eggs into a bowl and dip each fish finger in it. You might need a bit more egg depending on size.

Put the ground almonds, spices and some salt and pepper into a ziplock bag and mix well. Working in batches, add the fish to the plastic bag and make sure the fingers get covered on all sides with the almond mixture. Place on the lined baking tray and bake for 20 minutes, until the fish fingers are golden brown. Serve with hollandaise sauce.

PER 166G PORTION

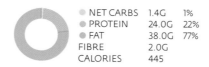

NET CARBS	1.4G	1%
PROTEIN	24.0G	22%
FAT	38.0G	77%
FIBRE	2.0G	
CALORIES	445	

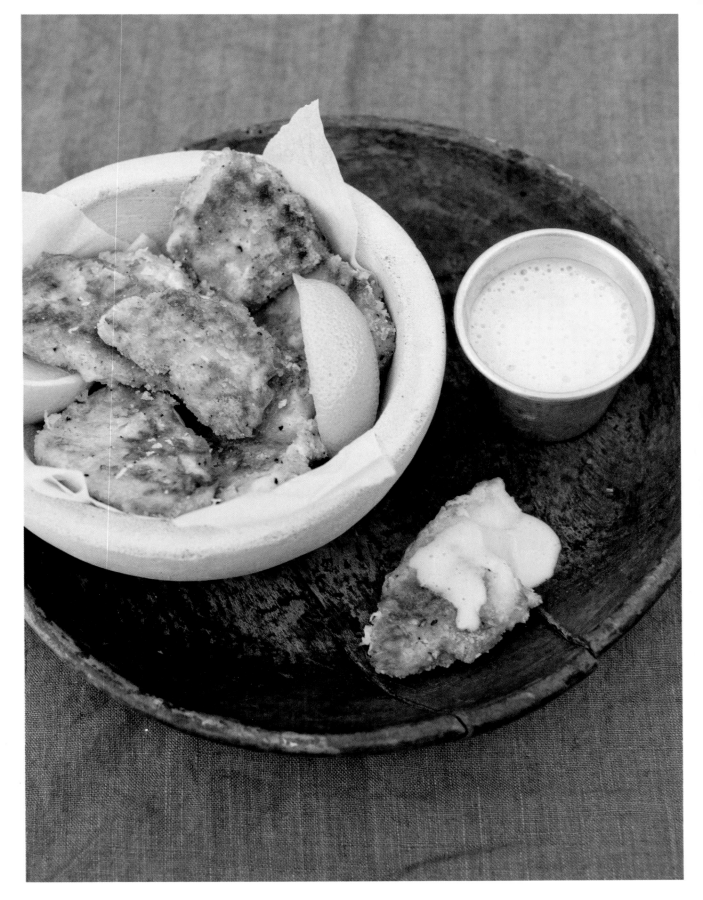

Meal Plan for Week 4 Day 28

RECIPE	QUANTITY		CALORIES	CARBS	PROTEIN	FAT
BREAKFAST						
Avocado, goats' cheese and spinach scramble	269g		609	2.7g	23.0g	55.0g
		Meal total:	609	2.7g	23.0g	55.0g
LUNCH						
Colourful salad	283g		697	3.6g	22.0g	65.0g
		Meal total:	697	3.6g	22.0g	65.0g
DINNER						
Anti-inflammatory chicken curry	280g		424	3.8g	22.0g	35.0g
½ portion cauliflower rice (page 297)	65g		138	1.7g	2.0g	13.5g
		Meal total:	562	5.5g	24.0g	48.5g
PLAN TOTAL:			1,868	11.8g	69.0g	168.5g

Macronutrient Analysis

	CARBOHYDRATE	PROTEIN	FAT	ALCOHOL
INTAKE	11.8g	69.0g	168.5g	0.7%g
	3% carbs	**15% protein**	**82% fat**	

Should you only buy organic ingredients? If you can afford it, go for it, but it's an unrealistic goal for most people. There are certain vegetables and fruit that tend to be more contaminated with pesticides than others. The Environmental Working Group in the US (www.ewg.org) is doing lots of research into this and has produced a list of the 'dirty dozen and clean fifteen'. The dirty dozen are the ones that should preferably be organic, while the clean fifteen tend to be less pesticide laden and can therefore be bought as conventional produce. On a ketogenic regime, some of these fruit and vegetables are excluded anyway but the list looks as follows:

Dirty ketogenic 'nine'	Clean ketogenic 'seven'
Apples	Avocados
Strawberries	Cabbage
Celery	Onions
Spinach	Asparagus
Sweet bell peppers	Eggplant
Cucumbers	Cauliflower
Cherry tomatoes	Sweet potatoes
Snap peas	
Kale/collard greens	

Heat the avocado oil in a frying pan, then scramble the eggs and fry the spinach until it's wilted. Put the avocado and goats' cheese on top, cover with a lid and leave for 2–3 minutes, until the avocado is warm and the goats' cheese has slightly melted. Season well with salt and pepper.

Avocado, goats' cheese and spinach scramble

2 tbsp avocado oil (28g)
3 eggs, beaten (150g)
30g (1.1 oz) spinach (30g)
220g (7.8 oz) avocado, cubed (220g)
100g (3.5 oz) full-fat goats' cheese rind (100g)
Salt and pepper (3g)

Serves 2

PER PORTION

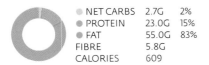

NET CARBS	2.7G	2%
PROTEIN	23.0G	15%
FAT	55.0G	83%
FIBRE	5.8G	
CALORIES	609	

Colourful salad

2 portions duck breast (leftovers from Day 26), thinly sliced (228g)

2 stalks of celery, sliced (120g)

30g (1.1 oz) carrot, grated (30g)

4 tbsp grated celeriac (32g)

6 tbsp alfalfa sprouts (18g)

55g (1.9 oz) chopped butterhead or cos lettuce (55g)

4 tbsp olive oil (52g)

2 tbsp cider vinegar (22g)

2 tsp Dijon mustard (8g)

Salt and pepper (3g)

Serves 4

You can use any kind of leftovers instead of the duck, but it works really nicely in this salad. I always heat the duck slices lightly if I'm at home for lunch, but it's also delicious as a cold salad if you use it as a packed lunch.

Gently heat the thinly sliced duck breast in a dry frying pan (there is enough fat and sauce in the duck that no oil should be needed). Toss the vegetables and sprouts in a bowl and mix with the lettuce leaves.

Whisk together the olive oil, vinegar, mustard and seasoning and pour the dressing over the salad, then place the sliced duck on top to serve.

PER PORTION

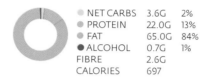

NET CARBS	3.6G	2%
PROTEIN	22.0G	13%
FAT	65.0G	84%
ALCOHOL	0.7G	1%
FIBRE	2.6G	
CALORIES	697	

Anti-inflam-matory chicken curry

3 good tbsp coconut oil (81g)

2 small red onions, chopped (100g)

3 garlic cloves, crushed (9g)

2 green chillies, deseeded and thinly sliced (40g)

1 tsp grated fresh ginger (5g)

1 tsp black mustard seeds (2g)

1 tsp ground coriander (2g)

1 tsp ground cumin (2g)

1 tsp ground turmeric (2.2g)

400g (14.1 oz) chicken thighs (400g)

375ml (1½c) homemade chicken stock (see the note on page 340) (375g)

90g (3.2 oz) spinach (90g)

Handful of cilantro leaves (10g)

Serves 4

At first sight this looks like a complicated dish because it has so many ingredients, but don't worry, most of them are herbs and spices that you just need to throw in.

Heat the coconut oil in a large frying pan and gently fry the onion, garlic, chilli and ginger. When they are soft, add all the spices and continue to cook until they become fragrant. Add the chicken thighs and stock. Bring to the boil, turn down the heat and simmer for 45–60 minutes, until the chicken is cooked through. Add the spinach and stir until it's wilted. Garnish with cilantro leaves and serve with a half portion of cauliflower rice (page 297).

PER PORTION

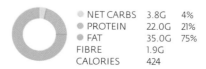

NET CARBS	3.8G	4%
PROTEIN	22.0G	21%
FAT	35.0G	75%
FIBRE	1.9G	
CALORIES	424	

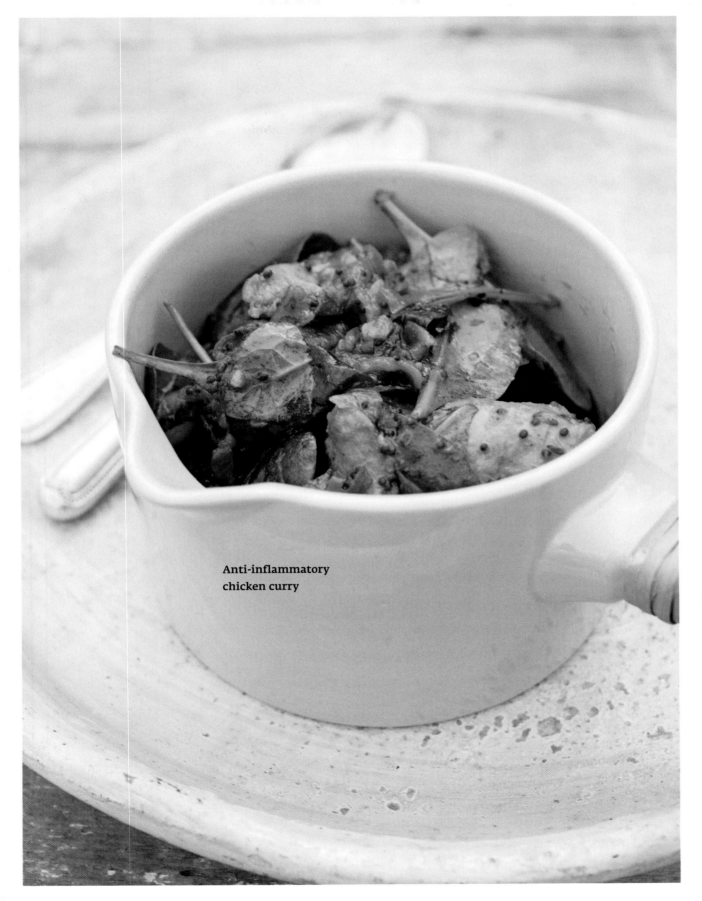

**Anti-inflammatory
chicken curry**

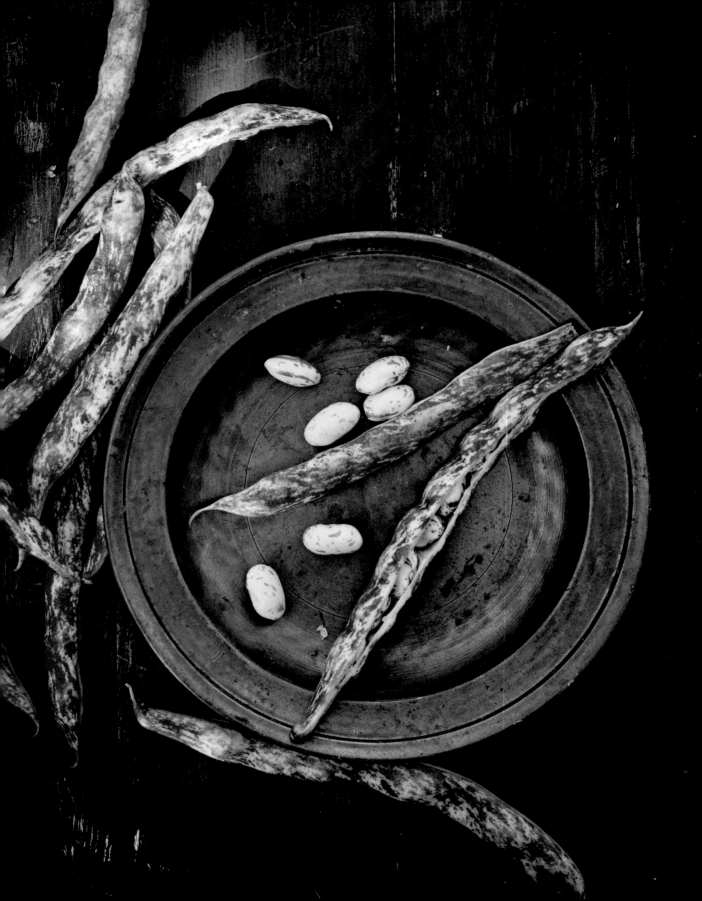

Part 4: In Times of Treatment and Recovery

Nourishing food

During treatment, food can become a great source of stress. Appetite sometimes vanishes and is replaced by nausea and diarrhoea. The patient's taste buds can change completely, which can make it challenging to eat any food.

Nobody denies that chemotherapy in particular is very toxic not only to cancer cells, but healthy cells too. There are studies that show that the effects can be long-lasting and damaging to overall health, which is why some people want to opt out of conventional treatments. But one area of research that is of particular interest to any complementary therapist is how we can help make treatments more effective or reduce their side effects. Domini and I recommend staying away from practitioners who claim that they can cure cancer with alternative treatments and that there is no need to do the 'toxic conventional' therapies.

In most hospitals, patients are unfortunately given very little time to prepare for treatment or to research their options. Of course it's important to take action and deal with the tumour as soon as possible after diagnosis, but the latest research shows that treatment could actually be made far more effective if certain things are taken into consideration before starting it.

On a visit to an integrated clinic in Switzerland a few years ago, I learned what it means to follow 'best practice'. Each patient goes for comprehensive tests straight after diagnosis, including blood tests and stool analysis. Some people are also sent for dental check-ups. Upon evaluation of the tests, nutrient deficiencies or overloads are corrected, supplements to balance the gut flora are prescribed and other steps are taken to prepare the patient for treatments in an optimal way.

The importance of the microbiome: The human gut as a world in itself

Emerging research (Iida et al, 2013; Viaud et al, 2013) stresses the importance of the gut microbiome (human digestive system) during cancer treatment. In other words, chemotherapy may not work as well when gut flora is compromised or beneficial bacteria are lacking. The mechanisms of these effects aren't fully understood yet. One possible explanation is that intestinal bacteria might gain the ability to enter the bloodstream and the lymph nodes, where they stimulate the immune system and enhance the body's ability to fight cancer.

The role of exercise

For a long time, cancer patients undergoing treatment were advised to 'take it easy' and rest as much as possible. But based on the latest research, exercise during cancer treatment is safe and feasible.

Patricia follows the research of Kerry Courneya, PhD, whom she met at a conference in Germany in 2014, very closely. His research confirms that fewer delays in chemotherapy treatments and sometimes even dose reductions were possible for breast cancer patients participating in a resistance-training programme.

For cancer patients who aren't active on a regular basis and for whom exercise is something completely new, they may need to start with very low-intensity exercise, such as walking, stretching and yoga. People who are on bed rest can benefit greatly from physical therapy to maintain strength and flexibility.

According to the American Cancer Society, the American College of Sports Medicine, the American Institute for Cancer Research and other organisations, the current guidelines for physical activity are as follows:

- At least **150 minutes** (2½ hours) per week of **moderate-intensity aerobic activity** (e.g. brisk walking); and
- At least **two to three sessions of strength training** per week (weights or resistance exercises with own body weight) that include exercises for all the major muscle groups; and
- **Stretching** of major muscle groups and tendons on days that other exercises are performed.
- Doing intermittent physical activity is better for regulating blood sugars, especially for older people. Walking 15 minutes three times a day, ideally after a meal, instead of doing a single 45-minute walk has shown better health benefits (DiPietro et al, 2013).

But if you're unable to meet the above goals for health reasons, please don't beat yourself up about it. Try to get moving and be physically active. It doesn't need to be in a gym or 'formal' exercise – any movement is positive. Take the stairs instead of the lift, even if it's just for one floor; park a bit further away from your destination and walk; take a yoga class (online is great too if you don't want to leave the house); or do some deep breathing and gentle stretching.

In any case, individuals undergoing treatment should obtain approval from their oncologist before starting an exercise programme, they should have their vital signs (temperature, pulse, blood pressure, respiration rate) monitored regularly and ideally they should exercise with a partner, caregiver or exercise professional for safety reasons.

Fasting and cancer treatment

Another area of research that is worth exploring is the link between cell growth, fasting and cancer. The current recommendation in most hospitals is to make sure cancer patients, especially those at risk of losing weight, consume high-calorie foods during treatment, even if they have no appetite. This can also include foods like scones, ice cream or Mars bars; it doesn't seem to matter as long as there are calories. Often, strong anti-nausea medication is given to ensure patients can keep eating during treatment.

But what is the evidence for this practice? On its website, the National Cancer Institute states that '[w]eight loss has been identified as an indicator of poor prognosis in cancer patients'. Cancer-induced weight loss can indeed be a problem, especially for certain cancer types like pancreatic or lung cancer. The fear of developing cachexia (the 'wasting' syndrome where cancer patients lose weight and muscle rapidly) is ever present. However, very recent research (Ghadjar et al, 2015) shows that weight loss before but not during treatment is associated with reduced survival.

According to Dr Claire Donohoe et al (2011), anorexia, inflammation, insulin resistance and increased muscle protein breakdown are frequently associated with cachexia. If we have this evidence, why does anybody recommend foods that raise blood sugars, which triggers an insulin response? The cells won't be responsive to this hormone (in insulin resistance, cells don't respond to insulin and therefore don't allow glucose to enter) and a situation arises whereby both blood glucose and insulin are high – not a good combination for cancer patients! We also know that sugar, refined and processed foods (like white flour in baked goods or processed meat) and trans fatty acids (in baked goods with margarine or vegetable oils) promote inflammation. Staying away from pro-inflammatory foods and adding anti-inflammatories like omega-3 from fish oils is therefore good advice for any cancer patient, but particularly for those at risk of losing weight.

Here is why scientists' attention is drawn to the effects of fasting and calorie restriction during treatment: chemo- and radiotherapy are particularly likely to damage rapidly dividing cells like cancer cells, but also healthy cells like hair roots (follicles) or osteoblasts (a type of bone cell). Studies have shown that when we are deprived of food for even quite a short period of time, our healthy cells respond by slowing down metabolism and going into repair/survival mode until food is available again.

Cancer cells work differently and follow their own rules – as usual! They will go on selfishly proliferating, whatever the circumstances in the environment. In this case, fasting can be an opportunity to make them more vulnerable to treatment (Lee et al, 2012) while healthy cells are 'hibernating' and at a lot less risk of being affected.

Valter Longo, Professor of Gerontology/Alzheimer's Research/Cancer Research, Biological Sciences at the University of Southern California, is considered one of the world's foremost experts in all things fasting, especially when it comes to prolonging lifespan and longevity. Longo and his team found that 'starvation-dependent' stress protects normal but not cancer cells against high-dose chemotherapy (Raffaghello et al, 2008). It's estimated that more than 20% of cancer-related deaths are precipitated or even caused by the toxic effects of chemotherapy. Toxicities don't only result in side effects, but also often reduce the overall effectiveness of the treatment because of dose or frequency reductions. Longo and his team also found that temporary nutrient restriction could increase stem cells' (undifferentiated cells that can differentiate into specialised cells) resistance to certain stressors. In their 2014 study, Cheng et al discovered the following:

'We show that prolonged fasting periods cause a major reduction in white blood cell number followed by its replenishment after refeeding. We discovered that this effect, which may have evolved to reduce energy expenditure during periods of starvation, is able to switch stem cells to a mode able to not only regenerate immune cells and reverse the immunosuppression caused by chemotherapy, but also rejuvenate the immune system of old mice.' (Cheng et al, 2014)

Another reason why fasting, or at least carbohydrate and sugar reduction, can be so effective is because it decreases blood glucose levels. A number of very recent medical papers demonstrate the detrimental effects of elevated blood sugar in patients undergoing cancer treatment (Derr et al, 2009; Mayer et al, 2014; McGirt et al, 2008). High glucose conditions not only promote cancer cell growth, but also reduce the effects of chemotherapy drugs (Zhao et al, 2015) and radiotherapy (Klement and Champ, 2014). It makes us wonder why we get tea and sugar-laden biscuits in hospital waiting rooms – are oncologists not aware that it won't help their work?

More research trials are currently underway that explore the benefits and practicalities of fasting for cancer patients, e.g. 'Short-Term Fasting Before Chemotherapy in Treating Patients with Cancer' at the Mayo Clinic. It appears that fasting *after* chemotherapy might also be important to reduce the risk of DNA damage by the chemotherapy drug, which could lead to secondary tumours and other toxicities. Further animal and clinical studies are now exploring the possible length of a post-chemotherapy fast. This will be calculated based on the half-life of the chemotherapy drug to minimise toxicity to normal cells when food is taken in again.

Fasting is definitely an area in cancer research that has a lot of potential once it's combined with other strategies. Valter Longo even founded a company called L-Nutra that received funds from the US National Cancer Institute to develop fasting-mimicking diets. The products were developed after many cancer patients were asking for diets that could substitute fasting. The plan is to make these available worldwide within the next few years.

Although this research is compelling, it's preliminary and we don't recommend embarking on a fasting regime without supervision. But maybe it also gives reassurance to everybody who is feeling very poorly during chemotherapy and the last thing they want to do is eat. There might be a very good reason that this mechanism kicks in. After Domini's story about how fasting worked for her (more by accident than anything, as it happens), you will find recipes to refuel yourself once your appetite returns. And it will, we promise.

Domini's story

Most of the information above only fell into my lap long after I had finished both chemotherapy and radiotherapy. I have always been a fairly intuitive person, and during treatment I really just wanted to 'listen' to my body and respond accordingly. But I also had to allow for the fact that I can be a lazy cow and rarely want to exercise. Sometimes I have to bully myself into being good.

My nausea was pretty grim, as it is for many, during chemo, and the anti-nausea tablets did me little good. During this time, I inadvertently fasted. I didn't sit on the couch eating junk food, which chemo can sometimes make you feel like doing. Some patients feel hung-over, and hung-over people generally crave carbs, salt, fat and sugar in varying degrees or pecking order. We read articles in glossy magazines and newspapers (especially around Christmastime) about 'best practice' after hangovers: don't tax your system, don't overeat, avoid big, heavy, greasy fry-ups the next day and eat lighter, stay hydrated and do a little exercise. As if!

Well, during chemo, I felt I should engage in less taxing habits, so I ate very lightly for those three or four days of grimness. As Patricia mentioned above, I avoided the ubiquitous sweet tea, sandwiches and biscuits on the trolleys being offered up to patients. Instead, I would eat an apple or mandarin and a few nuts, plus herbal tea. At home, I ate the crusts of toasted sourdough bread with butter and a little avocado, maybe a few blueberries and then some miso soup, plus lots of water and that was it. I just wanted to be kind and gentle to my system, which was being bombarded with cancer-killing chemicals. I felt that eating a burger with chips and ketchup was probably not the way to go.

It worked for me, and as soon as I could, I would start walking and then go back to jogging again. But go easy on yourself. I was in my forties when I got cancer and was reasonably fit and in okay shape. If I was in my seventies, I might want to lock the door and stay on the couch.

When I had radiotherapy, I found the time commitment considerable, just when you think you are nearly 'done' with treatment. It's like the final hill you have to climb and I was a bit narky about visiting the hospital every day for six weeks. So I made it part of my 'route' and would jog or cycle up, get my blast of radiotherapy and then head home. It stopped me being so resentful of the treatment, as it was part of my exercise routine as opposed to a distinct and unique expedition to the hospital.

I totally appreciate that this isn't possible for many people (I live very close to the hospital!), but if you can find a way to make it as seamless as possible, it helps. More and more evidence about exercise and radiotherapy is emerging, which Patricia mentioned above. Again, a bit like reducing sugar and carbohydrates during chemo, I exercised during radiotherapy. Both seemed to have done me no harm and hopefully some good. They certainly helped keep my spirits and energy up, which is a vital part of the endurance test that is cancer treatment. Like Patricia, I am alive because of the conventional treatments I was given: surgery, chemotherapy, mastectomy and radiotherapy. But enhancing and contributing to your well-being through diet and exercise must offer better results, no? I certainly think so.

Vitamin D

There's no getting away from information on vitamin D these days. TV ads, leaflets at the doctor's office and magazine articles serve as constant reminders of the importance of adequate vitamin D intake and levels. There's even evidence that some chemotherapy drugs work better in conjunction with vitamin D (Sherman et al, 2014). The problem is that vitamin D deficiency is incredibly common these days – some experts are even talking about a vitamin D deficiency pandemic.

So what exactly does this mean in practice? How can you ensure you're protected from the various diseases that are linked to a deficiency of this hormone-like vitamin?

You've probably heard that '15 minutes of morning sun' is sufficient to make sure your vitamin D levels are adequate, or that all you need is three servings of dairy to do the same. Unfortunately, those claims couldn't be further from the truth.

More a hormone than a vitamin, vitamin D plays a role in virtually every system in the body. Its main role is to maintain normal blood levels of calcium and phosphorous, but that's not all. It has crucial effects across most body systems, especially for bones, cardiovascular, endocrine (hormonal) and immune health and also for neural and brain function. Vitamin D actually regulates the activity of over 200 genes, which is a lot more than any other vitamin. Optimum levels (more about that below) have been shown to reduce the risk for cancer and also the likelihood of developing auto-immune disease.

Contrary to what a lot of people think, and thanks to clever marketing, dairy – and food in general – isn't the best source of vitamin D. Let's make a comparison.

A glass of milk contains about 100 IU (international units) of vitamin D. If you have pale skin and lie outside in a bathing suit (termed 'modest sun exposure' in the research, meaning skin was not burned but lightly pink 24 hours later) for 15–20 minutes or so, you'll make anywhere from 15,000 to 20,000 IU of vitamin D (Holick, 2011), and the darker your skin, the longer it takes to produce the vitamin. As you can see, 100 IU vs. 15,000–20,000 IU is quite a difference!

So the main source of this vitamin is sun exposure or supplementation. **In fact, sun exposure accounts for around 90% of vitamin D in the body in individuals who do not take supplements** (Holick, 2004). In other words, if you're not in the sun much or live in the Northern Hemisphere – and yes, that includes Ireland and the British Isles in general – you'll need a supplement to meet your needs. Above and below latitudes of approximately 33°, vitamin D3 synthesis in the skin is very low or absent during most of the winter (MacDonald et al, 2011).

Interestingly, skin tone also affects vitamin D production. People with dark skin may require three to six times more time in the sun to produce the same amount of vitamin D as a very pale person. Obviously, if you're putting on sun cream or cover up with protective clothing, you're not making much vitamin D either. Sunscreen with an SPF of 30 blocks 97% of UVB rays, but therefore reduces vitamin D production by 95% (www.skincancer.org/prevention/uva-and-uvb/understanding-uva-and-uvb). This is because the 'damaging' rays that we're always told to avoid around midday (between 10am and 2pm) are the ones that your skin uses to make vitamin D.

So what to do with all this conflicting advice while trying to make sure you get adequate vitamin D without compromising skin health?

There are two options. If you do go into the sun, the ideal scenario is that you get a little exposure on bare skin (without burning, of course!) before you cover up with sun cream or clothes. If you can do this on a regular basis during the summer months, you should be safe. Otherwise you can take a vitamin D3 supplement, which is more effective at maintaining blood levels of the vitamin than D2. The dosage depends on your vitamin D status, which can be tested in any hospital lab (see the section at the end of the book on blood tests). The current recommended intake is set at a paltry 600 IU for adults, but respected researchers and doctors like the US clinical endocrinologist Robert Heaney suggest that 7,000 IU per day from all sources is much more accurate. We strongly advise that you test your vitamin D levels twice a year and supplement accordingly under supervision of a healthcare professional.

What levels of vitamin D (25(OH)D, to be exact) are ideal is hotly debated among experts. After lots of research and consulting with colleagues and doctors, Patricia has come to the conclusion that we should aim for quite a tight range: between 50–65ng/ml (125–162 nmol/l), especially for cancer patients. Both high and low circulating vitamin D levels are associated with increased risk for certain types of cancer, according to the Memorial Sloan Kettering Cancer Center in New York. A study looking at vitamin D levels in free-living nomadic tribes in Africa gives us an idea about truly normal vitamin D status. Their mean vitamin D levels were just below 50 ng/ml (Luxwolda et al, 2012).

Foods for recovery

Like we said, when you're feeling poorly and/or are recovering from a bout of chemo, food can be the last thing on your mind. And even when you think you want it, when you do make the effort to get something down you, it can sometimes taste so grim that you might as well be eating sand. But eat we must, at least when we can, and it's best to make the food we do eat as healing, nutritious and gentle on our systems as possible so that we feel restored or at least relatively normal, treatment side effects notwithstanding.

The following recipes are all designed to be tasty on the tongue and gentle on your system. These are savoury, soothing flavours and textures that feel easy on the tum. Because energy is a factor too when you're feeling under the weather, they are also simple and quick to prepare. Even the bone broth, though it requires long cooking, is a very hands-off affair. You can just leave it to simmer while you have a nice lie-down. Job done.

I am very lucky to have a gas burner that has a pilot light on it, which means I can keep something cooking on the hob for 24 hours, no problem. This may not be feasible for you to do safely. My sister has adapted this recipe so that she lets it cook overnight in a warming oven set at 90°C–100°C (190°F–210°F), while Patricia uses a slow cooker, which is another excellent tool. Whatever you do will be better than nothing, so don't get disheartened. I was told to cook bone broth for 4 hours, then 8 hours, and now I'm told it should be 24 hours. Inevitably, in another three years we'll be told 1 hour is optimum. Until then, I'll follow the advice I'm given, which has been handed down from Korean mums to daughters who have been cooking this for generations. Now that's wisdom. Thank you, Doris!

Simmer your roast chicken bones in 3 litres (13c) of water with a splash of cider vinegar for at least 4 hours (preferably 8–24 hours), covered. Even though you have a lid on it, you might need to top it up so that the bones remain covered. After it has cooked for as long as you can let it, take the lid off and let it reduce down by a third. At this point, I spoon out the bones and throw them away. Then I cool the stock down by putting the pot in a cold 'bath' in my kitchen sink. After about an hour, it should be cold enough to be transferred into a smaller pot or bowl, which can then fit in your fridge.

When you're ready to finish your broth, it couldn't be faster. In a large saucepan, heat the broth and add all the other ingredients except the fresh herbs and miso. Simmer for 10 minutes to allow the flavours to infuse before stirring in the miso (which shouldn't be boiled) and serving with chopped fresh cilantro.

Asian flavoured bone broth

1 leftover chicken carcass (from a roast chicken)
Splash of raw cider vinegar
Small bunch of scallions
4 garlic cloves, crushed
Large knob of ginger, peeled and finely sliced
2 sticks of lemongrass (outer leaves removed), finely chopped
4 lime leaves
Juice of 2 limes
1 tbsp fish sauce
Salt and pepper
1 tbsp miso
Bunch of fresh cilantro, chopped

Serves 4

Miso broth

2 tbsp olive oil or liquid coconut oil

200–400g (7–14 oz) button mushrooms, sliced

2 carrots, peeled and diced

1 small rutabaga, peeled and finely diced

1 leek, finely sliced

8 garlic cloves, finely sliced

Big knob of ginger, peeled and grated

2.5 litres (10½c) water

4 tbsp miso paste

Small handful of dried seaweed, soaked in cold water and then drained and roughly chopped if necessary

Salt and pepper

Sesame seeds

Makes 8–10 portions

I made this miso broth for myself all throughout chemo. Miso and seaweed are staples of Asian cooking, and seaweed is thankfully becoming a lot more mainstream thanks to the many great recipes in which it now features. Sally McKenna's book *Extreme Greens*, which has a fantastic supply of dishes with seaweed, is no exception and is well worth buying. Unless I am completely mistaken, this superfood is in abundance, so you can enjoy as much of it as you want without any guilt.

This makes a really large batch (8–10 portions) that will keep you going all week. In summer I leave out the root vegetables, but coming into winter, it feels a lot more satisfying to get a bite of turnip or carrot rather than tofu. Use whatever seaweed is suitable for soups. Kelp, dillisk or carrageen are all good, but often you will see on the back of the packages the ones they recommend for sprinkling into soups.

Heat the oil in a very large saucepan and cook the mushrooms over a high heat to get some good colour on them. They may get soggy at first, but keep the heat up and make them start to get a little colour, then add the carrots, rutabaga and leek along with the garlic and ginger. Sauté for a few minutes, then add the water (or you could use bone broth or stock). Bring up to a gentle simmer and cook gently for 10–15 minutes. If the vegetables are small enough, they will cook quite quickly. Turn off the heat and let it cool down until it's the right temperature to drink.

Miso needs gentle cooking, so mix it well with some hot water in a small cup, using the back of a spoon to make a liquid paste before adding it to the soup base. Add the seaweed and check the seasoning. Serve with some sesame seeds on top and enjoy bowls of this all week. Avoid rapid boiling to help keep the miso in its optimum state.

'Flu soup' is as far from a visual showstopper as you can get. Try as we might, it proved nigh impossible to make it look like anything more than flavoured green broth in the photographs. But my, my, for those seeking something to soothe and cleanse, it would be hard to find better.

Garlic and ginger are the foundation of many wonderful dishes, but I think it's the aromatic herbs that do the real work here. Sweet, savoury sage has long been famous for its medicinal properties – in fact, its scientific name, *Salvia officinalis*, derives from the Latin word *salvere*, which means 'to be saved.' And thyme has a history as a remedy for coughs and colds. So if you're feeling a little under the weather, give this soup a try. To make it that bit more substantial, add some cooked chicken, scallions, seaweed and/or a poached egg.

Heat the olive oil and (this is crucial) *very* gently sauté the garlic and herbs – this is almost an infusion. Add the ginger and water and season well. Simmer gently for 5 minutes, then take off the heat and let it sit for 1 hour. Reheat and serve with a little more olive oil and a poached egg, finely chopped scallions and shredded seaweed.

Flu soup

2 tbsp olive oil
2 heads (yes, whole heads) of garlic, peeled and finely sliced
Bunch of parsley, chopped
5 sage leaves, sliced
1 tbsp thyme leaves
Knob of ginger, peeled and sliced
2 litres (8½c) water
Salt and pepper

Serves 2–4, depending on what you add to it

Nourishing chicken soup

1 chicken, giblets removed

3 carrots, peeled and cut in half

1 large onion, peeled and cut in half

2 heads of garlic, cloves peeled and
   cut in half

Big knob of ginger, peeled and sliced
   into thick chunks

Few splashes of Worcestershire
   sauce

Few sprigs of thyme

1 bay leaf

2 good tsp ground turmeric

Salt and pepper

2 tbsp raw apple cider vinegar
   (optional)

I included this recipe in my last book, *Dinner*, and I include it again here simply because it's so darned good. It really could not be easier. One of the keys to it is rapid boiling for a minute or two to help anything that needs to be skimmed to bubble up to the surface. Then you need to turn it down really low and let it gently hover around a simmer or even lower. Quantities are vague because it depends on the size of the saucepan you have at home. Needless to say, as long as the chicken would be comfortably submerged in water (if you held it down), then that's enough. You don't need to brown bones for this. All you need is a big pot, some vegetables, herbs and a teaspoon of turmeric to help give it a gorgeous golden colour.

Fill a big saucepan about halfway up with cold water. Carefully add the chicken, then add everything else except the vinegar. Wash your hands well if you've handled the raw chicken. Put on the heat and slowly bring to the boil. Turn up the heat and let it bubble away furiously for about 2 minutes, then turn the heat down a little and skim any scum or impurities from the surface with a big metal spoon. Turn the heat right down, partially cover with a lid and let it simmer gently for about 2½ hours.

Carefully remove the chicken into a bowl with a tongs. The chicken may just fall to pieces when you do this, but it doesn't really matter. Scoop out the veg and discard them. Continue to gently simmer the broth on its own. When the chicken carcass has cooled down enough to handle it, remove the skin and discard it, then set about removing every scrap of meat from the bones and carcass with your hands. Set the meat aside and throw the bones and carcass back into the broth along with a couple tablespoons of raw apple cider vinegar, if using. Ideally you would give it a few more hours to really draw the nutrients out.

Taste the soup and decide if it needs longer cooking/reducing or more seasoning. Drain over a colander and discard the bones, herbs and any lurking vegetables, then put the broth back into the saucepan. Add the cooked chicken pieces and serve straight away.

Stracciatella

Okay, here you go. If you've roasted a chicken some night, have torn all the meat off it so you have dinner sorted the next night and have made bone broth overnight from the bones, then this is the soup for you. In fact, I think I might go and make it tonight.

From the larger saucepan, take as many portions of bone broth as you need. Separately, sauté some leeks in butter or olive oil. Season with a little garlic, thyme and pepper, then add in the bone broth. Bring up to a gentle simmer, then whisk in 2 eggs per person and a generous handful of grated Parmesan and a bunch of scallions and parsley. Or not – leave out the green stuff for fussy young people.

Chuck in roast chicken that's left over – whatever is handy. And you're done!

Sweet potato chips (à la Patricia)

2 large sweet potatoes
50ml (3½tbsp) olive oil
3 tbsp red wine vinegar
2 tsp dried oregano
2 tsp salt
1 tsp ground black pepper

Makes 8 portions

I've always found that white potatoes are fabulous to deal with nausea – before I went keto, obviously! While they are a very nutritious food, they can unfortunately also drive your blood sugar levels up quickly. Try sweet potatoes or parsnips instead, which hit your bloodstream at a slower rate. They do contain mostly carbs, so quantities need to be limited.

Preheat the oven to 180°C (350°F). Line a baking tray with non-stick baking paper or tin foil.

Wash and scrub the potatoes to clean them and remove any dirt. Leave the skin on and cut into 2.5cm (1in) slices, then cut each slice into sticks (about 5cm × by 5cm × 10cm [2in × 2in × 4in]). Toss the sticks in a bowl with the oil and red wine vinegar. Add the oregano, salt and pepper and toss again, making sure the fries are well coated with the seasonings.

Spread the fries onto the lined tray in a single layer. Bake for 16–18 minutes, then cool for 10 minutes.

Many people ask about juicing because it's something many cancer patients 'discover' very quickly after a diagnosis. In my experience, a lot of people who get interested in nutrition inadvertently end up hearing about the wonders of juicing. In my opinion, juicing is certainly fabulous for anybody who has a compromised gut function (which is the case with many cancer patients going through chemotherapy, for instance) and therefore has a hard time absorbing nutrients from whole foods without suffering from bloating, diarrhoea or constipation. I also have a number of colon cancer patients who are advised by their consultant to stay off fibre completely, in which case juicing comes in really handy to provide them with nutrients without the fibre, which is removed during the juicing process.

However, I observe that most people mainly juice fruit like grapefruit, apples or oranges and throw in a few kale stems or broccoli. That's why we've created a green juice recipe that is very low in sugar but high in greens. Carbohydrates are a little bit over 2g per serving (150ml [⅝c]). The lemon will help take the bitterness out of the green vegetables and ginger is fabulous for combating nausea.

Put all the ingredients through a masticating juicer and serve.

Green juice

1 cucumber
3 stalks of celery
70g (2.5 oz) kale
1 large broccoli stem
½ lemon, peeled
½ thumb of ginger
3 large sprigs of parsley

Makes 4 servings (or 2 large ones)

Other ideas for meals and snacks during treatment

- Smoothies, e.g. the berry smoothie on page 261
- Simple salmon (or any fish) and broccoli without spices, maybe just a bit of butter
- Eggs scrambled in a little coconut oil or butter
- Pancakes or crêpes (pages 32, 299, 310 or 364)
- Different types of crackers (pages 31, 268 or 294), maybe with some butter or avocado, nut butter or any other spread you like
- Stewed apples with cinnamon (page 22) and coconut cream
- Hazelnut bread (376) with any of the pestos (page 192 or page 262) or tapenades (page 194)
- No-grain nut, kale and seed bread (page 48) with goats' cheese

If cravings kick in, turn to one of the desserts in the treats section (pages 198–220) to see if you can find something that you like.

References

Cheng, C.W. et al (2014) 'Prolonged fasting reduces IGF-1/PKA to promote hematopoietic stem cell-based regeneration and reverse immunosuppression', *Cell Stem Cell*, 14(6), pp. 810–823.

Derr, R.L. et al (2009) 'Association between hyperglycemia and survival in patients with newly diagnosed glioblastoma', *Journal of Clinical Oncology*, 27(7), pp. 1,082–1,086.

DiPietro, L. et al (2013) 'Three 15-min bouts of moderate postmeal walking significantly improves 24-h glycemic control in older people at risk for impaired glucose tolerance', *Diabetes Care*, 36(10), pp. 3,262–3,268.

Donohoe, C.L., Ryan, A.M. and Reynolds, J.V. (2011) 'Cancer cachexia: Mechanisms and clinical implications', *Gastroenterology Research and Practice*, 2011.

Ghadjar, P. et al (2015) 'Impact of weight loss on survival after chemoradiation for locally advanced head and neck cancer: Secondary results of a randomized phase III trial (SAKK 10/94)', *Radiation Oncology*, 10, p.21.

Holick, M.F. (2004) 'Sunlight and vitamin D for bone health and prevention of autoimmune diseases, cancers, and cardiovascular disease', *American Society for Clinical Nutrition*, 80(6 Suppl), pp. 1,678S–1,688S.

Holick, M.F. (2011) 'Vitamin D: A d-lightful solution for health', *Journal of Investigative Medicine*, 59(6), pp. 872–880.

Iida, N. et al (2013) 'Commensal bacteria control cancer response to therapy by modulating the tumor microenvironment,' *Science*, 342, pp. 967–970.

Klement, R.J. and Champ, C.E. (2014) 'Calories, carbohydrates, and cancer therapy with radiation: Exploiting the five R's through dietary manipulation', *Cancer Metastasis Review*, 33(1), pp. 217–229.

Lee, C. et al (2012) 'Fasting cycles retard growth of tumors and sensitize a range of cancer cell types to chemotherapy', *Science Translation Medicine*, 4(124).

Luxwolda, M.F. et al (2012) 'Traditionally living populations in East Africa have a mean serum 25-hydroxyvitamin D concentration of 115 nmol/l', *British Journal of Nutrition*, 23, pp. 1–5.

MacDonald, H.M. et al (2011) 'Skin color change in Caucasian postmenopausal women predicts summer-winter change in 25-hydroxyvitamin D: Findings from the ANSAViD cohort study', *Journal Clinical Endocrinology and Metabolism*, 96(6), pp. 1,677–1,686.

Mayer, A. et al (2014) 'Strong adverse prognostic impact of hyperglycemic episodes during adjuvant chemoradiotherapy of glioblastoma multiforme', *Strahlenther und Onkologie*, 190(10), pp. 933–938.

McGirt, M.J. et al (2008) 'Persistent outpatient hyperglycemia is independently associated with decreased survival after primary resection of malignant brain astrocytomas', *Neurosurgery*, 63(2), pp. 286–291.

Raffaghello, L. et al (2008) 'Starvation-dependent differential stress resistance protects normal but not cancer cells against high-dose chemotherapy', *Proceedings of the National Academy of Sciences of the United States of America*, 105(24), pp. 8,215–8,220.

Sherman, M.H. et al (2014) 'Vitamin D receptor-mediated stromal reprogramming suppresses pancreatitis and enhances pancreatic cancer therapy', *Cell*, 159(1), pp. 80–93.

Viaud, S. et al. (2013) 'The intestinal microbiota modulates the anticancer immune effects of cyclophosphamide,' *Science*, 342, pp. 971–976.

Zhao, W. et al (2015) 'High glucose promotes gastric cancer chemoresistance in vivo and in vitro', *Molecular Medicine Reports*, 12(1), pp. 843–850.

Appendices

Blood tests for the ketogenic diet: Baseline and monitoring

Even if you're in good health, it's always a good idea to ask your doctor to do some basic blood tests before starting a low-carb or ketogenic diet. Unless there are any significant abnormalities in cardiac, liver, kidney or hormonal functions, frequent clinical monitoring is usually not necessary.

If you're suffering from a chronic disease, chances are you get these blood tests done on a regular basis anyway, especially the full blood count, electrolytes and liver function test. But if you haven't had any bloods taken for a while, we recommend you ask for these very common routine tests, which can be performed at any hospital or in any laboratory.

Once the baseline tests are done, it's advisable to retest after six to eight weeks of being in nutritional ketosis and address any negative changes. If you're thriving on a ketogenic diet and your markers are all on track, testing every six to 12 months is sufficient in most cases for monitoring purposes.

1. Complete blood count
- Evaluation of white blood cells
- Evaluation of red blood cells
- Evaluation of platelets

2. Comprehensive metabolic panel
- Glucose (fasting)
- Calcium
- Proteins: albumin, total protein
- Electrolytes: sodium, potassium, bicarbonate, chloride
- Kidney: blood urea nitrogen (BUN), creatinine
- Liver: ALP, ALT, AST, bilirubin, GGT

3. Fasting lipid panel (preferably high-sensitivity tests)
- Total cholesterol
- HDL cholesterol
- LDL cholesterol
- Triglycerides

4. Thyroid panel (please note that the full panel is not available in some countries)
- TSH
- Free T4 and T3
- Total T4 and T3
- Reverse T3
- Anti-thyroglobulin antibodies
- Anti-thyroperoxidase (TPO) antibodies

5. Other useful tests
- C-reactive protein (systemic inflammation)
- Hb1Ac
- Vitamin D (25-hydroxy-vitamin D)
- Vitamin B12

See www.labtestsonline.org for more information.

Monitoring blood glucose and ketone levels

A word of comfort: blood monitoring is not difficult to do.

In fact, millions of people (mainly diabetics) do it every day. It takes just a couple of minutes, and the gadget you use is small enough to fit into any handbag (or manbag). Some of Patricia's clients – okay, it's mainly the men – love the gadgetry and precision of it so much that they very quickly adapt to using it, but in fact everyone gets used to it soon enough and then it becomes as second nature as brushing your teeth.

Right, now to the science bit. Jeff Volek (RD, PhD) and Stephen Phinney (MD, PhD) define nutritional ketosis as having beta-hydroxybutyrate (a ketone body) levels in the range of 0.5–3mM (mmol/l) (Volek and Phinney, 2011), but they don't give any indication as to what blood sugar levels should be.

In the case of cancer in particular, **the overall goal is to work towards a 1:1 ratio of blood glucose levels to ketone levels**, as outlined by Dr Thomas Seyfried (Boston College, author of *Cancer as a Metabolic Disease*) and his team. This ratio is also called **GKI (Glucose Ketone Index)**. In his latest paper (Medenbauer, Mukherjee and Seyfried, 2015), Dr Seyfried states that 'the zone of metabolic management is likely entered with **GKI values between 1 and 2** for humans. Optimal management is predicted for values approaching 1.0.'

Because there are three different types of ketone bodies, different testing devices are also available.

- **β-hydroxybutyrate (β-OHB):** This is what is measured with blood ketone strips.
- **Acetoacetate:** This is detected with urine ketone strips (Ketostix). They can be useful **in the initial stages** (i.e. the first two weeks) of the ketogenic diet before acetoacetate in urine decreases in most people. That's when a switch to blood ketone strips is necessary to get accurate results.
- **Acetone:** Acetone is a breakdown product of acetoacetate, which the body excretes via exhalation. Acetone is what the Ketonix tool, for instance, is measuring. Research is underway to see how useful breath testers can be for ketone testing.

Monitoring blood glucose and ketone levels is the gold standard. This can be done with a meter that can test for both glucose and ketones (with the same meter), which is typically used by diabetic patients. **Precision Xtra** by Abbott Laboratories seems to provide the most accurate readings, but names for the devices can differ in different countries.

You have **two different types of strips**: one type for ketones, the other one for glucose. Make sure you know which colour packaging is for what type of blood test! From the same drop of blood (you prick your finger with a lancet – and no, it's not painful), you can first test your ketones and then your blood sugar. Once you've written down your reading, you can test for blood glucose by inserting a glucose strip into the meter and using the same drop of blood.

Dr Seyfried's Glucose Ketone Index

The GKI doesn't rely on reaching a specific glucose or ketone range, but it looks at a **desirable ratio of glucose to ketone levels**. It tracks the relationship between these two metabolic markers in the blood in patients. Based on Dr Seyfried's research, most people make good progress if they achieve a 1:1 ratio.

The formula for the GKI is:

$$\frac{Blood\ glucose\ measurement\ (mmol)}{Blood\ ketone\ measurement\ (mmol)} = 1.0\ or\ below$$

Make sure you use the **same units for both measurements (mmol/l)**.

Please don't get too caught up in the ratio. Many factors apart from the food you eat influence your blood glucose and ketone levels, like stress, age, medication (especially steroid hormones, which can raise your blood glucose), surgery or treatments, sickness (for instance, a flu) and exercise, but also hormones. And don't forget that meters are only required to be accurate to +/−20%, so if you get a totally unexpected result, it may be a good idea to either retest or take your meter for an accuracy check. Ask your pharmacist to do this for you or match your reading with lab results, or take your glucose monitor along when you visit your doctor or have an appointment for lab work, for instance.

When is the best time to measure?

Blood glucose and ketone values should be measured **two to three hours after a meal**, **twice a day** if possible. Patricia recommends measuring after lunch and after dinner because **blood ketone concentrations tend to be lowest in the morning**, increase during the day and reach a maximum in the afternoon. This will allow you to connect your dietary intake to changes in your GKI.

However, we're aware that ketone strips are expensive and are not always covered by health insurance, unlike in the case of diabetes. If you can only afford to test once a day, that's fine. The longer you're in nutritional ketosis, the more tuned in you'll be to possible blood sugar rises or drops in ketones.

Ketogenic pantry

For the pantry: Jars, cartons and pans

Almond milk
Apple cider vinegar
Artichokes
Capers
Coconut aminos (instead of soy)
Coconut milk and/or cream
Fish sauce
Gherkins (low sugar)
Mustard
Nut butter (almond, Brazil, macadamia, hazelnut, pistachio)
Olives
Pestos
Sun-dried tomatoes in olive oil
Tahini (sesame paste)
Canned sardines, anchovies and salmon
Tomato passata/paste

For the pantry: Dry goods

Almond flour (ground blanched almonds)
Baking powder (gluten and aluminium free)
Baking soda
Cacao butter
Coconut flour
Dark chocolate (85–90% cocoa solids)
Desiccated coconut or coconut flakes (untoasted)
Herbal teas (camomile, elderberry, fennel, ginger/lemon, nettle, peppermint, rooibos)
Konjac noodles
Nuts (almonds, Brazil, hazelnuts, macadamias, pecans, walnuts)
Psyllium husks
Raw cacao powder
Seeds (chia, flax, hemp, pumpkin, sesame, sunflower)

Fats and oils

Almond oil
Avocado oil
Coconut oil (extra virgin, organic)
Flaxseed oil
Macadamia oil
Olive oil, extra virgin
Pistachio oil
Walnut oil

Herbs and spices

Fresh: Basil, bay leaf, chives, cilantro, ginger, lemongrass, mint, oregano, parsley, rosemary, tarragon, thyme, turmeric, wasabi
Dry: Black pepper, caraway, cardamom, cayenne, celery seed, chilli flakes, cinnamon, cloves, coriander, cumin, curry, dill, fennel, fenugreek, juniper berry, marjoram, nutmeg, oregano, paprika, rosemary, saffron, sage, sea salt, thyme, turmeric

Butcher and fishmonger

Bratwurst (no fillers)
Chorizo (small quantities)
Cooked or raw prawns
Duck (whole, half, legs)
Free-range, organic bacon
Free-range, organic chicken (whole, thighs, wings)
Grass-fed beef
Lamb (chops, loin, mince, roast, shank)
Oily fish (anchovies, herring, mackerel, pilchards, salmon, sardines, trout)
Organ meat (chicken/lamb liver, kidneys or sweetbreads)
Parma ham (small quantities)
White fish (cod, coley, haddock, monkfish, pollack, sea bass)
Venison and game (high protein)

handy at all times to put into pancakes, fat bombs, crackers or breads.

- **A good whisk** to make sauces, dressings, chocolate, fat bombs and other goodies. Use **spatulas** to make sure you're not wasting a thing!
- **A lemon squeezer** for making fresh lemon juice, which you can use to add flavour to all sorts of things.
- **A glass baking dish** to make quiches, shepherd's pies, roast vegetables and other keto-friendly meals. Glass is preferable to other non-stick options in terms of chemicals.
- For storing leftovers, nuts and other perishable foods, Patricia mainly uses **glass or mason jars**. The coconut oil she buys, for instance, comes in a 1 litre glass jar, which she always saves; 1 litre stores a lot of leftovers. Again, the issue with plastic containers is that they could potentially leach chemicals. It's nothing to be overly paranoid about – we're exposed to chemicals all the time, after all – but her mantra is 'every little helps'. If you can avoid small amounts of leaching/chemical exposure often enough and it's not a major effort, then do it.

Optional equipment

- **A small fold-up cooler bag** can be handy if it gets warmer and you want to take your fat bombs or homemade chocolate with you without ending up with a big melted blob. You can even put a small ice pack into the cooler bag if it's really hot outside.
- **A Thermos bottle** is great if you want to take some bone broth, homemade soup or tea with you. It can make for a great lunch option or a good alternative if you know you're going someplace with limited keto options.
- **An immersion blender** if you don't have a regular blender (which I would get if I were you, though!). It's

particularly handy for making your own homemade mayonnaise (if you can't live without mayonnaise, then an immersion blender would be an essential piece of kit!). You can get one with an add-on mini blender underneath so that you can quickly create chia puddings, whipped cream, pestos or chop onions. Patricia has a Philips blender, but there are lots of other good, reliable brands available.

- To some people a **microwave** is an absolute must-have, but Patricia has never owned one in her whole life. There are no published studies showing microwave ovens to be harmful and some even show that they are good at preserving nutrients (Jiménez-Monreal et al, 2009). It's one of these tricky questions that doesn't seem to have a black or white answer, but Patricia prefers to steam or bake her food.
- There are so many **other gadgets** that you could get to make the ketogenic lifestyle more palatable: a donut maker, waffle maker, SodaStream, bread maker, avocado cuber, garlic peeler, herb chopper, egg cooker, you name it. It's up to you.

References

Jiménez-Monreal, A.M. et al (2009) 'Influence of cooking methods on antioxidant activity of vegetables', *Journal of Food Science*, 74(3), pp. H97–H103.

Medenbauer, J., Mukherjee, P. and Seyfried, T. (2015) 'The glucose ketone index calculator: A simple tool to monitor therapeutic efficacy for metabolic management of brain cancer', *Nutrition & Metabolism*, 12, p. 12.

Volek, J. and Phinney, S. (2011) *The Art and Science of Low Carbohydrate Living: An Expert Guide to Making the Life-Saving Benefits of Carbohydrate Restriction Sustainable and Enjoyable*. Beyond Obesity LLC.

Index

About the authors

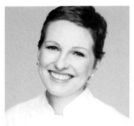

Barry McCall

DOMINI KEMP is an award-winning chef, food writer, and entrepreneur. In 2013, she was diagnosed with breast cancer, and since then she has shifted her focus towards healthier eating. She changed her column in *The Irish Times* to focus on healthier recipes and opened Alchemy Juice Co.—a juice and whole foods cafe. *The Ketogenic Kitchen* is her fifth cookbook and is focused on nutrition and well-being.

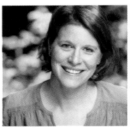

Rafal Kostrzewa

PATRICIA DALY is an experienced nutritional therapist and author specialising in cancer care and the ketogenic diet in particular. She has worked with hundreds of cancer patients in Ireland and abroad, lectures at the Irish Institute of Nutrition and Health and is a well-regarded speaker at conferences and in cancer centres. After writing three ebooks, *The Ketogenic Kitchen* is her first print book.